RECENT ADVANCES IN PLANT-BASED, TRADITIONAL, AND NATURAL MEDICINES

RECENT ADVANCES IN PLANT-BASED, TRADITIONAL, AND NATURAL MEDICINES

Edited by

Subramanyam Vemulpad, PhD, and Joanne Jamie, PhD

Apple Academic Press

TORONTO   NEW JERSEY

Apple Academic Press Inc.	Apple Academic Press Inc.
3333 Mistwell Crescent	9 Spinnaker Way
Oakville, ON L6L 0A2	Waretown, NJ 08758
Canada	USA

©2014 by Apple Academic Press, Inc.

First issued in paperback 2021

Exclusive worldwide distribution by CRC Press, a member of Taylor & Francis Group
No claim to original U.S. Government works

ISBN 13: 978-1-77463-335-9 (pbk)
ISBN 13: 978-1-77188-013-8 (hbk)

Library of Congress Control Number: 2013958423

Library and Archives Canada Cataloguing in Publication

Recent advances in plant-based, traditional, and natural medicines/edited by Subramanyam Vemulpad, PhD, and Joanne Jamie, PhD.

Includes bibliographical references and index.
ISBN 978-1-77188-013-8 (bound)

1. Medicinal plants. 2. Materia medica, Vegetable. 3. Traditional medicine.
4. Ethnopharmacology. I. Vemulpad, Subramanyam, editor of compilation II. Jamie, Joanne, editor of compilation

---

| RS164.R42 2014 | 615.3'21 | C2014-900068-5 |

Apple Academic Press also publishes its books in a variety of electronic formats. Some content that appears in print may not be available in electronic format. For information about Apple Academic Press products, visit our website at **www.appleacademicpress.com** and the CRC Press website at **www.crcpress.com**

ABOUT THE EDITORS

SUBRAMANYAM VEMULPAD, PhD

Prof. Vemulpad (BSc Bangalore University, 1973; MSc Faculty of Medicine, Madras University, 1976; PhD Faculty of Medicine, Delhi University, 1983) is a microbiologist, with research and academic experience in India and Malawi prior to migrating to Australia. He joined Sydney's Macquarie University in 2000 and currently is an Associate Professor in the Department of Chiropractic. He teaches medical microbiology, research methods, and biological effects of radiation. He has many years of experience in demystifying science by conducting hands-on science activities for school children in India. He is the current Chair of the University Biosafety Committee and has served on a variety of university committees, including Biosafety, Ethics (Human Research) and teaching and learning.

Along with co-editor Prof. Joanne Jamie, he is co-director of the Indigenous Science Education Program (which won the 2011 Australian Learning and Teaching Council Awards for University Teaching) and the Indigenous Bioresources Research Group at Macquarie University. The group's major objectives are to systematically document first-hand traditional medicinal plant knowledge of Indigenous people using best ethical practices and to apply this knowledge to identify medicinally important compounds following targeted chemical and biological studies. Prof. Vemulpad's research interests include infectious diseases, plant products as antimicrobial agents, rapid diagnostics, exemplary ethical practices in relation to traditional knowledge ownership and manual therapy. He has published 75 journal articles and 19 book chapters in these areas.

JOANNE JAMIE, PhD

Prof. Jamie was formally trained as a biological/organic chemist at the University of Queensland (BSc, Hons 1st class, 1987) and at the Australian National University (PhD 1992). She entered academia in 1994, following her appointment as Lecturer in biological/medicinal chemistry at the University of Wollongong, NSW, Australia, and has been at Macquarie University, Sydney, Australia, since her appointment in 2000 as Senior Lecturer in biological chemistry. In her academic positions, Prof. Jamie has directed a dynamic research team and conducted teaching in the areas of bioorganic, medicinal and natural products chemistry. Her current research, based at the Department of Chemistry and Biomolecular Sciences at Macquarie University, includes investigating the structure and function of medically important human enzymes and designing small molecule inhibitors of them for potential therapeutic use; studies on human lens chemistry to understand age-related nuclear cataract, which is a major cause of human blindness; and collaborative research with Indigenous people on traditional knowledge, including investigating medicinal flora, for cultural preservation and drug discovery. With co-editor Prof. Subramanyam Vemulpad, she co-directs the Indigenous Bioresources Research Group, and is committed to ensuring that true collaborative partnerships are in place for the Indigenous communities they work with, on traditional medicines.

Prof. Jamie has published journal articles on approaches to working with Indigenous people and documentation of their traditional knowledge; bioassay guided isolation and structural elucidation of bioactive compounds from traditional medicinal plants; development of new bioassays, including antimicrobial and enzyme assays for medium throughput screening; isolation, structural elucidation and total synthesis of new human lens (UV) filter compounds and model studies with UV filter compounds and human lens proteins to understand cataract formation; protein expression and purification; identification of proteins with novel function; and design and synthesis of new enzyme inhibitors for therapeutic use.

CONTENTS

ACKNOWLEDGMENT AND
HOW TO CITE

The editor and publisher thank each of the authors who contributed to this book, whether by granting their permission individually or by releasing their research as Open Source articles. The chapters in this book were previously published in various places in various formats. To cite the work contained in this book and to view the individual permissions, please refer to the citation at the beginning of each chapter. Each chapter was read individually and carefully selected by the editors. The result is a book that provides a nuanced study of the recent advances in plant-based, traditional, and natural medicine. Specifically:

- A holistic approach is required for understanding the true value of traditional knowledge and healing systems. Chapter 1 provides a sociological context, an often neglected aspect, to ethnopharmacological research.
- There is increasing evidence that inflammatory pathways underpin the proliferation associated with cancerous cells. This has led to an increased interest in investigating antiinflammatory substances for their ability to hinder cell proliferation. Chapter 2 has been chosen to illustrate the role of antiinflammatory agents for their antiproliferative activity.
- Unlike a large number of studies that have been published on the biological effects of fatty acids (FAs) of animal origin, not much is documented regarding the fatty acids of plant origin. In Chapter 3, the authors document the superiority of FAs from *Ranunculus* (a common medicinal plant across many cultures) in the down-regulation of pro-inflammatory cytokines.
- Edible mushrooms have been widely used due to their varied medicinal properties. Chapter 4 documents the utility of *Agaricus blazei* as a source of a potent antiallergen.
- Reactive oxygen species is a major cause of cytotoxicity. Therefore a lot of research has focused on antioxidants. Chapter 5 exemplifies the potential neuroprotective effect of flowers of a common Chinese medicinal plant, through antioxidant activity. While the roots of this plant (*Panax*) have been extensively studied, other parts of this plant have not received much attention. Hence, the demonstration of antioxidant activity of flowers is of interest.

- Biological effects of alkaloids from plants of the *Papaveraceae* family have been well characterised. Tubers of this family are widely used in European and Asian folk medicine. Chapter 6 is the first documentation of HeLa cell cytotoxicity of plant defense and pathogenicity related proteins obtained from *Corydalis cava* tubers.
- Chapter 7 documents the mechanism at the level of gene expression of inhibition of interferon gamma and interleukin 2 by arctigenin, isolated from the Chinese medicinal herb *Arctium lappa*.
- Induction of apoptosis and inhibition of angiogenesis are two important attributes of therapeutic agents with anticancer activity. Chapter 8 summarizes the current understanding of certain traditional Chinese medicines (*Scutellaria Baicalensis, Curcuma longa,* and *Artemisia absinthium*) in the context of these two mechanisms of anticancer activity.
- Turmeric (from *Curcuma longa)* is a widely used substance in Indian cuisine. The major phytochemical in it, curcumin, has been extensively studied for its antioxidant, antitoxic, antiinflammatory and potentially chemotherapeutic properties. Chapter 9 reviews the anticancer effects of *Curcumin* via cell cycle regulation.
- Chapter 10 evaluates the *in vitro* antioxidant and reactive oxygen species scavenging activities of the fruits of three medicinal plants commonly used in traditional Indian medicines: *Terminalia chebula, Terminalia belerica,* and *Emblica officinalis*.
- Chapter 11 is the first report of the antiHIV activity of the sea alga, *Sargassum fusiforme*. The aqueous extract of this sea alga has demonstrated potent inhibition of HIV-1 infection and replication in a variety of human cells including T cells. This dose dependent activity was similar to inhibition by the antiretroviral nucleoside analogue 2',3'- dideoxycytidine (ddC, zalcitabine).
- Chapter 12 is the first multidisciplinary study drawing on four different sources (taxonomic, phylogenetic, biogeographic and ethnobotanical) of information to explore new perspectives on bioactivity in plants.
- Chapter 13 describes a new approach, the application of 'omics', to the field of ethnobotany. It explores the field of 'ethnobotany genomics', a synthesis of the traditional knowledge and scientific knowledge systems, using two case studies with *Biophytum* and *Tripogon*.
- Chapter 14 describes a systematic analysis of several thousand TCM prescriptions for 30 types of cancers in Taiwan. In yet another approach to bringing the modern and traditional medicine together, the authors have attempted to statistically associate an ICD-9 coded cancer to a TCM prescription. Approaches like this pave the way for better understanding and integrating the traditional medicine with modern medical approaches.
- Chapter 15 has been included as a befitting conclusion to the theme of this book. This is an exposition of the person-centered medicine from the holistic perspective of traditional, complementary, and alternative medicine (TCAM). Salutogenesis as the fundamental principle of TCAM is explored in this paper.

LIST OF CONTRIBUTORS

Mauro Alivia
Charity Association for Person Centred Medicine, Via Siepelunga, 36/12, Bologna, 40141, Italy and Italian Society of Anthroposophic Medicine (SIMA), Milan, 20121, Italy

Jamal A. Al-Saghir
Department of Physiology, Faculty of Medicine, American University of Beirut, Beirut, Lebanon and Nature Conservation Center for Sustainable Futures (IBSAR), American University of Beirut, Beirut, Lebanon

Stanislaw Balcerkiewicz
Department of Plant Ecology and Environment Protection, Institute of Environmental Biology, Faculty of Biology, Adam Mickiewicz University, Umultowska 89, 61-614 Poznan, Poland

Wojciech Bialas
Department of Biotechnology and Food Microbiology, Poznan University of Life Sciences, Wojska Polskiego 48, 60-627 Poznan, Poland

Santanu Biswas
Division of Molecular Medicine, Bose Institute, P-1/12 CIT Scheme VIIM, Kolkata-700054, India

Mario Canki
Center for Immunology and Microbial Disease, Albany Medical College, Albany, NY, USA

João E. Carvalho
CPQBA, P.O. Box 6171, University of Campinas, 13083-970, Campinas, SP, Brazil

Chu-Ting Chang
Institute of Life Science, Fu-Jen University, Taipei, 24205, Taiwan

Shwu-Fen Chang
Graduate Institute of Medical Sciences, Taipei Medical University, Taipei, 11031, Taiwan

Jijun Chen
State Key Laboratory of Phytochemistry and Plant Resources in West China, Kunming Institute of Botany, Chinese Academy of Sciences, Kunming, Yunnan 650204, China

Anna Wing-Han Cheung
Center for Chinese Medicine and Department of Biology, Hong Kong University of Science and Technology, Clear Water Bay, Kowloon, Hong Kong SAR, China

Pei-Hsun Chiu
Institute of Systems Biology and Bioinformatics, National Central University, Chungli Taoyuan, Taiwan

Roy Chi-Yan Choi
Center for Chinese Medicine and Department of Biology, Hong Kong University of Science and Technology, Clear Water Bay, Kowloon, Hong Kong SAR, China

Bruce Clark
Center for Immunology and Microbial Disease, Albany Medical College, Albany, NY, USA and Department of Ob/Gyn, Albany Medical Center, Albany, NY, USA

Robin Cotter
Center for Immunology and Microbial Disease, Albany Medical College, Albany, NY, USA

Tanya Das
Division of Molecular Medicine, Bose Institute, P-1/12 CIT Scheme VII M, Kolkata, 700054, India

Paolo Roberti di Sarsina
High Council of Health, Ministry of Health, Rome, 00144, Italy, Charity Association for Person Centred Medicine, Via Siepelunga, 36/12, Bologna, 40141, Italy, and Observatory and Methods for Health, University of Milano-Bicocca, Milan, 20126, Italy

Heidi Dolder
Department of Anatomy, Cellular Biology, Physiology and Biophysics, Institute of Biology, P.O. Box 6109, University of Campinas, 13083-970, Campinas, SP, Brazil

Tina Tingxia Dong
Center for Chinese Medicine and Department of Biology, Hong Kong University of Science and Technology, Clear Water Bay, Kowloon, Hong Kong SAR, China

Linda K. Ellertsen
Department of Environmental Immunology, Norwegian Institute of Public Health, Oslo, Norway

Rima A. Ezzeddine
Department of Chemistry, Faculty of Arts and Sciences, American University of Beirut, Beirut, Lebanon and Nature Conservation Center for Sustainable Futures (IBSAR), American University of Beirut, Beirut, Lebanon

Mary A. Foglio
Department of Anatomy, Cellular Biology, Physiology and Biophysics, Institute of Biology, P.O. Box 6109, University of Campinas, 13083-970, Campinas, SP, Brazil

Félix Forest
Jodrell Laboratory, Royal Botanic Gardens, Kew, Richmond, United Kingdom

Sabreen F. Fostok
Department of Biology, Faculty of Arts and Sciences, American University of Beirut, Beirut, Lebanon and Nature Conservation Center for Sustainable Futures (IBSAR), American University of Beirut, Beirut, Lebanon

Louise Francis
Jodrell Laboratory, Royal Botanic Gardens, Kew, Richmond, United Kingdom

Qiang Fu
Center for Chinese Medicine and Department of Biology, Hong Kong University of Science and Technology, Clear Water Bay, Kowloon, Hong Kong SAR, China

Anna Gozdzicka-Jozefiak
Department of Molecular Virology, Institute of Experimental Biology, Faculty of Biology, Adam Mickiewicz University, Umultowska 89, 61-614 Poznan, Poland

Paola Guadagni
Charity Association for Person Centred Medicine, Via Siepelunga, 36/12, Bologna, 40141, Italy and Italian Society of Anthroposophic Medicine (SIMA), Milan, 20121, Italy

Julie A. Hawkins
School of Biological Sciences, University of Reading, Reading, United Kingdom

Bibhabasu Hazra
Division of Molecular Medicine, Bose Institute, P-1/12 CIT Scheme VIIM, Kolkata-700054, India

Geir Hetland
Department of Immunology and Transfusion Medicine, Oslo University Hospital, Ulleval, Oslo, Norway

Fadia R. Homaidan
Department of Physiology, Faculty of Medicine, American University of Beirut, Beirut, Lebanon and Nature Conservation Center for Sustainable Futures (IBSAR), American University of Beirut, Beirut, Lebanon

Hsin-Ying Hsieh
Institute of Systems Biology and Bioinformatics, National Central University, Chungli Taoyuan, Taiwan

Zhiyong Jiang
Center for Chinese Medicine and Department of Biology, Hong Kong University of Science and Technology, Clear Water Bay, Kowloon, Hong Kong SAR, China and State Key Laboratory of Phytochemistry and Plant Resources in West China, Kunming Institute of Botany, Chinese Academy of Sciences, Kunming, Yunnan 650204, China

Michael T. Klein
Center for Immunology and Microbial Disease, Albany Medical College, Albany, NY, USA

Bente B. Klitgaard
Herbarium, Library, Art and Archives, Royal Botanic Gardens, Kew, Richmond, United Kingdom

Yuh-Chi Kuo
Institute of Life Science, Fu-Jen University, Taipei, 24205, Taiwan

David Tai-Wai Lau
Center for Chinese Medicine and Department of Biology, Hong Kong University of Science and Technology, Clear Water Bay, Kowloon, Hong Kong SAR, China

David Y-W Lee
Bio-Organic and Natural Products Laboratory, Mailman Research Center, McLean Hospital, Harvard Medical School, Belmont, MA, USA

Tzong-Huei Lee
Graduate Institute of Pharmacology Science, Taipei Medical University, Taipei, 11031, Taiwan

Wen Li
Department of Microbiology and Immunology, Dartmouth Medical School, Lebanon, NH, USA

Xudong Lin
Center for Immunology and Microbial Disease, Albany Medical College, Albany, NY, USA

Gang Liu
Division of Molecular and Gene Therapies, School of Medical Science – Griffith Health, Gold Coast Campus, Griffith University, Brisbane, QLD 4222, Australia

Yanze Liu
Bio-Organic and Natural Products Laboratory, Mailman Research Center, McLean Hospital, Harvard Medical School, Belmont, MA, USA

Shao-Chun Lu
Department of Biochemistry and Molecular Biology, College of Medicine, National Taiwan University, Taipei, 10051, Taiwan

Nripendranath Mandal
Division of Molecular Medicine, Bose Institute, P-1/12 CIT Scheme VIIM, Kolkata-700054, India

Robert Nawrot
Department of Molecular Virology, Institute of Experimental Biology, Faculty of Biology, Adam Mickiewicz University, Umultowska 89, 61-614 Poznan, Poland

Steven G Newmaster
Botany Division, Centre for Biodiversity Genomics and Biodiversity Institute of Ontario Herbarium, University of Guelph, Guelph, Ontario, Canada

Harendra S. Parekh
The University of Queensland, School of Pharmacy, St Lucia QLD 4072, Brisbane, Australia

Elena E. Paskaleva
Center for Immunology and Microbial Disease, Albany Medical College, Albany, NY, USA

Fabricia S. Predes
Department of Anatomy, Cellular Biology, Physiology and Biophysics, Institute of Biology, P.O. Box 6109, University of Campinas, 13083-970, Campinas, SP, Brazil

Subramanyam Ragupathy
Botany Division, Centre for Biodiversity Genomics and Biodiversity Institute of Ontario Herbarium, University of Guelph, Guelph, Ontario, Canada

Victoria Reyes-García
ICREA and Institut de Ciència i Tecnologia Ambientals, Universitat Autònoma de Barcelona, 08193 Bellatera, Barcelona, Spain

Emily Roberge
Center for Immunology and Microbial Disease, Albany Medical College, Albany, NY, USA

Ana L.T.G. Ruiz
CPQBA, P.O. Box 6171, University of Campinas, 13083-970, Campinas, SP, Brazil

Gaurisankar Sa
Division of Molecular Medicine, Bose Institute, P-1/12 CIT Scheme VII M, Kolkata, 700054, India

Najat A. Saliba
Department of Chemistry, Faculty of Arts and Sciences, American University of Beirut, Beirut, Lebanon and Nature Conservation Center for Sustainable Futures (IBSAR), American University of Beirut, Beirut, Lebanon

Ralph G. Salloum
Nature Conservation Center for Sustainable Futures (IBSAR), American University of Beirut, Beirut, Lebanon and Department of Internal Medicine/Pediatrics, School of Medicine, Wayne State University, Detroit, MI 48201, USA

Rhitajit Sarkar
Division of Molecular Medicine, Bose Institute, P-1/12 CIT Scheme VIIM, Kolkata-700054, India

C. Haris Saslis-Lagoudakis
School of Biological Sciences, University of Reading, Reading, United Kingdom and Division of Biology, Silwood Park Campus, Imperial College London, Ascot, United Kingdom

Vincent Savolainen
Division of Biology, Silwood Park Campus, Imperial College London, Ascot, United Kingdom and Jodrell Laboratory, Royal Botanic Gardens, Kew, Richmond, United Kingdom

Rabih S. Talhouk
Department of Biology, Faculty of Arts and Sciences, American University of Beirut, Beirut, Lebanon and Nature Conservation Center for Sustainable Futures (IBSAR), American University of Beirut, Beirut, Lebanon

Wei-Jern Tsai
National Research Institute of Chinese Medicine, Taipei, 11221, Taiwan

Karl Wah-Keung Tsim
Center for Chinese Medicine and Department of Biology, Hong Kong University of Science and Technology, Clear Water Bay, Kowloon, Hong Kong SAR, China

Jean-Claude Veille
Center for Immunology and Microbial Disease, Albany Medical College, Albany, NY, USA and Department of Ob/Gyn, Albany Medical Center, Albany, NY, USA

Guei-Jane Wang
National Research Institute of Chinese Medicine, Taipei, 11221, Taiwan

Sun-Chong Wang
Institute of Systems Biology and Bioinformatics, National Central University, Chungli Taoyuan, Taiwan and Epigenetics Laboratory, Centre for Addiction and Mental Health, Toronto, Ontario, Canada

Zhengtao Wang
Institute of Chinese Materia Medica, Shanghai University of Traditional Chinese Medicine, 1200 Cailun Road, Zhangjiang Hi-Tech Park, Shanghai 201203, China

Ming Q. Wei
Division of Molecular and Gene Therapies, School of Medical Science – Griffith Health, Gold Coast Campus, Griffith University, Brisbane, QLD 4222, Australia

Elizabeth M. Williamson
School of Pharmacy, University of Reading, Reading, United Kingdom

Maria Wolun-Cholewa
Department of Cell Biology, University of Medical Sciences, Rokietnicka 5d, 60-806 Poznan, Poland

Danuta Wyrzykowska
Department of Molecular Virology, Institute of Experimental Biology, Faculty of Biology, Adam Mickiewicz University, Umultowska 89, 61-614 Poznan, Poland

Heidi Qun Xie
Center for Chinese Medicine and Department of Biology, Hong Kong University of Science and Technology, Clear Water Bay, Kowloon, Hong Kong SAR, China

Er K. Yu
Center for Immunology and Microbial Disease, Albany Medical College, Albany, NY, USA

INTRODUCTION

This book discusses the use of several medicinal plants and their wider applications in the domain of medicinal, clinical, and pharmaceutical treatment. The articles chosen serve as a useful source of ideas and inspiration for further cell and molecular biology research toward developing additional treatments from these traditional remedies. The book is divided into four parts. The first defends the importance of traditional knowledge to modern biological science. The second provides several case studies of various traditional medicines that have been used to treat disease. The third focuses on the molecular biology of several traditional remedies, and the final section offers an argument for person-centered medicine as a way to tie the chapters together.

Ethnopharmacology is at the intersection of the medical, natural, and social sciences. Despite its interdisciplinary nature, most ethnopharmacological research has been based on the combination of the chemical, biological, and pharmacological sciences. Far less attention has been given to the social sciences, including anthropology and the study of traditional knowledge systems. In Chapter 1, Reyes-García reviews the literature on traditional knowledge systems, highlighting its potential theoretical and methodological contributions to ethnopharmacology. The author discusses three potential theoretical contributions of traditional knowledge systems to ethnopharmacological research. First, while many plants used in indigenous pharmacopoeias have active compounds, those compounds do not always act alone in indigenous healing systems. Research highlights the holistic nature of traditional knowledge systems and helps understand plant's efficacy in its cultural context. Second, research on traditional knowledge systems can improve our understanding of how ethnopharmacological knowledge is distributed in a society, and who benefits from it. Third, research on traditional knowledge systems can enhance the study of the social relations that enable the generation, maintenance, spread, and devolution of cultural traits and innovations, including ethnopharmacological knowledge. At a methodological level, some ethnopharmacolo-gists have used anthropological tools to understand the context of plant use and local meanings of health and disease. The author discusses two more potential methodological contributions of research on traditional knowledge systems to ethnopharmacological research. First, traditional knowledge systems research has developed methods that would help eth-nopharmacologists understand how people classify illnesses and remedies, a fundamental aspect of folk medicinal plant selection criteria. Second, ethnopharmacologists could also borrow methods derived from cultural consensus theory to have a broader look at intracultural variation and at the analysis of transmission and loss of traditional ethnopharmacologi-cal knowledge. Ethical considerations in the ethnopharmacology of the 21st century should go beyond the recognition of the Intellectual Property Rights or the acquisition of research permits, to include considerations on the healthcare of the original holders of ethnopharmacological knowledge. Ethnopharmacology can do more than speed up to recover the traditional knowledge of indigenous peoples to make it available for the development of new drugs. Ethnopharmacologists can work with health care providers in the developing world for the local implementation of ethnopharmaco-logical research results.

Arctium lappa, known as burdock, is widely used in popular medicine for hypertension, gout, hepatitis and other inflammatory disorders. Phar-macological studies indicated that burdock roots have hepatoprotective, anti-inflammatory, free radical scavenging and antiproliferative activities. The aim of this study was to evaluate total phenolic content, radical scav-enging activity by DPPH and *in vitro* antiproliferative activity of differ-ent *A. lappa* root extracts. Hot and room temperature dichloromethanic, ethanolic and aqueous extracts; hydroethanolic and total aqueous extract of *A. lappa* roots were investigated in Chapter 2, by Predes and colleagues, regarding radical scavenging activity by DPPH, total phenolic content by Folin-Ciocalteau method and antiproliferative *in vitro* activity was evalu-ated in human cancer cell lines. The hydroethanolic extract analyzed by high-resolution electrospray ionization mass spectroscopy. Higher radical scavenging activity was found for the hydroethanolic extract. The higher phenolic contents were found for the dichloromethane, obtained both by Soxhlet and maceration extraction and hydroethanolic extracts. The HRE-

SI-MS demonstrated the presence of arctigenin, quercetin, chlorogenic acid and caffeic acid compounds, which were identified by comparison with previous data. The dichloromethane extracts were the only extracts that exhibited activity against cancer cell lines, especially for K562, MCF-7 and 786-0 cell lines. The hydroethanolic extracts exhibited the strongest free radical scavenging activity, while the highest phenolic content was observed in Soxhlet extraction. Moreover, the dichloromethanic extracts showed selective antiproliferative activity against K562, MCF-7 and 786-0 human cancer cell lines.

Medicinal plants represent alternative means for the treatment of several chronic diseases, including inflammation. The genus *Ranunculus*, a representative of the *Ranunculaceae* family, has been reported to possess anti-inflammatory, analgesic, antiviral, antibacterial, antiparasitic and antifungal activities, possibly due to the presence of anemonin and other compounds. Different studies have shown the occurrence of unusual fatty acids (FAs) in *Ranunculaceae*; however, their therapeutic role has not been investigated. The purpose of this study was to characterize potential anti-inflammatory bioactivities in *Ranunculus constantinopolitanus* D'Urv., traditionally used in Eastern Mediterranean folk medicine. In Chapter 3, by Fostok and colleagues, the aerial part of *R. constantinopolitanus* was subjected to methanol (MeOH) extraction and solvent fractionation. The bioactive fraction (I.2) was further fractionated using column chromatography, and the biologically active subfraction (Y2+3) was identified using infrared (IR) spectroscopy, nuclear magnetic resonance (NMR) and gas chromatography-mass spectrometry (GC-MS). The effects of I.2 and Y2+3 on cell viability were studied in mouse mammary epithelial SCp2 cells using the trypan blue exclusion method. To study the anti-inflammatory activities of I.2 and Y2+3, their ability to reduce interleukin (IL)-6 levels was assessed in endotoxin (ET)-stimulated SCp2 cells using enzyme-linked immunosorbent assay (ELISA). In addition, the ability of Y2+3 to reduce cyclooxygenase (COX)-2 expression was studied in IL-1-treated mouse intestinal epithelial Mode-K cells via western blotting. Data were analyzed by one-way analysis of variance (ANOVA), Student-Newman-Keuls (SNK), Tukey HSD, two-sample t-test and Dunnett t-tests for multiple comparisons. The chloroform fraction (I.2) derived from the crude MeOH extract of the plant, in addition to Y2+3, a FA mix isolated from this fraction and containing palmitic acid, C18:2 and C18:1 isomers and stearic acid (1:5:8:1 ratio), reduced ET-induced IL-6 levels in SCp2 cells without affecting cell viability or morphology. When compared to fish oil, conjugated linoleic acid (CLA) and to individual FAs as palmitic, linoleic, oleic and stearic acid or to a mix of these FAs (1:5:8:1 ratio), Y2+3 exhibited higher potency in reducing ET-induced IL-6 levels within a shorter period of time. Y2+3 also reduced COX-2 expression in IL-1-treated Mode-K cells. The studies demonstrate the existence of potential anti-inflammatory bioactivities in *R. constantinopolitanus* and attribute them to a FA mix in this plant.

Agaricus blazei Murill (AbM) is an edible Brazilian mushroom that has been used in traditional medicine for a range of diseases. It has been shown to have anti-infection and anti-tumor properties in the mouse, which are due to induction of Th1 responses. On the other hand, IgE-mediated allergy is induced by a Th2 response. Since according to the Th1/Th2 paradigm an increased Th1 response may promote a reduced Th2 response, the aim of Ellertsen and Hetland in Chapter 4 was to examine whether AbM had anti-allergy effects. A mouse model for allergy was employed, in which the mice were immunized s.c. with the model allergen ovalbumin (OVA). Additionally, the animals were given a mushroom extract, AndoSan™, mainly (82%) containing AbM, but also *Hericium erinaceum* (15%) and *Grifola frondosa* (3%), or PBS p.o. either a day before or 19 days after the immunization. The mice were sacrificed on day 26, and anti-OVA IgE (Th2 response) and IgG2a (Th1 response) antibodies were examined in serum and Th1, Th2 and Treg cytokines in spleen cells cultures. It was found that the AndoSan™ extract both when given either before or after OVA immunization reduced the levels of anti-OVA IgE, but not IgG2a, in the mice. There was a tendency to reduced Th2 relative to Th1 cytokine levels in the AndoSan™ groups. This particular AbM extract may both prevent allergy development and be used as a therapeutical substance against established allergy.

Radix notoginseng is used in Chinese medicine to improve blood circulation and clotting; however, the pharmacological activities of other parts of Panax notoginseng have yet to be explored. Chapter 5, by Choi and colleagues, reports the anti-oxidative effects of various parts of *Panax notoginseng*. Various parts of *Panax notoginseng*, including the biennial

flower, stem-leaf, root-rhizome, fiber root and sideslip, were used to pre-
pare extracts and analyzed for their anti-oxidation effects, namely suppressing xanthine oxidase activity, H_2O_2-induced cytotoxicity and H_2O_2-
induced ROS formation. Among various parts of the herb (biennial flower,
stem-leaf, root-rhizome, fiber root and sideslip), the water extract of the
biennial flower showed the strongest effects in (i) inhibiting the enzymatic activity of xanthine oxidase and (ii) protecting neuronal PC12 cells
against H_2O_2-induced cytotoxicity. Only the water extracts demonstrated
such anti-oxidative effects while the ethanol extracts did not exert significant effects in suppressing xanthine oxidase and H_2O_2-induced neuronal
cytotoxicity. The present study demonstrates the biennial flower of Panax
notoginseng to have a neuroprotection effect on cultured neurons and the
underlying protection mechanism may involve anti-oxidation.

    Corydalis cava Schweigg. & Koerte is a plant of numerous pharmaco-
logical activities. Along with *Chelidonium majus* L. (Greater Celandine),
it belongs to the family *Papaveraceae*. The plant grows in Central and
South Europe and produces the sizeable subterraneous tubers, empty inside, which are extremely resistant to various pathogen attacks. The *Corydalis* sp. tubers are a rich source of many biologically active substances,
with the extensive use in European and Asian folk medicine. They have
analgetic, sedating, narcotic, anti-inflammatory, anti-allergic and anti-
tumour activities. On the other hand, there is no information about possible biological activities of proteins contained in *Corydalis cava* tubers.
In Chapter 6, Narwot and colleagues isolated nucleolytic proteins from the
tubers of *C. cava* by separation on a heparin column and tested for DNase
activity. Protein fractions showing nucleolytic activity were tested for cytotoxic activity in human cervical carcinoma HeLa cells. Cultures of HeLa
cells were conducted in the presence of three protein concentrations: 42,
83 and 167 ng/ml during 48 h. Viability of cell cultures was appraised using the XTT colorimetric test. Protein fractions were separated and protein
bands were excised and sent for identification by mass spectrometry (LC-
ESI-MS/MS). The studied protein fractions showed an inhibiting effect on
mitochondrial activity of HeLa cells, depending on the administered dose
of proteins. The most pronounced effect was obtained with the highest
concentration of the protein (167 ng/ml) - $43.45 \pm 3\%$ mitochondrial activity of HeLa cells were inhibited. Mass spectrometry results for the proteins

of applied fractions showed that they contained plant defense- and patho-genesis-related (PR) proteins. The cytotoxic effect of studied proteins to-ward HeLa cell line cells has been evident and dependent on increasing dose of the protein. The present study, most probably, represents the first investigations on the effect of purified PR proteins from tuber extracts of a pharmacologically active plant on cell lines.

Arctium lappa (Niubang), a Chinese herbal medicine, is used to treat tissue inflammation. Chapter 7, by Tsai and colleagues, investigates the effects of arctigenin (AC), isolated from *A. lappa*, on anti-CD3/CD28 Ab-stimulated cell proliferation and cytokine gene expression in primary human T lymphocytes. Cell proliferation was determined with enzyme immunoassays and the tritiated thymidine uptake method. Cytokine pro-duction and gene expression were analyzed with reverse transcription-polymerase chain reaction. AC inhibited primary human T lymphocytes proliferation activated by anti-CD3/CD28 Ab. Cell viability test indicated that the inhibitory effects of AC on primary human T lymphocyte prolif-eration were not due to direct cytotoxicity. AC suppressed interleukin-2 (IL-2) and interferon-γ (IFN-γ) production in a concentration-dependent manner. Furthermore, AC decreased the IL-2 and IFN-γ gene expression in primary human T lymphocytes induced by anti-CD3/CD28 Ab. Re-porter gene analyses revealed that AC decreased NF-AT-mediated reporter gene expression. AC inhibited T lymphocyte proliferation and decreased the gene expression of IL-2, IFN-γ and NF-AT.

Although traditional Chinese medicine has benefitted one fifth of the world's population in treating a plethora of diseases, its acceptance as a real therapeutic option by the West is only now emerging. In light of a new wave of recognition being given to traditional Chinese medicine by health professionals and regulatory bodies in the West, Parekh and colleagues argue in Chapter 8 that an understanding of their molecular basis and highlighting potential future applications of a proven group of traditional Chinese medicine in the treatment of a variety of cancers is crucial—this is where their calling holds much hope and promise in both animal and hu-man trials. Furthermore, the rationale for combining conventional agents and modern biotechnological approaches to the delivery of traditional Chinese medicine is an avenue set to revolutionize the future practice of cancer medicine—and this may well bring on a new dawn of therapeutic strategies where East truly meets West.

Increasing knowledge on the cell cycle deregulations in cancers has promoted the introduction of phytochemicals, which can either modulate signaling pathways leading to cell cycle regulation or directly alter cell cycle regulatory molecules, in cancer therapy. Most human malignancies are driven by chromosomal translocations or other genetic alterations that directly affect the function of critical cell cycle proteins such as cyclins as well as tumor suppressors, e.g., p53. In this respect, cell cycle regulation and its modulation by curcumin are gaining widespread attention in recent years. Extensive research has addressed the chemotherapeutic potential of curcumin (diferuloylmethane), a relatively non-toxic plant derived poly-phenol. The mechanisms implicated are diverse and appear to involve a combination of cell signaling pathways at multiple levels. In Chapter 9, Sa and Das discuss how alterations in the cell cycle control contribute to the malignant transformation and provide an overview of how curcumin targets cell cycle regulatory molecules to assert anti-proliferative and/or apoptotic effects in cancer cells. The purpose of this article was to present an appraisal of the current level of knowledge regarding the potential of curcumin as an agent for the chemoprevention of cancer via an under-standing of its mechanism of action at the level of cell cycle regulation. Taken together, this review sought to summarize the unique properties of curcumin that may be exploited for successful clinical cancer prevention.

Cellular damage caused by reactive oxygen species (ROS) has been implicated in several diseases, and hence natural antioxidants have signifi-cant importance in human health. Chapter 10, by Hazra and colleagues, was carried out to evaluate the *in vitro* antioxidant and reactive oxygen species scavenging activities of *Terminalia chebula, Terminalia belerica* and *Emblica officinalis* fruit extracts. The 70% methanol extracts were studied for *in vitro* total antioxidant activity along with phenolic and fla-vonoid contents and reducing power. Scavenging ability of the extracts for radicals like DPPH, hydroxyl, superoxide, nitric oxide, hydrogen perox-ide, peroxynitrite, singlet oxygen, hypochlorous acid were also performed to determine the potential of the extracts. The ability of the extracts of the fruits in exhibiting their antioxative properties follow the order *T. chebula* > *E. officinalis* > *T. belerica*. The same order is followed in their flavonoid content, whereas in the case of phenolic content it becomes *E. officinalis* > *T. belerica* > *T. chebula*. In the studies of free radicals' scavenging, where the activities of the plant extracts were inversely proportional to their IC50 values, *T. chebula* and *E. officinalis* were found to be taking the leading role with the orders of *T. chebula* >*E. officinalis* > *T. belerica* for superoxide and nitric oxide, and *E. officinalis* > *T. belerica* > *T. chebula* for DPPH and peroxynitrite radicals. Miscellaneous results were observed in the scavenging of other radicals by the plant extracts, viz., *T. chebula* > *T. belerica* > *E. officinalis* for hydroxyl, *T. belerica* > *T. chebula* >*E. officinalis* for singlet oxygen and *T. belerica* > *E. officinalis* > *T. chebula* for hypochlorous acid. Overall, the studied fruit extracts showed quite good efficacy in their antioxidants and radical scavenging abilities, compared to the standards. The evidences as can be concluded from the study of the 70% methanol extract of the fruits of *Terminalia chebula, Terminalia belerica* and *Emblica officinalis*, imposes the fact that they might be useful as potent sources of natural antioxidants.

The high rate of HIV-1 mutation and increasing resistance to currently available antiretroviral (ART) therapies highlight the need for new antiviral agents. Products derived from natural sources have been shown to inhibit HIV-1 replication during various stages of the virus life cycle, and therefore represent a potential source of novel therapeutic agents. To expand our arsenal of therapeutics against HIV-1 infection, in Chapter 11 Paskaleva and colleagues investigated the aqueous extract from *Sargassum fusiforme* (*S. fusiforme*) for its ability to inhibit HIV-1 infection in the periphery, in T cells and human macrophages, and for its ability to inhibit in the central nervous system (CNS), in microglia and astrocytes. The *S. fusiforme* extract blocked HIV-1 infection and replication by over 90% in T cells, human macrophages and microglia, and it also inhibited pseudo-typed HIV-1 (VSV/NL4-3) infection in human astrocytes by over 70%. Inhibition was mediated against both CXCR4 (X4) and CCR5 (R5)-tropic HIV-1, was dose dependant and long lasting, did not inhibit cell growth or viability, was not toxic to cells, and was comparable to inhibition by the nucleoside analogue 2',3'-didoxycytidine (ddC). *S. fusiforme* treatment blocked direct cell-to-cell infection spread. To investigate at which point of the virus life cycle this inhibition occurs, we infected T cells and CD4-negative primary human astrocytes with HIV-1 pseudotyped with envelope glycoprotein of vesicular stomatitis virus (VSV), which bypasses the HIV receptor requirements. Infection by pseudotyped HIV-1 (VSV/NL4-3) was also inhibited in a dose dependant manner, although up to 57% less, as compared to inhibition of native NL4-3, indicating post-entry interferences. This is the first report demonstrating *S. fusiforme* to be a potent inhibitor of highly productive HIV-1 infection and replication in T cells, in primary human macrophages, microglia, and astrocytes. Results with VSV/NL4-3 infection, suggest inhibition of both entry and post-entry events of the virus life cycle. Absence of cytotoxicity and high viability of treated cells also suggest that *S. fusiforme* is a potential source of novel naturally occurring antiretroviral compounds that inhibit HIV-1 infection and replication at more than one site of the virus life cycle.

The study of traditional knowledge of medicinal plants has led to discoveries that have helped combat diseases and improve healthcare. However, the development of quantitative measures that can assist our quest for new medicinal plants has not greatly advanced in recent years. Phylogenetic tools have entered many scientific fields in the last two decades to provide explanatory power, but have been overlooked in ethnomedicinal studies. Several studies show that medicinal properties are not randomly distributed in plant phylogenies, suggesting that phylogeny shapes ethnobotanical use. Nevertheless, empirical studies that explicitly combine ethnobotanical and phylogenetic information are scarce. In Chapter 12, Saslis-Lagoudakis and colleagues borrowed tools from community ecology phylogenetics to quantify significance of phylogenetic signal in medicinal properties in plants and identify nodes on phylogenies with high bioscreening potential. To do this, the authors produced an ethnomedicinal review from extensive literature research and a multi-locus phylogenetic hypothesis for the pantropical genus *Pterocarpus* (Leguminosae: Papilionoideae). They demonstrate that species used to treat a certain conditions, such as malaria, are significantly phylogenetically clumped and we highlight nodes in the phylogeny that are significantly overabundant in species used to treat certain conditions. These cross-cultural patterns in ethnomedicinal usage in Pterocarpus are interpreted in the light of phylogenetic relationships. This study provides techniques that enable the application of phylogenies in bioscreening, but also sheds light on the processes that shape cross-cultural ethnomedicinal patterns. This community phylogenetic approach demonstrates that similar ethnobotanical uses can arise in parallel in different areas where related plants are available. With a vast amount of ethnomedicinal and phylogenetic information available, we predict that this field, after further refinement of the techniques, will expand into similar research areas, such as pest management or the search for bioactive plant-based compounds.

Newmaster and Ragupathy present in Chapter 13 the first use of DNA barcoding in a new approach to ethnobotany they coined "ethnobotany genomics". This new approach is founded on the concept of 'assemblage' of biodiversity knowledge, which includes a coming together of different ways of knowing and valorizing species variation in a novel approach seeking to add value to both traditional knowledge (TK) and scientific knowledge (SK). The authors employed contemporary genomic technology, DNA barcoding, as an important tool for identifying cryptic species, which were already recognized ethnotaxa using the TK classification systems of local cultures in the Velliangiri Hills of India. This research is based on several case studies in the authors' lab, which define an approach to that is poised to evolve quickly with the advent of new ideas and technology. The results show that DNA barcoding validated several new cryptic plant species to science that were previously recognized by TK classifications of the Irulas and Malasars, and were lumped using SK classification. The contribution of the local aboriginal knowledge concerning plant diversity and utility in India is considerable; this study presents new ethnomedicine to science. Ethnobotany genomics can also be used to determine the distribution of rare species and their ecological requirements, including traditional ecological knowledge so that conservation strategies can be implemented. This is aligned with the Convention on Biological Diversity that was signed by over 150 nations, and thus the world's complex array of human-natural-technological relationships has effectively been re-organized.

Targeted cancer therapies, with specific molecular targets, ameliorate the side effect issue of radiation and chemotherapy and also point to the development of personalized medicine. Combination of drugs targeting multiple pathways of carcinogenesis is potentially more fruitful. Traditional Chinese medicine (TCM) has been tailoring herbal mixtures for individualized healthcare for two thousand years. A systematic study of the patterns of TCM formulas and herbs prescribed to cancers is valuable. In Chapter 14, Chiu and colleagues analyzed a total of 187,230 TCM prescriptions to 30 types of cancer in Taiwan in 2007, a year's worth of collection from the National Health Insurance reimbursement database (Taiwan). They found that a TCM cancer prescription consists on average of two formulas and four herbs. They show that the percentage weights of TCM formulas and herbs in a TCM prescription follow Zipf's law with an exponent around 0.6. TCM prescriptions to benign neoplasms have a larger Zipf's exponent than those to malignant cancers. Furthermore, the study shows that TCM prescriptions, via weighted combination of formulas and herbs, are specific to not only the malignancy of neoplasms but also the sites of origins of malignant cancers. From the effects of formulas and natures of herbs that were heavily prescribed to cancers, that cancers are a 'warm and stagnant' syndrome in TCM can be proposed, suggesting anti-inflammatory regimens for better prevention and treatment of cancers. The authors show that TCM incorporated relevant formulas to the prescriptions to cancer patients with a secondary morbidity. They compared TCM prescriptions made in different seasons and identified temperatures as the environmental factor that correlates with changes in TCM prescriptions in Taiwan. Lung cancer patients were among the patients whose prescriptions were adjusted when temperatures drop. The findings of this study provide insight to TCM cancer treatment, helping dialogue between modern western medicine and TCM for better cancer care.

Traditional, complementary and alternative medical (TCAM) systems contribute to the foundation of person-centered medicine (PCM), an epistemological orientation for medical science which places the person as a physical, psychological and spiritual entity at the center of health care and of the therapeutic process, and is the subject of Chapter 15, by di Sarsina and colleagues. PCM wishes to broaden the bio-molecular reductionistic approach of medical science towards an integration that allows people, doctors, nurses, health-care professionals and patients to become the real protagonists of the health-care scene. The doctor or caregiver needs to act out of empathy to meet the unique value of each human being, which unfolds over the course of a lifetime from conception to natural death. Knowledge of the human being should not be instrumental to economic or political interests, ideology, theories or religious dogma. Research needs to be broadened with methodological tools to investigate person-centred medical interventions. Salutogenesis is a fundamental principle of PCM, promoting health and preventing illness by strengthening the individual's self-healing abilities. TCAM systems also give tools to predict the insurgence of illness and treat it before the appearance of overt organic disease. A task of PCM is to educate people to take better care of their physical, psychological and spiritual health. Health-care education needs to be broadened to give doctors and health-care workers of the future the tools to act in innovative and highly differentiated ways, always guided by deep respect for individual autonomy, personal culture, religion and beliefs.

PART I

RELEVANCE OF TRADITIONAL KNOWLEDGE TO BIOLOGICAL TESTING

CHAPTER 1

THE RELEVANCE OF TRADITIONAL KNOWLEDGE SYSTEMS FOR ETHNOPHARMACOLOGICAL RESEARCH: THEORETICAL AND METHODOLOGICAL CONTRIBUTIONS

VICTORIA REYES-GARCÍA

1.1 BACKGROUND

Ethnopharmacology is, by definition, at the intersection of the medical, natural, and social sciences [1]. Despite the interdisciplinary nature of ethnopharmacology, much of its research has been exclusively based on the combination of the chemical, biological, and pharmacological sciences. Less attention has been given to the potential contributions of the social sciences, including anthropology and the study of traditional knowledge systems (but see, for example, the work of Giovannini and Heinrich [2], Thomas, Vandebroek, and colleagues [3,4], Pieroni and colleagues [5], Albuquerque and Oliveira [6], Pardo-de-Santayana and colleagues [7] among others). When anthropological expertise and tools have been used, the main purpose has been to obtain catalogues of medicinal

This chapter was originally published under the Creative Commons Attribution License. Reyes-García V. The Relevance of Traditional Knowledge Systems for Ethnopharmacological Research: Theoretical and Methodological Contributions. Journal of Ethnobiology and Ethnomedicine **6**,*32 (2010), doi:10.1186/1746-4269-6-32.*

plant uses, which were often abstracted from their cultural contexts and subject to little analysis or interpretation [8-10]. Furthermore, more often than not—and especially when working among indigenous peoples—the sole purpose of obtaining those lists and catalogues has been to facilitate the intentional and focused discovery of active compounds. In sum, with some remarkable exceptions and without undervaluing researchers who have catalogued the often threatened knowledge of medicinal plant uses, to date many ethnopharmacologists have limited themselves to document indigenous pharmacopoeias in the search for pharmacologically unique principles that might result in the development of commercial drugs [11] or nutraceuticals [12].

Several reviews of the development of the discipline have warned against the disciplinarily bias in ethnopharmacology. For example, in a review of articles published in one of the flagship journals of the discipline, the Journal of Ethnopharmacology, Etkin and Elisabetsky [1] stated:

> Mission statement notwithstanding, during the first two decades of its existence most of the articles published in the JEP were not interdisciplinary. Two retrospective content analyses of the journal revealed for the periods 1979-1996 and 1996-2000 an increasing number of articles dedicated exclusively or primarily to pharmacology and pharmacognosy. More significant to the present discussion is the consistently small number of multi- or interdisciplinary articles, 4-6% of the total published (pg 24).

Almost a decade later, the situation seem not to have changed much, as the editorial of a 2010 issue of the same journal [13] states that

> [Since its origins] numerous studies in the Journal dealing with medicinal and other useful plants as well as their bioactive compounds have used a multitude of concepts and methodologies. In many cases these were interdisciplinary or multidisciplinary studies combining such diverse fields as anthropology, pharmacology, pharmacognosy.... pharmaceutical biology, natural product chemistry, toxicology, clinical research, plant physiology and others (see Soejarto, D.D., 2001, Journal of Ethnopharmacology

74: iii). However, many studies still only pay lip service to such interdisciplinary research and there still remains an urgent need to further strengthen the contributions made by anthropology and other social and cultural sciences as well as to explore the political and social implication of our research.

That ethnopharmacologists are growing aware of theoretical and methodological biases in the discipline is an important first step. Even more important is that the growing awareness on those biases has paralleled a more fundamental change in the goals of ethnopharmacology. Namely, the initial bias towards the chemical, biological, and pharmacological sciences closely related to the understanding that the overarching goal of ethnopharmacology is the search of biologically active compounds of plants, fungi, animals, and mineral substances used in traditional medicines. But, as this new field of research grows, ethnopharmacologists become more conscious that finding active compounds should only be one of the goals of the discipline. Many ethnopharmacologists have been—and still are—pushing for changes in how the goals of ethnopharmacology are conceptualized [14-18]. For instance, in a relatively recent article, Etkin and Elisabetsky argued that the discipline now "strives for a more holistic, theory-driven, and culture- and context sensitive study of the pharmacologic potential of (largely botanical) species used by indigenous peoples for medicine, food, and other purposes"[1]. But ethnopharmacology can not achieve these new goals without simultaneously adopting theoretical and methodological contributions from the social sciences. Here, I aim to contribute to that effort by reviewing the potential theoretical and methodological contributions to ethnopharmacological research of a branch of a social science discipline: research on traditional knowledge systems.

1.1.1 THEORETICAL CONTRIBUTIONS OF THE STUDY OF TRADITIONAL KNOWLEDGE SYSTEMS TO ETHNOPHARMACOLOGY

I use the terms traditional knowledge and traditional knowledge systems to refer to the knowledge of resource and ecosystem dynamics and associated management practices existing among people of communities that, on a daily basis and over long periods of time, interact for their benefit and livelihood with ecosystems [19,20]. The term does not merely refer to information about human uses of plants and animals [20]. Rather, it includes a system of classifications, a set of empirical observations about the local environment, and a system of resource use and management. It also includes believes in non-human beings (i.e., spirits, ancestors, ghosts, gods) and on how they relate to society. The study of TKS parallels ethnopharmacology in that both fields of research initially emphasized descriptive accounts, but they are now moving towards a more hypotheses-driven research. Here I will focus on three theoretical contributions from research on TKS, highlighting their relation to ethnopharmacological research.

1.1.2 TK AS A HOLISTIC SYSTEM OF KNOWLEDGE

The first theoretical contribution relates to the holistic nature of traditional knowledge systems. As mentioned, TK, rather than a compilation of information about plants and animals, is a way to understand the world, or what we understand as "culture". Anthropologists state that culture patterns human behavior and—through it—affects human health and well-being. In traditional societies, an essential function of culture has been to establish and transmit a body of knowledge, practices, and believes regarding the use of locally available natural resources to improve health and nutritional status. Quantitative research on the topic highlights the effects of locally developed traditional knowledge on adult and infant health and nutritional status. For example, in my collaborative research among the Tsimane', a hunter-horticulturalist society in the Bolivian Amazon, we have found that the level to which an individual shares the knowledge of the group is associated to own nutritional status [21] and offspring's health [22]. That is, people who share larger amounts of the traditional knowledge developed by the group display better health—measured through objective and subjective indicators—than people who do not share as much knowledge.

Ethnopharmacology can draw two important theoretical conclusions from those research findings. First, notice that those findings are based in a broad measure of traditional knowledge, not on the targeted study of a plant or a group of plants with active compounds. That is, we did not conduct a pharmacological study of local medicinal plants and then include those with active compounds in our questionnaire. Furthermore, our measure of TK was not limited to medicinal plants. Rather, our measure included questions on a wide range of useful plants (medicinal, but also edible, construction, dyes, and plants with other uses). We interpret the positive association between our broad measure of TK and objective and subjective indicators of health as indications that medicinal knowledge systems are not built of isolated pieces of information, but rather constitute a complex body of knowledge linked to a larger coherent ensemble. The implication is then that identifying active compounds in a plant might be of good use for the pharmacological industry, but it might be of limited use for knowledge holders, because it is possible that for a given medicine to be effective in the local context, it requires the accompanying practices and beliefs that provide the medicinal "meaning" to the plant (sensu Moerman, see bellow). The first point I want to stress here, then, is that, while it is evident that many plants used in indigenous pharmacopoeias do have active compounds, it is also likely that those active compounds do not act alone in indigenous healing systems, but they partially act because they have a shared medicinal cultural meaning [23]. And, as it has been highlighted by previous researchers [10,23], the efficacy of a medicinal plant should be measured in a culturally appropriated way, and the failure to consider the cultural context within which plants are used can result in misunderstandings of a plant's efficacy. So, it is the complex system, rather than the intake of particular plants with active compounds, that might shape the health and well-being of TK holders.

The second related lesson to be drawn from the example above relates to the indigenous understanding of health. Indigenous peoples have sophisticated ideas of health and well-being. As also recognized for the World Health Organization, for many indigenous peoples, health is not merely absence of disease [24]. Health is a state of spiritual, communal, and ecosystem equilibrium and wellbeing [25], which probably explains why traditional pharmacopeias include remedies both to cure physical ailments (whether caused by spiritual or magical beings, or by the physical world) and to improve one's well-being (i.e., to protect infants from witches or evil spirits or to enhance hunting abilities). Furthermore, among indigenous peoples, the choice of a medical treatment is often explained by this complex understanding of health and the perceived causes of illness. For example, the Tsimane' choice of medical treatment is often related to the perceived cause of the illness. Common illnesses, caused by the natural world, can be cured by medicinal plants or drugs, whereas illnesses caused by spiritual beings can only be cured by the intervention of a traditional healer [26]. When a person gets sick, she is often first treated as if she suffered from a common illness. Plants (or pharmaceutical) remedies are administered sequentially or simultaneously, often without consultation from any expert. If the condition persists, the Tsimane' start being suspicious that the illness is caused by witchcraft, in which case, they seek the help of a traditional healer. So, physical symptoms are only one of the clues to be used when selecting a treatment and the perceived (natural or spiritual) causes of the illness might be more relevant in the selection of the treatment. In that sense, as Moerman and Jonas have highlighted [23,27,28], even plants without active compounds can have healing effects, in the same way that placebo medicines have healing effects in Western culture. Plants and medicines might be effective, not because of their pharmacology, but because of the cultural "meaning" (sensu Moerman 2007) assigned to them. To put it in Moerman's [23] words:

> However, the effectiveness of these plants as medicines is not simply a consequence of their pharmacology; they are not pills disguised as herbs. Botanical medicinal effectiveness is inevitably some varying combination of pharmacology and meaning. Neglecting either aspect of this effectiveness is to provide only a partial, and thereby an erroneous, view of the subject (pg. 459).

In sum, research on TKS and its relation to the health of indigenous people suggests that the medicinal uses of plants, animals, fungi, and minerals are better understood if studied as a domain of knowledge embedded in the large body of cultural knowledge, practices, and beliefs of a group. The focus on testing the active compounds of indigenous pharmacopoeias conveys the idea that local medicines become meaningful only when pharmacologically validated, and thus diminishes traditional knowledge systems and indigenous explanations of the world. Thus, an important task ahead for ethnopharmacology is to contextualize uses and cultural perceptions of plants as a way to acknowledge that the intangible attributes of a species may be as important criteria for inclusion in indigenous pharmacopeias as its tangible attributes.

1.1.3 THE DISTRIBUTION OF TRADITIONAL KNOWLEDGE

The second theoretical contribution from research on TK that can help in the ethnopharmacological enterprise relates to the distribution of knowledge within a group. Recently, Heinrich and colleagues [29] claimed that "minimally, any [ethnopharmacological] field study should examine how plant knowledge is distributed in a society, and include some sort of consensus analysis to highlight the difference between common and specialist knowledge" (pg. 9). The legitimate question is "why?"

From research initiated in the 1970s and continued to this day, we know that there are differences in the amount of cultural knowledge that individuals' hold [30-34]. For instance, in a study in the Brazilian Amazon, Wayland [35] shows that knowledge and use of medicinal plants is concentrated among women because of their role as managers of household health. Some other variables that have been shown to correlate with intra-cultural variation of TK include market integration [36,37], kinship affiliation [38], age [39], schooling [40], positions in a social network [41], and—of course—level of specialization on the domain of knowledge [42-45]. For example, in a now classic study in a Tarascan community in Mexico, Garro [42] found important differences in the level of medical knowledge of curers and laypeople. Overall curers and laypeople shared a single system of beliefs, however, curers showed higher agreement among themselves in expressing this system than non-curers.

The implications of intra-cultural differences on how laypeople and specialists understand the causes, symptoms, and treatments of illnesses have been addressed in medical [46], but not so much in ethnopharmacological research. Three decades ago, Kleinman and colleagues [46] suggested that the models of sickness held by laypersons and specialists may differ in terms of perceptions of what caused the ailment, why it started, when it did, what it did to the person, how severe it was, what were the treatment options, what results were expected from treatment, and what were the fears about the illness. They stressed the critical importance of understanding potential differences between laypersons and specialists for the successful resolution of health problems. As they argued, the different understanding of illness between patients and specialists may be at the root of medical problems, particularly because different understanding of illnesses might result in patient lack of adherence to medical regimens.

Folk healers (i.e., herbalists, curers, shamans, and the like) have been the typical focus of ethnopharmacological research. Ethnopharmacologists have focused on folk healers under the assumption that they concentrate most ethnopharmacological knowledge. However, specialists have often been studied in isolation, giving little attention to how specialists relate, interact, and contrast with non-specialists. But if—as we have learned from research on the distribution of TK—specialists and non-specialists do not necessarily share the same body of knowledge, nor the same understanding on how to cure diseases, then the focus on specialists knowledge necessarily biases the type of information being collected in ethnopharmacological studies. Furthermore, this focus on specialists limits the possibility of understanding how the patterned distribution of ethnopharmacological knowledge within a society affects the health of the group.

Thus, the patterned distribution of TK has two important implications for ethnopharmacological research. The first implication relates, of course, to the selection of informants. If TK is unequally distributed, the amount and quantity of information one can obtain clearly depends on how much and what type of knowledge is held by the selected informants. Researchers have highlighted differences between laypersons and specialists, but—as in other domains of traditional knowledge—most likely other patterned differences exist. For example, men can give different explanations to illnesses symptoms and treatments than women, or young people might use different treatments than elders. Thus, minimally understanding how knowledge is distributed in a community should be an important consideration in ethnopharmacological research, which so heavily relies on locally provided information.

The second implication of the patterned distribution of knowledge for ethnopharmacological research is more theoretical. If ethnopharmacological knowledge is unevenly distributed, and if this uneven distribution is patterned, then one should expect that people in certain characteristics should benefit more from the ethnopharmacological knowledge of the group than people without those characteristics. It also implies that similarities and differences in the belief systems of specialists and non-specialists are likely to affect how treatment alternatives are perceived and utilized. All important issues that ethnopharmacology could potentially address.

1.1.4 TRANSMISSION OF TRADITIONAL KNOWLEDGE

A third theoretical contribution from research on TK to ethnopharmacological research relates to the study of the social relations that enable the generation, maintenance, spread, and devolution of cultural traits and innovations, including ethnopharmacological knowledge. Researchers have hypothesized that, unlike biological traits, largely transmitted by a vertical path through genes, cultural information can be transmitted through at least three distinct—but not mutually exclusive—paths: 1) from parent-to-child (vertical transmission), 2) between any two individuals of the same generation (horizontal transmission), and 3) from non-parental individuals of the parental generation to members of the filial generation (oblique transmission) [47]. Oblique transmission can take the form of (a) one-to-many, when one person (e.g., a teacher) transmits information to many people of a younger generation or (b) many-to-one, when the person learns from older adults other than the parents [47].

So the question is "how is ethnopharmacological knowledge transmitted?" Some anthropologists have stated that folk biological knowledge, including knowledge about what constitutes an illness and how to cure it, is mainly transmitted by parents to offspring [48,49]. For example, in a study of a rural population in Argentina, Lozada and colleagues [50] analyzed the transmission of knowledge of medicinal and edible plants and concluded that family members (especially mothers) were the most important source of medicinal knowledge. Other researchers have argued that parent-child transmission might not be the dominant mode of cultural learning, at least when a person's total lifespan is considered [51]. Quantitative studies on oblique transmission of ethnobotanical knowledge are scarce and focus on the transmission of knowledge from one-to-many. For example, Lozada and colleagues [50] found that experienced traditional healers outside the family are the second important source for the acquisition of knowledge of medicinal plants. Last, several authors have argued that there are also social and evolutionary reasons to expect intra-generational transmission of some types of cultural knowledge [52,53]. Observational studies suggest that, in some domains, children learn a considerable amount from age-peers [48,54]. For example, children regularly teach each other tasks and skills during the course of their daily play [48]. In a study in Mexico [54], Zarger showed that siblings pass along extensive information to one another about plants, including where to find them, their uses, or how to harvest or cultivate them. In my own fieldwork, I have often observed children using plants for medicinal purposes, both for themselves and for they playmates, which would suggest that children also pass to each other information on curative plants. Research also suggests that, later in life, young adults turn to age-peers rather than parents for information. Specifically in situations of cultural change, age-peers—not elders—are most likely to have tracked changes and should provide the best information to navigate in the new context; information that sometimes updates or replaces information previously acquired from parents [47,51]. In sum, although previous empirical research has outlined the importance of the vertical path in the transmission of TK, theoretical models and empirical evidence from fields other than anthropology suggest that the importance of vertical transmission may be overstated [51], and that neither vertical nor oblique transmission should be expected to dominate across all domains [55,56].

The studies cited here also highlight that the selection of one type of transmission over another might depend both on the cultural group and the domain of knowledge examined. For example, medicines to cure illnesses from the natural world might be transmitted by a different channel than medicines to cure illnesses caused by spirits. Understanding the strategy selected by a society for the transmission of ethnopharmacological knowledge is important because each of those transmission pathways—or the way they are combined—affect differently the distribution, spread, and therefore maintenance of knowledge. For example, as is the case for other cultural traits [47], ethnopharmacological information vertically transmitted (i.e., from the parent to the child, or from one selected adult in the parent generation to one selected young, as many iniciatic systems) would be highly conservative. That is, because it is less shared, information vertically transmitted may maintain individual variation across generations. Furthermore, innovations and new information would experience slower rates of diffusion in a population when compared with horizontal or oblique transmission. By contrast, horizontal transmission might lead to fast diffusion of new information or innovations if contact with transmitters is frequent. Furthermore, vertical transmission is based in two models, whereas oblique and horizontal transmissions are based on larger samples, and larger samples might provide more accurate (less biased) information [57]. The combination of horizontal and oblique transmission involving many transmitters to one receiver would generate the highest uniformity in ethnopharmacological knowledge within a social group, while allowing for generational cultural change.

It is also possible that the strategies to transmit TK change over time. Theoretical modeling suggests that changing social contexts, as the ones that experience many indigenous societies nowadays with globalization and market integration, favor reliance on oblique rather than on vertical transmission [55]. For example, with increasing exposure to market economy and commercial drugs, ethnopharmacological knowledge might need to be used in new situations or in interaction with new products. To navigate cultural shifts, individuals might opt to select information that has been effective from a wider subset of the population (like non-parental adults). This shift might help ethnopharmacologists understand why indigenous pharmacopoeias heavily reliant on vertical transmission are threatened by modernization in a much deeper way that indigenous pharmacopoeias that have traditionally been transmitted through other pathways.

Last, research on the transmission of TK can also help ethnopharmacologists understand the different paths through which different types of knowledge are transmitted. For example, research among the Tsimane' suggests that ethnobotanical knowledge (such as names or traits used for plant recognition) and skills (or how to put this knowledge into practice) are not transmitted through the same paths [56]. Ethnobotanical knowledge might be easier to acquire than ethnobotanical skills and is mainly acquired during childhood. The acquisition of knowledge relies on cumulative memory and individuals can learn quickly and effectively through relatively few interactions; therefore, individuals can acquire ethnobotanical knowledge from many sources. The acquisition of skills might require higher investments by the learner. Acquiring skills is more costly in time and might require a number of direct observations and repetition within a particular context. So, individuals might be more conservative in selecting models for the transmission of skills and place more weight on information acquired from older or more experienced informants.

To sum up, a focus on understanding how ethnopharmacological knowledge is transmitted would open new research possibilities in ethnopharmacology. Specifically, quantitative data on the mechanisms of transmission of cultural traits could be useful in predicting within-group variability and stability of traditional pharmacopeias over time and space.

I now move to discuss how methodological contributions in the study of TKS can help in ethnopharmacological research.

1.1.5 METHODOLOGICAL CONTRIBUTIONS OF THE STUDY OF TRADITIONAL KNOWLEDGE SYSTEMS TO ETHNOPHARMACOLOGY

Ethnopharmacology has drawn on many tools from anthropology. The broad contributions of anthropology to ethnopharmacological research have been the subject of previous reviews [58] and critical assessments [59]. So here I would just make a general consideration on those tools, referring the reader to previous work for detailed information.

Previous researchers with anthropological training have argued that anthropology can make a unique contribution to ethnopharmacological research by providing the conceptual and practical tools that would allow ethnopharmacologists to develop the ethnography of plant use and of health and disease in sufficient depth to correlate with laboratory investigations of plant constituents and activities [58]. Among the many tools that anthropology can—and has—contributed to ethnopharmacology, researchers have highlighted that detailed ethnographic research is crucial in understanding traditional medical practices. As argued before, traditional medical systems are holistic in nature and often consider illness, healing, and human physiology as a series of interrelationships among nature, spirits, society, and the individual [60,61]. As Elisabetsky argued [62]

> Traditional remedies, although based on natural products, are not found in "nature" as such; they are products of human knowledge. To transform a plant into a medicine, one has to know the correct species, its location, the proper time of collection [...], the part to be used, how to prepare it [...], the solvent to be used [...], the way to prepare it [...], and, finally, posology [...]. Needless to say, curers have to diagnose and select the right medicine for the right patients (pg. 10).

Ethnographic research—based on extensive field studies—has proven key to understand those relations and to assess how local people perceive, understand, classify, and use resources in their environments. Specifically, some of the qualitative and ethnographic methods more commonly used in ethnopharmacological research include participant observation, interviews with key informants, focus groups, structured and unstructured interviews, survey instruments and questionnaires, lexical and semantic studies, and discourse and content analysis (see [58,59,63,64].

In sum, although still underused [14], some of the anthropological tools that ethnopharmacologists can add to their toolkit to reveal the cultural construction of health and healing in diverse cultures have been already discussed by other researches. I would like to move now to discuss two methods frequently used in research on TKS whose contributions to ethnopharmacological research are not so commonly known: 1) folk classification and 2) cultural consensus analysis.

1.1.6 ETHNOCLASSIFICATION

In its broadest sense, ethnoclassification, or folk taxonomy, refers to how traditional communities identify, classify, categorize, and name the world around them. Ethnobiologists place folk taxonomies within the broader analysis of TK because folk taxonomies are considered to be reflections of how people organize their knowledge of the universe [32,65-68], and have large impacts on people's perceptions and actual behaviors [66]. Food taboos, for example, reflect local knowledge and perceptions of edible and inedible foods, which in turn impact subsistence, technology, the construction of social landscapes, social interactions, notions of prestige, and gender distinctions, among other behaviors [69]. Consequently, studies on folk taxonomy can provide insights into ethnopharmacology because folk taxonomy not only organizes and condenses information about the natural world, but it also provides a powerful systematic tool to examine the distribution of biological and ecological properties of organisms [66].

Studies on ethnoclassification have mostly documented how different cultural groups classify the environment, especially plants and animals. A seminal work on the topic is the research by Berlin, Breedlove, and Raven in the 1970s [67,70]. Based on ethnobotanical studies in Central and South America, those authors elaborated general principles of folk taxonomy and drew convincing parallels with Linnaean taxonomy. According to Berlin [71], humans respond to plant and animal diversity in their environment by grouping living organisms 1) into named categories that express differences and similarities between them and 2) into hierarchical classificatory categories of greater or lesser inclusion. Because native taxonomies differentiate taxa by broad morphological traits, there is often a strong correspondence between Linnaean and other folk taxonomies at the "generic-species" level [66,71]. Thus, folk classificatory systems retain a vast store of information about biology, ecology, and ethology of animals and plants. Berlin's principles, though not without critics, have been tested by other authors (e.g., [30,72]), and many studies throughout the world suggest that the folk classification of animals and plants are not arbitrary, but determined by some degree of biological reality or universal cognition.

But people do not only organize plants and animals into categories. One area where ethnoclassification can inform ethnopharmacological research relates to the classification of illnesses and medicines, and how this classification affects the selection of curative and preventive substances [9,10,73]. I will illustrate the point of how ethnoclassification can contribute to ethnopharmacological research through the example of the hot-cold humoral system.

Humoral folk medicinal models rest on the idea that illnesses are a consequence of some imbalance of intangible qualities of the body (or humors). Under this classificatory system, illnesses should be treated (or prevented) with medicines with opposite qualities [34,74]. For example, under the hot-cold system, a humoral folk medicinal model common in areas as diverse as Latin America [34] or China [74], health is believed to be a balance between hot and cold elements in the body, and illnesses appear when the body is too "hot" or too "cold." If the body is too "hot", balance can be restored by treatment with "cold" foods, remedies, or medicines, and viceversa. Under this humoral system, then, medicines are selected, not exclusively by their particular active properties, but also depending on where they fit in people's classification system.

Thus, understanding how people classify illnesses and remedies on humoral systems is key in ethnopharmacological research because those classifications are a fundamental—although not exclusive—part of medicinal plant folk selection criteria. For example, Ankli and colleagues [75,76] investigated hot/cold classifications and taste and smell perceptions of Yucatec Maya medicinal and non-medicinal plants. Their results show that non-medicinal plants were more often reported to have no smell or taste than medicinal plants: good odor was a sign of medicinal use and a large percentage of medicinal plants were reported to be astringent or sweet. Non-medicinal plants were rarely classified humorally and medicinal plants humoral qualities appeared to refer to a plant's classification. Ankli and colleagues found correlations between Mayan perceptions of taste and smell and known chemical constituents [75,77], but no specific group(s) of compounds was associated with alleged hot or cold properties of plants. Ankli and her colleagues concluded that taste and smell are important selection criteria for medicinal plants among the Maya, but they are not a central unifying principle of Maya medicinal plant classification. Shephard [78] has also documented the role of the senses in medicinal plant selection.

In sum, it is evident that there are often biological bases for medicinal plant selection, but folk classification also constitutes a fundamental part of medicinal plant folk selection criteria. A bigger emphasis in ethnoclassification would help ethnopharmacology to move from a narrow focus on "what plants are included in indigenous pharmacopeias?" to broader questions such as "why are those plants selected and used?"

1.1.7 CULTURAL CONSENSUS ANALYSIS

The second set of methods commonly used in research on TKS that offers interesting possibilities in ethnopharmacological research are methods derived from cultural consensus theory [79]. Cultural consensus theory was developed by anthropologists trying to estimate culturally correct answers for different domains of local knowledge [80]. The cultural consensus theory rests on several assumptions. First, there is a culturally correct answer for every question. Whatever the cultural reality is, it is the same for all informants and is defined as the answer given by most people [81]. Second, knowledge consists of agreement between informants. The level of agreement between informants reflects their joint agreement [38,82]. Third, the probability that an informant will answer a given question correctly is a result of that informant's competence in that domain of knowledge. Competence refers to the share of correct answers by the informant.

Information for the cultural consensus model consists of responses by informants to multiple-choice questions. A computer software, ANTHRO-PAC [83], calculates each informant's competence and establishes whether the domain of knowledge being analyzed is consensual. The cultural consensus model has been largely used in TKS research (see [84] for a review) and has also been used to analyze folk medical beliefs [44,85-88] and humoral classifications of illness [34]. However, and despite the importance that consensual responses have in ethnopharmacological research [23,89,90], cultural consensus analysis is still not widely used in ethnopharmacology.

Cultural consensus analysis would allow ethnopharmacologists a broader look at intracultural variation and at the analysis of transmission and loss of traditional ethnopharmacological knowledge. Cultural consensus analysis differs from other ways of examining consensual responses in a group in that it reflects the patterning of responses and variation around the cultural norm. Under the traditional knowledge-testing approach, informant's knowledge is described in terms of deviance from the bio-medical model, but it does not allow distinguishing between errors that are due to a lack of biomedical knowledge and those that are due to different explanatory models. In contrast, cultural consensus analysis can identify items that are part of a group's explanatory model. In that sense, cultural consensus analysis could complete the traditional knowledge-testing approach. The traditional knowledge-testing approach allows researchers to assess individual performance in terms of biomedically correct answers; the cultural consensus analysis allows researchers to identify items that are part of a group's explanatory model.

1.2 CONCLUSIONS

In this article I have tried to highlight theoretical and methodological, actual and potential, contributions of research on TKS to ethnopharmacological research. Let me now orient this last part to discuss the future of the discipline through the lenses of an anthropologist who specializes in the study of TK.

In commenting on a previous version of this paper, Moerman, Pieroni, and McClatchey highlighted to me the fact that there has not been a drug added to the Northern pharmacopoeia by any ethnobotanical or ethnopharmacological lead in probably half a century (Moerman, comm. pers., [91]) Furthermore, despite much ethnopharmacological research conducting bioevaluation of traditional drugs, traditional medicines and herbal drugs available on global and local markets are not—in large parts—isolated molecules resulting from bioevaluation, but rather raw dried herbs and plant-based extracts and fractions (Pieroni, comm. pers.) Yet the romance of ethnopharmacology as a pathway to develop new drugs out of the evaluation of traditional remedies persists in the minds of many. And one can not help but wonder whether this romance is just an attempt to justify the existence of a discipline that failed to meet its original goals.

Through the lenses of an anthropologist, that is, through the lenses of someone who is not necessarily interested in the bioevaluation of traditional medicines, there are, however, other possible futures for ethnopharmacology. In this article I have tried to discuss several research venues where ethnopharmacologists could contribute to improve our understanding cultural differences in perceptions, uses, and management of traditional remedies. Let me conclude by emphasizing the public health application that derives from the research suggestions made here.

While indigenous pharmacopoeias have historically contributed to the development of allopathic and herbal drugs thus adding to improve health in the global north, rarely ethnopharmacological expertise and findings are used to improve the long-run health in the regions of study. The consequence is that nowadays indigenous peoples suffer from the worst health status around the word [92-97].

Ethnopharmacologists have been fundamental in the widespread awareness of the ethical issues associated with documenting indigenous pharmacopoeias. Ethnopharmacologists and anthropologists have been among the first ones raising concerns about the compensation to indigenous people for the commercial uses of their traditional knowledge by pharmaceutical industries, about the need to develop appropriated mechanisms for the protection of indigenous people's intellectual property, and about the importance of conducting research in an ethical way (including issues such as asking for Prior Informed Consent and other relevant research permits granted by universities and governmental organizations [11,16,98-103]). That is, ethnopharmacologists, with ethnobiologists, have raised their hands against the commodification of the sacred, to use Posey's words [20]. As a response, international legal frameworks, such as the one established by the Convention of Biological Diversity, have been developed to safeguard the intellectual property of cultures and individuals with specialist knowledge.

As the discipline considers expanding its objectives from the intentional search of biologically active compounds of substances used in the traditional medicines to a more holistic and culture-sensitive study of the pharmacologic potential of those substances, ethnopharmacology should also incorporate new ethical considerations related to the new knowledge developed. Those considerations should go beyond the recognition of the Intellectual Property Rights of indigenous peoples or the acquisition of appropriated research permits, to include the healthcare of the original holders of ethnopharmacological knowledge. Many authors have highlighted the importance of culturally appropriate health services for indigenous peoples. In some regions of the world including Australia, New Zealand, Canada, Colombia, Ecuador, and Peru, new medical services are being implemented where indigenous medicine is practiced alongside allopathic medicine [93,95]. Ethnopharmacologists can be instrumental in working with health care providers in the developing world for practical implementation of ethnopharmacological research results.

In sum, ethnopharmacology can do more than speed up to recover the traditional knowledge of indigenous peoples to try to make it available for the development of new drugs in the North. Ethnopharmacology has the potential to contribute to the improvement of the health of indigenous peoples.

Let me finish quoting the words of Nina Etkin [14], as a tribute to someone who not only did invaluable, theoretical, methodological, and ethical contributions to the discipline, but also as a tribute to someone who was an inspiration to make ethnopharmacology more meaningful for local populations.

> Today, the interest that many pharmaceutical companies have in primarily developing-world diseases has more to do with implications for Western travelers than with indigenous populations who cannot afford expensive prophylaxis and therapy. Ethnopharmacologists could accept a challenge to turn this around. It would be provident at this juncture to address how the results of sophisticated medical ethnography and rigorous bioassays can be meaningfully integrated, translated, and applied to the traditional populations who use those plants (pg. 182).

This should be, in my opinion, a primary goal of the discipline.

REFERENCES

1.   Etkin NL, Elisabetsky E: Seeking a transdisciplinary and culturally germane science: The future of ethnopharmacology. Journal of Ethnopharmacology 2005, 100:23-26.
2.   Giovannini P, Heinrich M: Xki yoma' (our medicine) and xki tienda (patent medicine)-Interface between traditional and modern medicine among the Mazatecs of Oaxaca, Mexico. Journal of Ethnopharmacology 2009, 121:383-399.

3. Thomas E, Vandebroek I, Sanca S, Van Damme P: Cultural significance of medicinal plant families and species among Quechua farmers in Apillapampa, Bolivia. Journal of Ethnopharmacology 2009, 122:60-67.

4. Vandebroek I, Calewaert J, De jonckheere S, Sanca S, Semo L, Van Damme P, Van Puyvelde L, De Kimpe N: Use of medicinal plants and pharmaceuticals by indigenous communities in the Bolivian Andes and Amazon. Bulletin of the World Health Organization 2004, 84:243-250.

5. Pieroni A, Quave C, Villanelli M, Mangino P, Sabbatini G, Santini L, Boccetti T, Profili M, Ciccioli T, Rampa LG, Antonini G, Girolamini C, Cecchi M, Tomasi M: Ethnopharmacognostic survey on the natural ingredients used in folk cosmetics, cosmeceuticals and remedies for healing skin diseases in the inland Marches, Central-Eastern Italy. Journal of Ethnopharmacology 2004, 91:331-344.

6. Albuquerque UP, de Oliveira RF: Is the use-impact on native caatinga species in Brazil reduced by the high species richness of medicinal plants? Journal of Ethnopharmacology 2007, 113:156-170.

7. Pardo De Santayana M, Blanco E, Morales R: Plants known as te' in Spain: An ethno-pharmaco-botanical review. Journal of Ethnopharmacology 2005, 98:1-19.

8. Ellen R: Putting plants in their place: anthropological approaches to understanding the ethnobotanical knowledge of rainforest populations. In Tropical rainforest research: current issues. Edited by Edwards DS, Booth W, Choy S. Dordrecht: Kluwer Academic Publishers; 1996::457-465.

9. Waldstein A, Adams C: The interface between medical anthropology and medical ethnobiology. Journal of the Royal Anthropological Institute 2006, 12(Suppl 1):95-118.

10. Etkin NL: Ethnopharmacology - Biobehavioral Approaches in the Anthropological Study of Indigenous Medicines. Annual Review of Anthropology 1988, 17:23-42.

11. Ten Kate K, Laird S: The Commercial Use of Biodiversity: Access to Genetic Resources and Benefit-Sharing. London: Earthscan; 1999.

12. Pieroni A, Price L: Eating and Healing. Traditional Foods as Medicine. New York: The Haworth Press; 2006.

13. Heinrich M: Editorial. Journal of Ethnopharmacology 2010., 131

14. Etkin NL: Perspectives in ethnopharmacology: forging a closer link between bioscience and traditional empirical knowledge. Journal of Ethnopharmacology 2001, 76:177-182.

15. Elisabetsky E: Sociopolitical, economical, and ethical issues in medicinal plant research. Journal of Ethnopharmacology 1991, 32:235-239.

16. Laird S: Biodiversity and Traditional Knowledge: Equitable Partnerships in Practice. London: Earthscan; 2002.

17. Heinrich M, Gibbons S: Ethnopharmacology in drug discovery: an analysis of its role and potential contribution. Journal of Pharmacy and Pharmacology 2001, 53:425-432.

18. Balick M: Ethnology and the Identification of Therapeutic Agents from the Rainforest. In Bioactive Compounds from Plants Edited by Chadwick D, Marsh J. 1990.

19. Berkes F, Colding J, Folke C: Rediscovery of traditional ecological knowledge as adaptive management. Ecological Applications 2000, 10:1251-1262.

20. Posey DA: Commodification of the sacred through intellectual property rights. Journal of Ethnopharmacology 2002, 83:3-12.
21. Reyes-Garcia V, McDade T, Vadez V, Huanca T, Leonard WR, Tanner S, Godoy R: Non-market returns to traditional human capital: Nutritional status and traditional knowledge in a native Amazonian society. Journal of Development Studies 2008, 44:217-232.
22. McDade T, Reyes-García V, Leonard W, Tanner S, Huanca T: Maternal ethnobotanical knowledge is associated with multiple measures of child health in the Bolivian Amazon. Proceedings of the National Academy of Sciences of the United States of America 2007, 104:6134-6139.
23. Moerman DE: Agreement and meaning: Rethinking consensus analysis. Journal of Ethnopharmacology 2007, 112:451-460.
24. Browner CH, Demontellano BRO, Rubel AJ: A Methodology for Cross-Cultural Ethnomedical Research. Current Anthropology 1988, 29:681-702.
25. Bristow F, Stephens C, Nettleton C: Utz W'achil: Health and wellbeing among Indigenous peoples. London: Health Unlimited/London School of Hygiene and Tropical Medicine; 2003.
26. Calvet-Mir L, Reyes-Garcia V, Tanner S, TAPS study team: Is there a divide between local medicinal knowledge and Western medicine? A case study among native Amazonians in Bolivia. Journal of Ethnoecology and Ethnomedicine 2008, 4:18.
27. Moerman DE: The meaning response and the ethics of avoiding placebos. Evaluation & the Health Professions 2002, 25:399-409.
28. Moerman DE, Jonas WB: Deconstructing the placebo effect and finding the meaning response. Annals of Internal Medicine 2002, 136:471-476.
29. Heinrich M, Edwards S, Moerman DE, Leonti M: Ethnopharmacological field studies: A critical assessment of their conceptual basis and methods. Journal of Ethnopharmacology 2009, 124:1-17.
30. Hays T: An empirical method for the identification of cover categories in ethnobiology. American Ethnologist 1976, 3:489-507.
31. Gardner P: Birds, words and a requiem for the omniscient informant. American Ethnologist 1976, 3:446-468.
32. Ellen R: Omniscience and ignorance. Variation in Nuaulu knowledge, identification and classification of animals. Language in Society 1979, 8:337-364.
33. Mathews H: Context specific variation in humoral classification. American Anthropologist 1983, 85:826-846.
34. Weller SC: New Data on Intracultural Variability - the Hot-Cold Concept of Medicine and Illness. Human Organization 1983, 42:249-257.
35. Wayland C: Gendering local knowledge: Medicinal plant use and primary health care in the Amazon. Medical Anthropology Quarterly 2001, 15:171-188.
36. Reyes-Garcia V, Vadez V, Byron E, Apaza L, Leonard WR, Perez E, Wilkie D: Market economy and the loss of folk knowledge of plant uses: Estimates from the Tsimane' of the Bolivian Amazon. Current Anthropology 2005, 46:651-656.
37. Godoy R, Brokaw N, Wilkie D: Of trade and cognition: Markets and the loss of folk knowledge among the Tawahka Indians of the Honduran rain forest. Journal of Anthropological Research 1998, 54:219-233.

38. Boster JS: Exchange of varieties and information between Aguaruna manioc cultivators. American Anthropologist 1986, 88:429-436.
39. Caniago I, Siebert SF: Medicinal plant economy, knowledge and conservation in Kalimantan, Indonesia. Economic Botany 1998, 52:229-250.
40. Zent S: Acculturation and Ethnobotanical Knowledge Loss among the Piaroa of Venezuela: Demonstration of a Quantitative Method for the Empirical Study of Traditional Ecological Knowledge Change. In On Biocultural Diversity: Linking Language, Knowledge, and the Environment. Edited by Maffi L. Smithsonian Institution Press. Washington D.C; 2001::190-211.
41. Boster JS, Johnson J, Weller S: Social position and shared knowledge: Actors' perception of status, role and social structure. Social Networks 1987, 9:375-387.
42. Garro L: Intracultural variation in folk medicinal knowledge: A comparison between groups. American Anthropologist 1986, 88:351-370.
43. Boster JS, Johnson J: Form or function: A comparison of expert and novice judgments of similarity among fish. American Anthropologist 1989, 91:866-889.
44. Baer RD, Weller SC, Garcia JGD, Rocha ALS: Cross-cultural perspectives on physician and lay models of the common cold. Medical Anthropology Quarterly 2008, 22:148-166.
45. Baer RD, Weller SC, Garcia JGD, Glazer M, Trotter R, Pachter L, Klein RE: A cross-cultural approach to the study of the folk illness nervios. Culture Medicine and Psychiatry 2003, 27:315-337.
46. Kleinman A, Eisenberg L, Good B: Culture, illness and care: Clinical lessons from anthropological and cross- cultural research. Annals of Internal Medicine 1978, 88:251-258.
47. Cavalli-Sforza LL, Feldman M: Cultural Transmission and Evolution: A Quantitative Approach. Princeton: Princeton University Press; 1981.
48. Lancy D: Playing on the Mother-Ground: Cultural Routines for Children's Development. New York: Guilford Press; 1999.
49. Hewlett B, De Silvestri A, Guglielmino C: Semes and genes in Africa. Current Anthropology 2002, 43:313-321.
50. Lozada M, Ladio AH, Weigandt M: Cultural transmission of ethnobotanical knowledge in a rural community of Northwestern Patagonia, Argentina. Economic Botany 2006, 60:374-385.
51. Aunger R: The life history of culture learning in a face-to-face society. Ethos 2000, 28:1-38.
52. Boyd R, Richerson P: Culture and the Evolutionary Process. Chicago: University of Chicago Press; 1985.
53. Harris J: The Nurture Assumption: Why Children Turn Out The Way They Do. London: Bloomsbury; 1999.
54. Zarger R: Acquisition and Transmission of Subsistence Knowledge by Q'eqchi' Maya in Belize. In Ethnobiology and Biocultural Diversity. Edited by Stepp JR, Wyndham FS, Zarger R. Athens GA: International Society of Ethnobiology; 2002::592-603.
55. McElreath R, Strimling P: When natural selection favors imitation of parents. Current Anthropology 2008, 49:307-316.
56. Reyes-Garcia V, Broesch J, Calvet-Mir L, Fuentes-Pelaez N, Mcdade TW, Parsa S, Tanner S, Huanca T, Leonard W, Martínez-Rodríguez M: Cultural transmission

of ethnobotanical knowledge and skills: an empirical analysis from an Amerindian society. Evolution and Human Behaviour 2009, 30:274-285.

57. Henrich J, Boyd R: The Evolution of Conformist Transmission and the Emergence of Between-Group Differences. Evolution and Human Behaviour 1998, 19:215-241.

58. Etkin NL: Anthropological Methods in Ethnopharmacology. Journal of Ethnopharmacology 1993, 38:93-104.

59. Edwards S, Nebel S, Heinrich M: Questionnaire surveys: Methodological and epistemological problems for field-based ethnopharmacologists. Journal of Ethnopharmacology 2005, 100:30-36.

60. Fabrega H: Need for An Ethnomedical Science. Science 1975, 189:969-975.

61. Fabrega H: Disease and social behavior: An interdisciplinary perspective. Cambridge: M.I.T. Press; 1974.

62. Elisabetsky E: Folklore, tradition, or know-how? Cultural Survival Quarterly 1991, 15:9-13.

63. Etkin NL: Ethnopharmacology: The Conjunction of Medical Ethnography and the Biology of Therapeutic Action. In Medical Anthropology: Contemporary Theory and Method. Edited by Sargent C, Johnson TM. Praeger Publishers; 1996::151-163.

64. Lipp FJ: Methods for Ethnopharmacological Field Work. Journal of Ethnopharmacology 1989, 25:139-150.

65. Seixas CS, Begossi A: Ethnozoology of fishing communities from Ilha Grandes (Atlantic Forest Coast, Brazil). Journal of Ethnobiology 2001, 21:107-135.

66. Atran S: Folkbiology and the anthropology of science: Cognitive universals and cultural particulars. Behavioral and Brain Sciences 1998, 21:547-609.

67. Berlin B, Breedlove DE, Laughlin RM, Raven PH: Cultural significance and lexical retention in Tzeltal-Tzotzil ethnobotany. In Meaning in Mayan Languages. Ethnolinguistic studies. Edited by Edmonson MS. The Hague: Mounton Black, M.J; 1973.

68. Hunn ES: The utilitarian factor in folk biological classification. American Anthropologist 1982, 84:830-847.

69. Ross EB: Food Taboos, Diet, and Hunting Strategy - Adaptation to Animals in Amazon Cultural Ecology. Current Anthropology 1978, 19:1-36.

70. Berlin B, Breedlove DE, Raven PH: Principles of Tzeltal Plant Classification: An Introduction to the Botanical Ethnography of a Mayan Speaking Community in Highland Chiapas. New York: Academic Press; 1974.

71. Berlin B: Ethnobotanical Classification: Principles of Categorization of Plants and Animals in Traditional Societies. Princeton: Princeton University Press; 1992.

72. Hays T: Utilitarian/adaptationist explanations of folk biological classifications: Some cautionary notes. Journal of Ethnobiology 1982, 2:89-94.

73. Ngokwey N: Naming and Grouping Illnesses in Feira (Brazil). Culture Medicine and Psychiatry 1995, 19:385-408.

74. Anderson EN: Why Is Humoral Medicine So Popular. Social Science & Medicine 1987, 25:331-337.

75. Ankli A, Sticher O, Heinrich M: Medical ethnobotany of the Yucatec Maya: Healers' consensus as a quantitative criterion. Economic Botany 1999, 53:144-160.

76. Ankli A, Sticher O, Heinrich M: Yucatec Maya medicinal plants versus nonmedicinal plants: Indigenous characterization and selection. Human Ecology 1999, 27:557-580.

77. Brett JA, Heinrich M: Culture, perception and the environment: The role of chemo-sensory perception. Journal of Applied Botany-Angewandte Botanik 1998, 72:67-69.

78. Shepard GH: A sensory ecology of medicinal plant therapy in two Amazonian societies. American Anthropologist 2004, 106:252-266.

79. Romney AK, Weller S, Batchelder W: Culture as consensus: A theory of culture and informant accuracy. American Anthropologist 1986, 88:313-338.

80. Weller SC: Cultural consensus theory: Applications and frequently asked questions. Field Methods 2007, 19:339-368.

81. Romney AK, Weller S: Predicting informant accuracy from patterns of recall among informants. Social Networks 1984, 6:59-77.

82. Boster JS: Requiem for the omniscent informant: There's life in the old girl yet. In Directions in Cognitive Anthropology. Edited by Dougherty J. Urbana: University of Illinois Press; 1985::177-197.

83. Borgatti SP: ANTHROPAC 4.0. Natick, MA: Analytic Technologies; 1996.

84. Reyes-Garcia V, Marti Sanz N, McDade T, Tanner SN, Vadez V: Concepts and methods in studies measuring individual ethnobotanical knowledge. Journal of Ethnobiology 2007, 27:182-203.

85. Garro L: Explaining high blood pressure: Variation in knowledge about illness. American Ethnologist 1988, 15:98-119.

86. Baer RD, Weller SC, Garcia JGD, Rocha ALS: A comparison of community and physician explanatory models of AIDS in Mexico and the United States. Medical Anthropology Quarterly 2004, 18:3-22.

87. Pachter LM, Weller SC, Baer RD, de Alba-Garcia JE, Trotter RT, Glazer M, Klein R: Variation in asthma beliefs and practices among mainland Puerto Ricans, Mexican-Americans, Mexicans, and Guatemalans. Journal of Asthma 2002, 39:119-134.

88. Weller SC, Baer RD: Intra- and intercultural variation in the definition of five illnesses: AIDS, diabetes, the common cold, Empacho, and Mal De Ojo. Cross-Cultural Research 2001, 35:201-226.

89. Ankli A, Sticher O, Heinrich M: Medical ethnobotany of the Yucatec Maya: Healers' consensus as a quantitative criterion. Economic Botany 1999, 53:144-160.

90. Heinrich M, Ankli A, Frei B, Weimann C, Sticher O: Medicinal plants in Mexico: Healers' consensus and cultural importance. Social Science and Medicine 1998, 47:1859-1871.

91. McClatchey W: Medicinal bioprospecting and ethnobotany research. Ethnobotany Research and Applications 2005, 3:189-190.

92. Anderson I, Crengle S, Kamaka ML, Chen TH, Palafox N, Jackson-Pulver L: Indigenous Health 1 - Indigenous health in Australia, New Zealand, and the Pacific. Lancet 2006, 367:1775-1785.

93. Kuper A: Indigenous people: an unhealthy category. Lancet 2005, 366:983.

94. Montenegro RA, Stephens C: Indigenous health 2 - Indigenous health in Latin America and the Caribbean. Lancet 2006, 367:1859-1869.

95. Ohenjo N, Willis R, Jackson D, Nettleton C, Good K, Mugarura B: Indigenous health 3 - Health of Indigenous people in Africa. Lancet 2006, 367:1937-1946.

96. Pincock S: Indigenous health in Australia still lagging. Lancet 2008, 372:18.

97. Stephens C, Porter J, Nettleton C, Willis R: Indigenous health 4 - Disappearing, displaced, and undervalued: a call to action for Indigenous health worldwide. Lancet 2006, 367:2019-2028.

98. Brush SB: Indigenous knowledge of biological resources and intellectual property rights: The role of anthropology. Am Anthropol 1993, 93:653-686.

99. Colchester M: Towards indigenous intellectual property rights? Seedling 1994., 11

100. Posey D: Intellectual property rights and just compensation for indigenous knowledge. Anthropology Today 1990, 6:13-16.

101. Elisabetsky E: Sociopolitical, Economical and Ethical Issues in Medicinal Plant Research. Journal of Ethnopharmacology 1991, 32:235-239.

102. Berlin B, Berlin EA: NGOs and the process of prior informed consent in bioprospecting research: the Maya ICBG project in Chiapas, Mexico. International Social Science Journal 2003, 55:629-638.

103. Heinrich M, Edwards S, Moerman DE, Leonti M: Ethnopharmacological field studies: A critical assessment of their conceptual basis and methods. Journal of Ethnopharmacology 2009, 124:1-17. |

CHAPTER 2

ANTIOXIDATIVE AND *IN VITRO* ANTIPROLIFERATIVE ACTIVITY OF *ARCTIUM LAPPA* ROOT EXTRACTS

FABRICIA S. PREDES, ANA L.T.G. RUIZ, JOÃO E. CARVALHO, MARY A. FOGLIO, and HEIDI DOLDER

2.1 BACKGROUND

Arctium lappa L. (Asteraceae) is a Japanese plant and introduced in Brazil, which is widely used in popular medicine worldwide, as a diuretic and antipyretic tea as well as for hypertension, gout, hepatitis and other inflammatory disorders [1,2]. The root has long been cultivated as a popular vegetable for dietary use and folk medicine [3,4]. *A. lappa* tea has become a promising and important beverage, because of ample therapeutic activity [3]. In the literature, many health benefits have been reported due to different classes of bioactive secondary metabolites. These classes include, among others, flavonoids and lignans, for which *A. lappa* is an important natural source [5]. Pharmacological studies and clinical trials indicated that burdock roots have hepatoprotective [3,6], anti-inflammatory [7] and free radical scavenging activities [7,8] attributed to the presence of caffeoylquinic acid derivatives [9]. Recently, antiproliferative and apoptotic effects of lignans from *A. lappa* were described for leukemic cells [10]

Originally printed under the terms of the Creative Commons Attribution License. Predes FS, Ruiz ALTG, Carvalho JE, Foglio MA, and Dolder H. Antioxidative and in vitro Antiproliferative Activity of Arctium lappa *Root Extracts.* BMC Complementary and Alternative Medicine **11**,25 (2011). doi:10.1186/1472-6882-11-25.

as well as antitumor effects of arctigenin on pancreatic cancer cell lines [11]. Consumption of dietary antioxidants from plant materials has been associated with lower incidence of diseases due to reduction of oxidative stress. Thus the aim of this study was to determine the total phenolic content by the Folin-Ciocalteau method, to evaluate the the antiradicalar properties based on their ability to quench the stable radical 2, 2-diphenyl-1-picrylhydrazyl (DPPH) and *in vitro* antiproliferative activity of eight different *A. lappa* root extracts.

2.2 METHODS

2.2.1 PLANT MATERIAL

The roots of *A. lappa* (Asteraceae) were collected at CPQBA, University of Campinas (UNICAMP), experimental field (Paulínia, Brazil) in August 2007. Dr. Glyn Mara Figueira was responsible for identification of the plant species. A voucher specimen was deposited at UNICAMP Herbarium under number 146021.

2.2.2 EXTRACTION 1

Fresh milled roots (770 g) were extracted successively in a Soxhlet apparatus with dichloromethane, 95% ethanol and water (2:1 solvent/plant ratio), for 6 hours each solvent. The extracts were concentrated under vacuum (Buchi RE 215) until complete elimination of the organic solvent and subsequently freeze-dried for water elimination, providing dichloromethane (DHE), ethanolic (EHE) and aqueous hot extract (AHE).

2.2.3 EXTRACTION 2

Fresh milled roots (276 g) were successively extracted by dynamic maceration with dichloromethane, 95% ethanol and water (1:5 plant/solvent ratio, 3 times each solvent), at room temperature, in an oscillating agitator (FANEM). The extracts were concentrated under vacuum (Buchi RE 215) until complete elimination of the organic solvent and subsequently freeze-dried for water elimination, providing dichloromethane (DE), ethanolic (EE) and aqueous (AE) extracts.

2.2.4 EXTRACTION 3

Fresh milled roots (100 g) were extracted three times consecutively in Soxhlet extractor with water (1:5 plant/solvent ratio). The aqueous extract was freeze-dried, providing the total aqueous extract (TAE).

2.2.5 EXTRACTION 4

Fresh milled roots (594 g) were extracted three times with 70% ethanol (1:5 plant/solvent ratio) under reflux, for 6 hours. The filtrates obtained were combined and concentrated under vacuum. The remaining water was freeze-dried resulting in the hydroethanolic extract (HE).

2.2.6 HIGH-RESOLUTION ELECTROSPRAY IONIZATION MASS SPECTROMETRY (HRESI-MS) OF HYDROETHANOLIC EXTRACT

HRESI-MS was recorded on a Q-Tof Mass Spectrometer (Micromass - U.K.) using direct infusion of a 10 µL.min-1 MeOH + 0.1% formic acid solution and ionization by electrospray in the negative ion mode. Major operation conditions were as follows: capillary voltage of 3.5 kV, source temperature of 100°C, desolvation temperature of 100°C and cone voltage of 35 V.

2.2.7 2, 2-DIPHENYL-1-PICRYLHYDRAZYL (DPPH) RADICAL SCAVENGING ACTIVITY

Microplate DPPH assay was performed as described by Brand-Williams et al. [12], modified by Brem et al. [13]. Briefly, in a 96-well plate, successive sample dilutions (100 μL/well, 0.25, 2.5, 25 and 250 μg/mL), tested in triplicate, received DPPH solution (40 μM in methanol, 100 μL/well) and absorbance was measured at 550 nm with a microplate reader (VERSA Max, Molecular Devices). Results were determined every 5 min up to 150 min in order to evaluate the kinetic behavior of the reaction. The percentage of remaining DPPH was calculated as follows: % DPPH rem = 100 × ([DPPH] sample/[DPPH] blank). A calibrated Trolox standard curve was also made. The percentage of remaining DPPH against the standard concentration was then plotted in an exponential regression, to obtain the amount of antioxidant necessary to decrease the initial DPPH concentration by 50% (EC_{50}). The time needed to reach the steady state for EC_{50} is defined as TEC_{50}. The antiradical efficiency [14], was calculated as follows: $AE = 1/(EC_{50} \times TEC_{50})$.

2.2.8 TOTAL PHENOLIC CONTENT

The total phenolic content was performed as described by Prior et al. [15], with small modifications in order to use a microplate reader. Briefly, an aliquot (10 μL) of the sample (1 mg/mL) was diluted in distilled water (600 μL). Then, this solution was applied in a 96-well plate (150 μL per well), in triplicate, and received Folin-Ciocalteau solution (12.5 μL), sodium carbonate (37.5 μL, 1 M) and water (50 μL). After incubation at 37°C for 2 h, absorbance was measured at 725 nm with a microplate reader (VERSA Max, Molecular Devices). A calibrated gallic acid standard curve was made and results were expressed as mg equivalents in gallic acid per gram of sample.

2.2.9 IN VITRO ANTIPROLIFERATIVE ACTIVITY ASSAY

Human tumor cell lines UACC-62 (melanoma), MCF-7 (breast), NCI-ADR/RES (ovarian expressing phenotype multiple drug resistance), 786-0 (renal), NCI-H460 (lung, non-small cells), PC-3 (prostate), OVCAR-3 (ovarian), HT-29 (colon), K562 (leukemia) were kindly provided by Frederick Cancer Research & Development Center - National Cancer Institute - Frederick, MA, USA. Stock cultures were grown in 5 mL of RPMI 1640 (GIBCO BRL, Life Technologies) supplemented with 5% fetal bovine serum. Penicilin: streptomycin (1000 μg/mL:1000 UI/mL, 1 mL/L) were added to the experimental cultures. Cells in 96-well plates (100 μL cells/well) were exposed to each extract in DMSO (0.25, 2.5, 25 and 250 μg/mL) at 37°C, 5% of CO_2 for 48 h. The final concentration of DMSO did not affect the cell viability. Then, a 50% trichloroacetic acid solution was added and after incubation (30 min at 4°C), washing and drying, cell proliferation was determined by spectrophotometric quantification (540 nm) of cellular protein content using sulforhodamine B assay. Using the concentration-response curve for each cell line the TGI (= concentration that produces total growth inhibition or a cytostatic effect) were determined through non-linear regression analysis using the software ORIGIN 7.5 (OriginLab Corporation) and corresponded to the test extract concentration necessary to inhibit proliferation of the cells.

2.3 RESULTS AND DISCUSSION

The yields of the different extraction for *A. lappa* are listed in Table 1. The extraction efficiency of the solvents in the successive extractions increased in the order: ethanol > water > dichloromethane. The aqueous and hydroethanolic extraction exhibited the greatest yields.

TABLE 1: Yield of the different solvent extractions of *A. lappa* root

Extract	Yield
Dichloromethane hot extract	0.12%
Ethanolic hot extract	6.39%
Aqueous hot extract	2.87%
Dichloromethanic extract	0.10%
Ethanolic extract	4.45%
Aqueous extract	3.51%
Total aqueous extract	10.56%
Hydroethanolic extract	10.25%

The phenolic compounds are ubiquitous phytochemicals present in plant foods with various biological activities including antioxidant properties. They exert properties such as free radical scavenging and inhibiting the generation of reactive species [16,17]. Phenolic compounds constitute a group of secondary metabolites that are quite widespread in nature with several therapeutical properties [17,18]. Their antioxidant activity is mainly due to their redox properties, which allow them to act as reducing agents, hydrogen donors, free radical scavengers, singlet oxygen quenchers and metal chelators [18].

TABLE 2: DPPH radical scavenging of *A. lappa* extract (mean ± SEM)

Sample	EC50 (µg/ml)	TEC50 (min)	AE
HE	4.79 ± 0.15	5	0.0418 ± 0.001
Lycopene	21.28 ± 0.11	0.1	0.47 ± 0.002
Trolox	1.13 ± 0.1	0.1	8.98 ± 0.84

Total phenolic content of all extracts are shown in Figure 1. The present study showed that the highest phenolic compound concentrations were obtained for Soxhlet extraction with dichloromethane (79.45 mg gallic acid/g extract) and ethanol (77.26 mg gallic acid/g extract) rather than extraction at room temperature. Whereas, the hydroethanolic extract (HE) showed a considerable phenolic content (72.61 mg gallic acid/g extract). A previous study with *A. lappa* roots reported that the extraction with a chloroform and ethanol (1:1) mixture resulted in higher concentration to phenolic compounds (85.15 ± 0.55 mg gallic acid/g dry extract), besides a great quantity of flavonoid (12.57 ± 0.05 mg quercetin/g extract) in the chloroformic extract; moreover, they reported a phenolic content (65.92 ± 0.36 mg gallic acid/g extract) [18] for the ethanol extract which is similar to that described herein. Also, researchers [19] described that *Arctium minus* ssp *minus* leaves aqueous extract exhibited a total phenolic content of 58.93 ± 2.72 mg gallic acid/g of extract, while the ethanolic extract gave 48.29 ± 0.21 mg gallic acid/g of extract.

Many authors have reported a direct relationship between total phenolic content and antioxidant activity in various seeds, fruits and vegetables

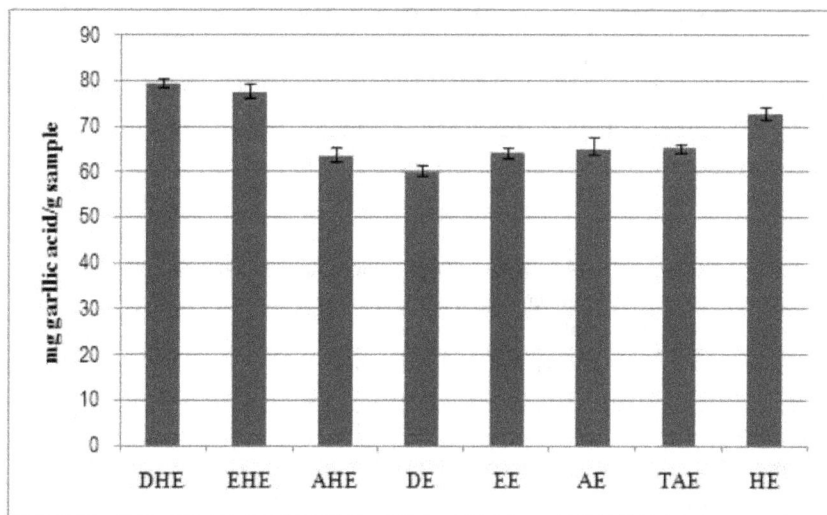

FIGURE 1: Total phenolic compounds of *A. lappa* extracts. DHE: dichloromethane hot extract; EHE: ethanolic hot extract; AHE: aqueous hot extract; DE: dichloromethane extract; EE: ethanolic extract; AE: aqueous extract; TAE: total aqueous extract; HE: hydroethanolic extract. The black bars represent standard deviation.

[20-22]. Antioxidant properties, especially radical scavenging activities, are very important due to the deleterious role of free radicals in foods and in biological systems. The DPPH radical has been widely accepted as a tool for estimating free radical scavenging activities of various compounds and plant extracts [19,21]. Although the present study evaluated the scavenging activity of all extracts, only hydroethanolic extract showed strong antiradicalar activity compared to the commercial standards used, licopene and trolox. Table 2 shows the scavenging effect of extracts and reference substances.

The hydroethanolic extract of *A. lappa* was then analyzed by high-resolution electrospray ionization mass spectroscopy and the presence of quercetin, arctigenin, chlorogenic acid and caffeic acid was demonstrated. These substances were identified by comparison of their calculated and measured high resolution deprotonated mass (Table 3). Phenolic compounds such as chlorogenic acid, caffeic acid [4], and caffeoylquinic acid derivatives [9] were isolated from *A. lappa* roots. Also, flavonoids such as quercetin and rutin were isolated from leaves [19] and roots [23] of *A. lappa*. Therefore, antioxidant properties of this plant could be attributed to these compounds. Moreover, Erdemoglu et al [19] reported that *A. minus* leaves aqueous extract had antioxidant activity attributed to flavonoids thus corroborating our results for *A. lappa*.

TABLE 3: High-resolution eletrospray ionization mass spectrometry (HRESI-MS) data of Quercetin, Arctigenin, Chlorogenic acid, and Caffeic acid identified in the hydroethanolic extract of *Arctium lappa* root

Compound	Molecular Formule	Calculated [M-H]- mass	Experimental [M-H]- mass	E (ppm)
Quercetin	$C_{15}H_{10}O_7$	301.0348	301.0293	18.27
Arctigenin	$C_{21}H_{24}O_6$	371.1495	371.1542	12.66
Chlorogenic acid	$C_{16}H_{18}O_9$	353.0872	353.0896	6.80
Caffeic acid	$C_9H_8O_4$	179.0344	179.0305	21.78

TABLE 4: Tumor growth inhibition (TGI) (µg/mL) induced by *A. lappa* extracts

	U	M	A	7	4	P	O	H	K
Doxo	3.22	0.16	16.79	0.20	0.05	0.34	>25	1.51	0.03
DHE	>250	>250	>250	155.79	>250	>250	>250	>250	17.06
DE	>250	41.12	>250	60.32	50.47	62.28	81.99	61.43	3.62

U = UACC-62 (melanoma), M = MCF-7 (breast), A = NCI-ADR/RES (expressing multiple drug resistance phenotype), 7 = 786-0 (renal), 4 = NCI-H460 (lung, non-small cells), P = PC-3 (prostate), O = OVCAR-3 (ovarian), H = HT-29 (colon), K = K562 (leukemia).

The antiproliferative properties of the eight extracts of *A. lappa* roots were assessed by using nine human cancer cell lines, and the chemotherapeutic drug, doxorubicin, as a positive control. Among all extracts evaluated, dichloromethane extracts were the only ones with antiproliferative activity. The most active extract (DE) presented a moderate activity for all cell lines with selectivity for K562 (TGI = 3.6 µg/mL) and MCF-7 (TGI = 41.1 µg/mL) (Table 4) while DHE extract displayed the lowest activity with selectivity for K562 (TGI = 17.0 µg/mL) and 786-0 (TGI

= 155.7 µg/mL) (Table 4). The difference in the antiproliferative effects between hot and room temperature extractions may have resulted from the different bioactive substances contained in the extracts due to the sensitivity to heat treatment. An antiproliferative activity study, using prostate cancer cells (LNCaP), attributed the inhibitory activity of *A. lappa* seeds hydromethanolic extract to the presence of compounds lappaol A, C and F [24]. A study performed with *A. lappa* showed that dichloromethane seed extract inhibits cancer cell viability under nutrient-deprived conditions, as observed in pancreatic cancer and hepatoma cell lines at 50 µg/ml concentration. The authors also reported the isolation of arctigenin which exhibits cytotoxicity by inducing necrosis in cancer cells [10]. Researchers [11] also reported that hydromethanolic extract of *A. lappa* fruits shows potent antiproliferative activity against B cell hybridoma cells (MH60) attributed to the presence of arctigenin. Ferracane et al [5] recently isolated arctiin from *A. lappa* root, which demonstrated, according to other research groups, a strong cytotoxic effect on human hepatoma cell line (HepG2) [25], human lung cancer (A549), human ovarian cancer (K-OV-3), human skin cancer (SK-MEL-2); human CNS cancer (XF498) and human colon cancer (HCT15) [26].

A. lappa is plant popularly used in the diet as a vegetable and in alternative medicine because it has ample therapeutic action. Moreover, this plant is a component of Flor-Essence® and Essiac®, which is two of the most widely used herbal products by cancer patients [27-29]. Several experimental studies have shown evidence of biological activity of *A. lappa* extracts or active compounds including antioxidant, anti-inflammatory, free radical-scavenging, antibacterial and hepatoprotective actions [2]. Thus the current study contributes to the growing literature which demonstrates that *A. lappa* show antioxidant and human tumor cell antiproliferative activities *in vitro*. Although, several studies demonstrated biological properties of *A. lappa in vitro*, further research is needed to elucidate the in vivo activities.

2.4 CONCLUSIONS

Our results demonstrated that hydroethanolic extracts exhibited the strongest free radical scavenger activity while the highest phenolic content was observed in Soxhlet extraction with dichloromethane, ethanol and hydro-ethanolic mixture. Moreover, the dichloromethanic extracts are the most important for this research in that they showed selective antiproliferative activity against K562, MCF-7 and 786-0 human cancer cell lines. On the other hand, the hydroethanolic extract had the greatest yield and shows free radical scavenger activity and high phenolic content, making this extract the best adapted for future "in vivo" studies.

REFERENCES

1. Pereira J, Bergamo D, Pereira J, França S, Pietro R, Silva-Sousa Y: Antimicrobial activity of *Arctium lappa* constituents against microorganisms commonly found in endodontic infections. Braz Dent J 2005, 16(3):192-196.
2. Predes F, Matta S, Monteiro J, Oliveira T: Investigation of liver tissue and biochemical parameters of adult wistar rats treated with *Arctium lappa* L. Braz Arch Biol Technol 2009, 52(2):335-340.
3. Lin S, Lin C, Lin C, Lin Y, Chen C, Chen I, Wang L: Hepatoprotective effects of *Arctium lappa* linne on liver injuries induced by chronic ethanol consumption and potentiated by carbon tetrachloride. J Biomed Sci 2002, 9(5):401-409.
4. Chen F, Wu A, Chen C: The influence of different treatments on the free radical scavenging activity of burdock and variations of its active components. Food Chem 2004, 86(4):479-484.
5. Ferracane R, Graziani G, Gallo M, Fogliano V, Ritieni A: Metabolic profile of the bioactive compounds of burdock (*Arctium lappa*) seeds, roots and leaves. J Pharm Biomed Anal 2010, 51(2):399-404.
6. Lin S, Chung T, Lin C, Ueng T, Lin Y, Lin S, Wang L: Hepatoprotective effects of *Arctium lappa* on carbon tetrachloride-and acetaminophen-induced liver damage. Am J Chin Med 2000, 28(2):163-173.
7. Lin C, Lin J, Yang J, Chuang S, Ujiie T: Anti-inflammatory and radical scavenge effects of *Arctium lappa*. Am J Chin Med 1996, 24(2):127-137.
8. Duh P: Antioxidant activity of burdock (*Arctium lappa* Linne): its scavenging effect on free-radical and active oxygen. J Am Oil Chem Soc 1998, 75(4):455-461.
9. Maruta Y, Kawabata J, Niki R: Antioxidative caffeoylquinic acid derivatives in the roots of burdock (*Arctium lappa* L.).J Agric Food Chem 1995, 43(10):2592-2595.
10. Awale S, Lu J, Kalauni S, Kurashima Y, Tezuka Y, Kadota S, Esumi H: Identification of arctigenin as an antitumor agent having the ability to eliminate the tolerance of cancer cells to nutrient starvation. Cancer Res 2006, 66(3):1751-1757.
11. Matsumoto T, Hosono-Nishiyama K, Yamada H: Antiproliferative and apoptotic effects of butyrolactone lignans from *Arctium lappa* on leukemic cells. Planta medica 2006, 72(3):276-278.
12. Brand-Williams W, Cuvelier M, Berset C: Use of a free radical method to evaluate antioxidant activity. LWT-Food Sci Technol 1995, 28(1):25-30.

13. Brem B, Seger C, Pacher T, Hartl M, Hadacek F, Hofer O, Vajrodaya S, Greger H: Antioxidant dehydrotocopherols as a new chemical character of Stemona species. Phytochemistry 2004, 65(19):2719-2729.

14. Jiménez-Escrig A, Jiménez-Jiménez I, Sánchez-Moreno C, Saura-Calixto F: Evaluation of free radical scavenging of dietary carotenoids by the stable radical 2, 2-diphenyl-1-picrylhydrazyl. J Sci Food Agricul 2000, 80(11):1686-1690.

15. Prior R, Wu X, Schaichs K: Standardized methods for the determination of antioxidant capacity and phenolics in foods and dietary supplements. J Agric Food Chem 2005, 53(10):4290-4302.

16. Zhang Y, Seeram N, Lee R, Feng L, Heber D: Isolation and identification of strawberry phenolics with antioxidant and human cancer cell antiproliferative properties. J Agric Food Chem 2008, 56(3):670-675.

17. Gülçin I: Antioxidant activity of caffeic acid (3, 4-dihydroxycinnamic acid). Toxicology 2006, 217(2-3):213-220.

18. Gilioli AMHH, Missau FC, Brighente IMC, Marques MCA, Pizzolatti MG: Avaliação do teor de fenólicos e flavonóides em extratos de *Arctium lappa*. 30ª Reunião Anual da Sociedade Brasileira de Química 2007, :177.

19. Erdemoglu N, Turan N, Akkol E, Sener B, AbacIoglu N: Estimation of anti-inflammatory, antinociceptive and antioxidant activities on Arctium minus (Hill) Bernh. ssp. minus. J Ethnopharmacol 2009, 121(2):318-323.

20. Carvalho M, Ferreira P, Mendes V, Silva R, Pereira J, Jerónimo C, Silva B: Human cancer cell antiproliferative and antioxidant activities of Juglans regia L. Food Chem Toxicol 48(1):441-447.

21. Gulcin I, Tel A, Kirecci E: Antioxidant, Antimicrobial, Antifungal, and Antiradical Activities of Cyclotrichium Niveum (BOISS.) Manden and Scheng. Inter J Food Prop 2008, 11(2):450-471.

22. Gülçin : The antioxidant and radical scavenging activities of black pepper (Piper nigrum) seeds. Int J Food Sci Nutrit 2005, 56(7):491-499.

23. Scorzoni LBT, Barizan WS, França SC, Pietro RCLR, Januária AH: Estudo fitoquímico de *Arctium lappa* (Compositae). 30ª Reunião Anual da Sociedade Brasileira de Química 2007, :20.

24. Ming D, Guns E, Eberding A, Towers N: Isolation and characterization of compounds with anti-prostate cancer activity from *Arctium lappa* L. using bioactivity-guided fractionation. Pharmaceutical Biology 2004, 42(1):44-48.

25. Moritani S, Nomura M, Takeda Y, Miyamoto K: Cytotoxic components of bardanae fructus (goboshi). Biol Pharm Bull 1996, 19(11):1515-1517.

26. Ryu S, Ahn J, Kang Y, Han B: Antiproliferative effect of arctigenin and arctiin. Arch Pharm Res 1995, 18(6):462-463.

27. Tai J, Cheung S, Wong S, Lowe C: *In vitro* comparison of Essiac® and Flor-Essence® on human tumor cell lines. Oncol Rep 2004, 11(2):471-476.

28. Tamayo C, Richardson M, Diamond S, Skoda I: The chemistry and biological activity of herbs used in Flor-EssenceTM herbal tonic and Essiac. Phytother Res 2000, 14(1):1-14.

29. Leonard S, Keil D, Mehlman T, Proper S, Shi X, Harris G: Essiac tea: Scavenging of reactive oxygen species and effects on DNA damage. J Ethnopharmacol 2006, 103(2):288-296.

CHAPTER 3

INTERLEUKIN-6 AND CYCLOOXYGENASE-2 DOWNREGULATION BY FATTY-ACID FRACTIONS OF *RANUNCULUS CONSTANTINOPOLITANUS*

SABREEN F. FOSTOK, RIMA A. EZZEDDINE,
FADIA R. HOMAIDAN, JAMAL A. AL-SAGHIR,
RALPH G. SALLOUM, NAJAT A. SALIBA, AND RABIH S. TALHOUK

3.1 BACKGROUND

Dietary supplements are used as preventive means to maintain a healthy state. Among them, polyunsaturated fatty acids (PUFAs), specifically members of the omega (n)-3 series and conjugated linoleic acid (CLA), have become the focus of extensive nutritional research in the last decade [1-6] due to their reported anti-inflammatory properties. Indeed, CLA and the n-3 eicosapentaenoic acid (EPA) and docosahexaenoic acid (DHA) were found to reduce the levels of many inflammatory mediators, including cytokines: interleukin (IL)-1, IL-6 and tumor necrosis factor (TNF)-α, eicosanoids: prostaglandins (PGs), thromboxanes (TXs) and leukotrienes (LTs), enzymes: cyclooxygenase (COX)-2 and 5-lipoxygenase (LOX), adhesion molecules: E-selectin, intercellular adhesion molecule (ICAM)-1 and vascular cell adhesion molecule (VCAM)-1 and ma-

This chapter was originally published under the Creative Commons Attribution License. Fostok SF, Ezzeddine RA, Homaidan FR, Al-Saghir JA, Salloum RG, Saliba NA, and Talhouk RS. Interleukin-6 and Cyclooxygenase-2 Downregulation by Fatty-Acid Fractions of Ranunculus constantinopolitanus. BMC Complementary and Alternative Medicine *9,44 (2009). doi:10.1186/1472-6882-9-44.*

trix metalloproteinases (MMPs) [7-10]. Clinically, reports have suggested that supplementation with n-3 fatty acids (FAs) has beneficial effects in chronic inflammatory diseases such as inflammatory bowel disease (IBD), rheumatoid arthritis (RA) and psoriasis [11]. Moreover, adding n-3 FAs to the diet of patients with hypertriglyceridemia is now recognized as an efficient triglyceride-lowering therapeutic measure [12]. CLA has been shown to possess similar effects, though the safety and efficacy of CLA dietary supplements is still under investigation [9,13,14].

In contrast to the numerous reports investigating the protective effects of animal-derived PUFAs in inflammation, the literature describing anti-inflammatory bioactivities in plant-derived FAs, and particularly those existing in the Ranunculaceae family, used as a medicinal herb, is poor. This family, comprising around 2500 species distributed all over the world, is especially widespread in slow streams, ditches and shallow ponds of muddy mineral-rich water. *Ranunculus*, a representative genus of the Ranunculaceae family, has been established as an anti-inflammatory, analgesic, antiviral, antibacterial, antiparasitic and antifungal agent [15-20]. Such properties of this genus could be due to the presence of anemonin, a dimerization product of the γ-lactone protoanemonin, both of which have been shown to possess several pharmacological effects [18,21-23]. In this paper, the effect of a FA mix extracted from *Ranunculus constantinopolitanus* D'Urv., an Eastern Mediterranean plant that extends as far as Armenia, on endotoxin (ET)-induced IL-6 and IL-1-induced COX-2 in SCp2 and Mode-K cells, respectively, is investigated. This effect is subsequently compared to the activities of over-the-counter products reported to modulate inflammation, including fish oil and CLA.

3.2 METHODS

3.2.1 CELL CULTURE

Mouse mammary epithelial cell strain, SCp2 cells (kindly provided as a gift by P.Y. Desprez, Geraldine Brush Cancer Research Institute, California

Pacific Medical Center, San Francisco, CA, USA) were cultured as previously described by Saliba et al. (2009) [24]. Briefly, cells were grown on 100-mm tissue culture plates (BD Falcon, Franklin Lakes, NJ, USA) in growth medium (GM) consisting of Dulbecco's Modified Eagle's Medium Nutrient Mixture/F12 Ham (DMEM/F12; Gibco, Paisley, Scotland) supplemented with 5% heat-inactivated fetal bovine serum (FBS; Gibco), insulin (5 µg/ml; Sigma, St. Louis, MO, USA) and 1% penicillin/streptomycin mixture (Gibco) in a humidified incubator (95% air 5% CO_2; VWR Scientific, West Chester, PA, USA) at 37°C. Upon confluency, cells were detached by trypsinization and replated in GM either on 100-mm tissue culture plates for maintenance or on 6-well plates (BD Falcon) at 1×10^6 cells/well to be used in different experiments. On the second day after plating, cells were shifted to differentiation medium (DM) consisting of DMEM/F12 supplemented with insulin (5 µg/ml), hydrocortisone (1 µg/ml; Sigma), ovine prolactin (3 µg/ml; Sigma) and 1% penicillin/streptomycin. On the third day, unless otherwise indicated, plant and ET treatments were performed in triplicates.

Murine intestinal epithelial cell type Mode-K cells were cultured as previously described by Homaidan et al. (2003) [25]. Briefly, cells were maintained in DMEM containing 1 g/L glucose and 10 mM sodium pyruvate (Invitrogen, Carlsbad, CA, USA) and supplemented with 10% FBS (Invitrogen), 1% non-essential amino acids (Invitrogen) and 0.5% penicillin/streptomycin (Invitrogen). At 70-80% confluency, cells were detached by trypsinization and replated on tissue culture flasks (BD Falcon) for maintenance or on 6-well plates at 2×10^5 cells/well to be used in different experiments. On the second day after plating, cells were starved. Plant and IL-1 treatments were performed on the second and third days.

3.2.2 EXTRACTION OF PLANT MATERIAL

3.2.2.1 COLLECTION AND DRYING

Ranunculus constantinopolitanus was collected from Yanta, Lebanon, located at an altitude of 1395 m. A voucher specimen of the plant (voucher number: 72) was deposited at the Post Herbarium of the American University of Beirut, Beirut, Lebanon. Following collection, the aerial part (stems, leaves and flowers) of *R. constantinopolitanus* was dried by leaving the plant sample in the shade for two weeks before grinding it into approximately 10-mm pieces using a blender. Ground samples were subjected to solvent extraction using methanol (MeOH) or else they were stored at -20°C for later use.

3.2.2.2 METHANOL EXTRACTION AND FRACTIONATION

The crude MeOH extract was subjected to further solvent fractionation as previously described by Saliba et al. (2009) [24]. In brief, the dried plant material was subjected to extraction through soaking in MeOH (1:10 w/v) for 16 hr. Incubation on a shaker at 20°C occurred in the first 2 hr, and then the plant sample was left in MeOH for the remaining time. The MeOH extract was filtered using a cheese cloth (sterile gauze sponges 30 × 30 cm) to give a solid phase (R-I) and a filtrate numbered "I" and referred to as "crude MeOH extract". R-I was soaked in ethyl acetate (EtOAc) at a ratio of 10:1 (w/v). It was then separated by filtration into a solid phase and a filtrate numbered "I.1". The crude MeOH extract (I) was evaporated to 1/10 of its volume at less than 40°C, acidified to pH 2 by concentrated H_2SO_4 and then separated into an aqueous and an organic layer using a mixture of $CHCl_3$ and H_2O (2:1 v/v). The organic layer was collected and labelled as "I.2". The aqueous layer was basified to pH 10 by the addition of concentrated NH_4OH and was then resuspended in a mixture of $CHCl_3$ and MeOH (3:1 v/v) (the total volume of $CHCl_3$:MeOH is equal to four times the volume of the aqueous layer) to be later separated into an organic layer and an aqueous layer labelled as "I.3" and "I.4", respectively. I.1, I.2, I.3 and I.4 were evaporated to dryness under vacuum, weighed, dissolved in 100% ethanol (EtOH) and stored in dark bottles at -20°C. The fractions were subsequently screened for potential biological activities, and the active ones were selected for further purification.

3.2.2.3 SEPARATION AND IDENTIFICATION OF SUBFRACTION Y_{2+3}

Biologically active fraction I.2 (6 g) was re-dissolved in a minimum volume of petroleum ether (P.ether):CHCl$_3$:EtOAc mixture (2:2:1) and was applied to a column chromatography consisting of 800 g of silica gel. A gradient elution was performed using P.ether:CHCl$_3$:EtOAc (2:2:1) (6500 ml), followed by P.ether:CHCl$_3$:EtOAc (1:3:1) (4000 ml), CHCl$_3$:EtOAc:MeOH (3:3:1) (4200 ml) and MeOH, successively. Subfraction Y_{2+3} was collected using P.ether:CHCl$_3$:EtOAc (2:2:1) as a mobile phase.

Y_{2+3}, which had the highest biological activity, was purified via solid phase extraction (SPE). Spectroscopic data using infrared (IR) spectroscopy and nuclear magnetic resonance (NMR) showed that Y_{2+3} was a mixture of FAs. The mixture was consequently converted to FA methyl esters (FAMEs) and resolved into individual components using gas chromatography-mass spectrometry (GC-MS). GC analysis was performed using a Trace™ gas chromatograph equipped with HP-5 capillary column (30 m long, 250 μm i.d and 0.25 μm film thickness), Helium as a carrier at a flow rate of 1 ml/min. The maximum temperature was 350°C. The column was heated from 35°C to 290°C. The injector temperature was set at 300°C in a splitless mode. Results were recorded as percent of total peak areas. The mass spectrometer employed in the GC-MS analysis was a Polarization Q series mass selective detector in the electron impact (EI) ionization mode (70 eV). Using appropriate reference standards of FAMEs, Y_{2+3} was identified as a mixture of four FAs: palmitic acid (C16:0), isomers of C18:2 and C18:1 and stearic acid (C18:0) in the corresponding proportion 1:5:8:1.

3.2.3 TREATMENT OF CELLS WITH PLANT EXTRACTS AND FATTY ACIDS

Plant extracts, fish oil, CLA, the FAs: palmitic, linoleic (cis-9, cis-12-octadecadienoic acid), oleic (cis-9-octadecenoic acid) and stearic acid and a mix of the four FAs (1:5:8:1 ratio) were all diluted in 100% EtOH and stored at -20°C. On day 3 after plating, SCp2 cells were treated with plant extracts or other FA compounds at different concentrations in DM supplemented with 1% FBS up to a final volume of 1 ml/well. Following treatment, cells were incubated at 37°C for different time points (24 or 48 hr) to assess cytotoxicity or for 30 min (short-term treatment) before ET treatment. For other experiments, media were supplemented with plant extracts or other FA compounds at different concentrations for 3 days as of the plating day (long-term treatment), and cells were treated with ET on day 3.

For Mode-K cells, on day 2 after plating, cultures were pretreated with Y_{2+3} or a synthetic FA mix at different concentrations in the absence of FBS up to a final volume of 1 ml/well. Following treatment, cells were incubated at 37°C for 8 or 12 hr before IL-1 treatment on day 3. Another method involved the cotreatment of Mode-K cells with Y_{2+3} or a synthetic FA mix and IL-1 on day 3 for 8 hr under similar conditions.

3.2.4 INDUCTION OF INFLAMMATION

3.2.4.1 ENDOTOXIN TREATMENT OF SCP2 CELLS

ET treatment was performed as previously described by Saliba et al. (2009) [24]. *Salmonella typhosa* ET (Sigma) was dissolved in DM, filter-sterilized using 0.2 μm non-pyrogenic sterile-R filter and stored at -20°C. On day 3 after plating, cells were treated with ET at 10 μg/ml and then incubated at 37°C for 9 hr.

3.2.4.2 INTERLEUKIN-1 TREATMENT OF MODE-K CELLS

IL-1 treatment was performed as previously described by Homaidan et al. (2003) [25]. IL-1α (US Biological, Swampscott, MA, USA) was dissolved in 1% bovine serum albumin (BSA; Invitrogen) and stored at -20°C. On

day 3 after plating, cells were treated with IL-1 at 10 ng/ml and then incubated at 37°C for 6 or 8 hr.

3.2.4.3 TRYPAN BLUE EXCLUSION METHOD

Twenty-four or 48 hr post plant treatment, viable and dead SCp2 cells
were counted using the trypan blue exclusion method. It involves the trypsinization of the attached cells and washing them using the same treatment medium, which contains dead cells, to form a suspension of the total
treated cells. An aliquot of 50 µl is taken from this suspension and mixed
with an equal volume of trypan blue (Gibco). Dead cells stain blue, while
viable cells appear bright. The percentage of viability is calculated relative
to the control.

3.2.5 ENZYME-LINKED IMMUNOSORBENT ASSAY (ELISA)

3.2.5.1 SAMPLE COLLECTION

Media of SCp2 cells were sampled from triplicate wells 9 hr post ET treatment. Forty µl of complete protease inhibitors [one tablet dissolved in 2 ml
of double distilled water (DDW); Roche Diagnostics GmbH, Mannheim,
Germany] was added to each 1 ml of sample. Samples were stored at
-80°C until the day of the assay.

3.2.5.2 INTERLEUKIN-6 ASSAY

A two-site (sandwich) ELISA was performed for the quantitative determination of mouse IL-6 (mIL-6) present in SCp2 cell culture media, using
mIL-6 ELISA immunoassay kit (BioSource International, Inc., Camarillo,
CA, USA). The IL-6 assay was performed according to manufacturers'

instructions. All standards and samples were run in duplicates on high-binding 96-well microtiter plates (Thermo Labsystems, Philadelphia, PA, USA). The optical density was measured at a wavelength of 450 nm by an ELISA microplate reader (Multiskan Ascent, Thermo Labsystems). Concentrations were calculated using the Ascent software and were expressed in pg/ml.

3.2.6 WESTERN BLOTTING

Mode-K cells were washed twice with phosphate-buffered saline (PBS) and scraped in 2× electrophoresis sample buffer (SB) containing 0.25 M Tris-HCl (pH 6.8; Amersham Biosciences, San Diego, CA, USA), 4% w/v sodium dodecyl sulfate (SDS; Amersham Biosciences), 20% w/w glycerol (Amersham Biosciences), 0.1% bromophenol blue and 40 µl/ml protease inhibitor cocktail (Biomol, Plymouth Meeting, PA, USA). Samples were then collected in microfuge tubes, boiled for 5 min, centrifuged and the supernatant representing total soluble protein extract was collected and stored at -80°C.

Total protein extracts were run on a 12% SDS-polyacrylamide gel (BioRad, Hercules, CA, USA), and the gels were transferred to polyvinylidene difluoride (PVDF) membranes (Amersham Biosciences) overnight at 4°C. Following transfer, membranes were washed once with TPBS wash buffer (PBS containing 0.1% Tween 20) and then blocked in 5% non-fat dry milk for 2 hr at room temperature. Rabbit polyclonal COX-2 antibody (Cayman Chemical, Ann Arbor, MI, USA) was then added to the membranes and incubated for 2 hr at room temperature. Unbound antibodies were washed three times with TPBS. Horse-raddish peroxidase (HRP)-conjugated anti-rabbit IgG (Santa Cruz Biotechnology, Santa Cruz, CA, USA) was added at 1:5000 dilution for 1 hr at room temperature. Membranes were washed, incubated with luminol reagents (Santa Cruz Biotechnology) and directly exposed to autoradiography.

3.2.7 STATISTICAL ANALYSIS

Data were expressed as mean ± S.D. The effectiveness of plant treatments was analyzed by one-way analysis of variance (ANOVA). To check for treatments with similar effects, Student-Newman-Keuls (SNK) and Tukey HSD tests were performed. The effect of each treatment, if any, was then compared to the control using two-sample t-test or Dunnett t-tests for multiple comparisons. All statistical analyses were carried out using statistical program for social sciences (SPSS) 11.5, except for t-test, which was performed using Excel. Statistical probability of $P < 0.05$ was considered significant.

3.3 RESULTS

3.3.1 EFFECT OF R. CONSTANTINOPOLITANUS EXTRACTS ON ENDOTOXIN-INDUCED INTERLEUKIN-6 LEVELS IN SCP2 CELLS

Ranunculus constantinopolitanus (Figure 1), known for its folk medicinal value, was subjected to chemical extraction and purification. The crude MeOH extract (I) from this plant was cytotoxic to SCp2 cells. Accordingly, I.2, the chloroform fraction derived from that extract, was tested for its biological activity on SCp2 cells. To determine the maximum concentration of I.2 that can be used without affecting cell viability or morphology, SCp2 cells were treated with I.2 at different concentrations (10, 25, 50 or 100 µg/ml) or EtOH, as a vehicle control, and viable cell counts were determined. None of the tested concentrations affected cell morphology 24 hr post-treatment (Data not shown), and cell viability for all concentrations did not vary significantly from the control treatment (Figure 2A). Thus, the ability of I.2 to inhibit ET-induced IL-6 was studied to evaluate its potential anti-inflammatory activities. SCp2 cells pretreated with I.2 at the different concentrations (10, 25, 50 or 100 µg/ml) showed, in a concentration-dependent manner, a significant reduction in IL-6 levels stimulated by ET (Figure 2B). Basal IL-6 levels were noted in cells pretreated with 100 µg/ml.

Treatment of SCp2 cells with Y_{2+3} at different concentrations (10, 20 or 30 µg/ml) or EtOH, as a vehicle control, did not alter cell morphology at any of the tested concentrations for up to 48 hr post-treatment (Data not shown). In addition, cell counts performed at the same time point showed that cell viability for each concentration was similar to that of the control treatment (Figure 3A). Consequently, Y_{2+3} was used at concentrations not exceeding 30 µg/ml in all subsequent experiments.

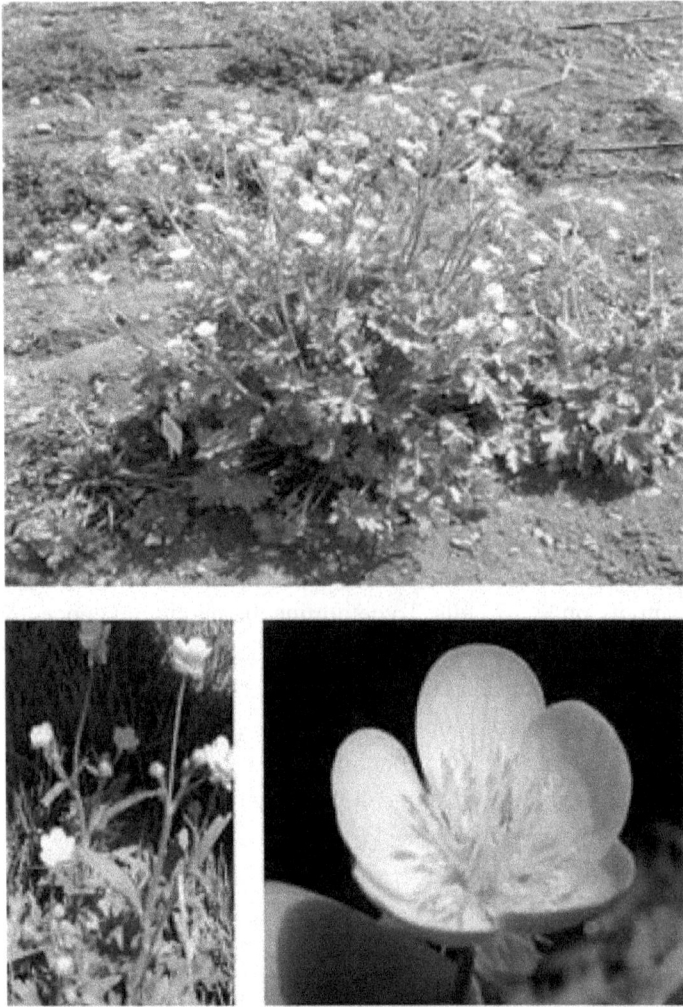

FIGURE 1: *Ranunculus constantinopolitanus. Ranunculus constantinopolitanus* (Arabic name: Hawdhan fa'ri) is an Eastern Mediterranean plant that grows in Aintab and extends from Hasbayya to Jazzin. Description: "Villous below, appressed-hairy above. Root-fibers descending directly from neck. Root-leaves triangular-ovate, ternate, with obovate, cut, and coarsely toothed lobes. Carpels large, ovate, striate, smooth, ending abruptly in a very short, hooked beak". Its flowering season falls between April and June [41]. The plant has been identified by Dr. Nada Sinno-Saoud, and a voucher specimen (voucher number: 72) was deposited at the Post Herbarium of the American University of Beirut, Beirut, Lebanon. Photos courtesy of Mr. Khaled Sleem (2004), Crop Production and Protection Department, Faculty of Agricultural and Food Sciences, American University of Beirut, Beirut, Lebanon.

A

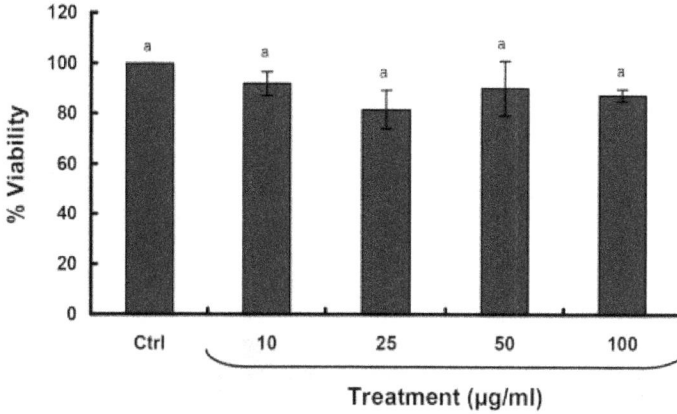

B

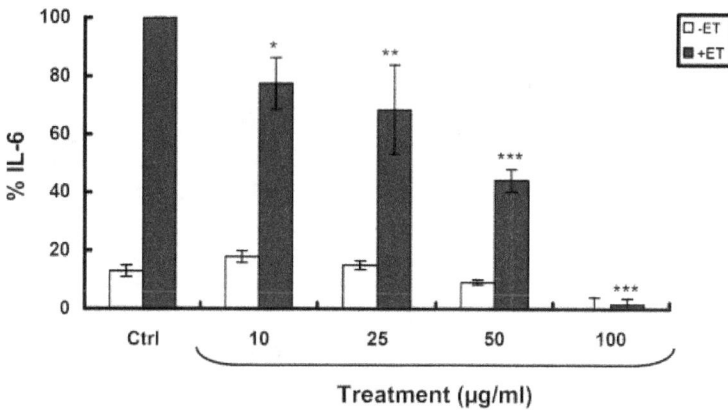

FIGURE 2: Exposure of SCp2 cells to *R. constantinopolitanus* fraction I.2 at noncytotoxic concentrations reduces, in a concentration-dependent manner, ET-induced IL-6 levels. SCp2 cells were treated on day 3 of culture with EtOH (Ctrl) or I.2 at different concentrations in DM supplemented with 1% FBS: (A) Twenty-four hr later, trypan blue assay was performed. (B) Thirty min later, cells were treated with ET at 10 μg/ml and their media collected 9 hr post-ET. The values depicted are the means (± S.D.) of a triplicate treatment. Means with the same letter are not significantly different. Statistical significance of the difference from Ctrl+ET is with *P < 0.05, **P < 0.01 or ***P < 0.001. (Ctrl, control; ET, endotoxin; IL-6, interleukin-6). -ET (white square); +ET (black square).

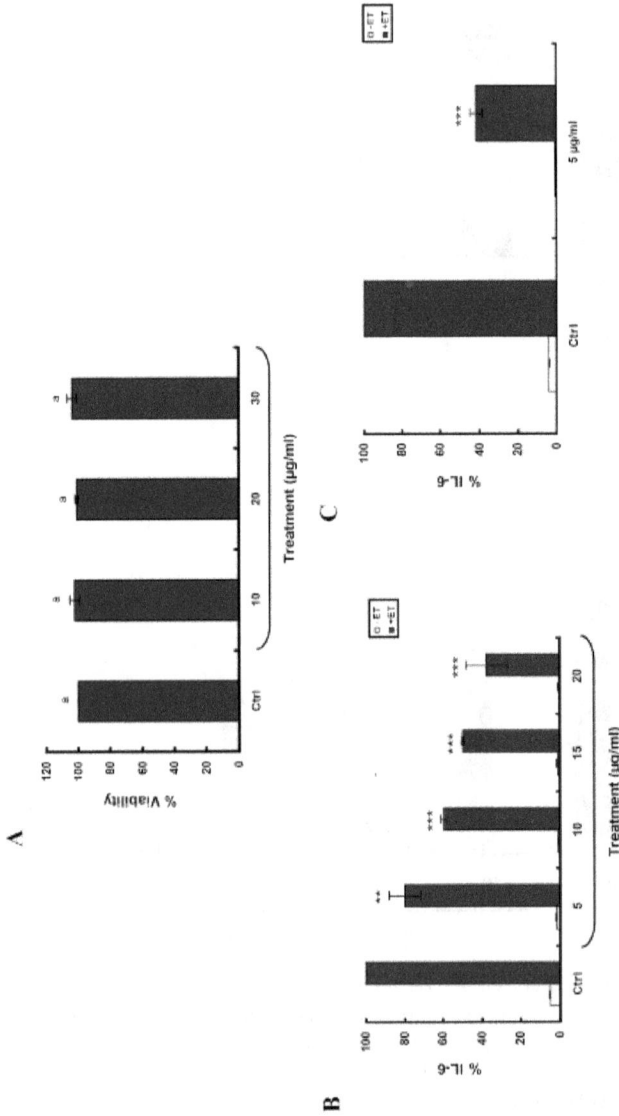

FIGURE 3: Exposure of SCp2 cells to Y$_{2+3}$ at noncytotoxic concentrations reduces, in a concentration-dependent manner, ET-induced IL-6 levels. (A) SCp2 cells were treated on day 3 of culture with EtOH (Ctrl) or Y$_{2+3}$ at different concentrations in DM supplemented with 1% FBS. Forty-eight hr later, trypan blue assay was performed. SCp2 cells were treated (B) on day 3 of culture 30 min before ET (short-term exposure) or (C) for 3 days (long-term exposure), as of day 1 of culture, with EtOH (Ctrl) or Y$_{2+3}$ at different concentrations. Cells were treated on day 3 with ET at 10 µg/ml in DM supplemented with 1% FBS and their media collected 9 hr post-ET. The values depicted are the means (± S.D.) of a triplicate treatment. Means with the same letter are not significantly different. Statistical significance of the difference from Ctrl+ET is with **P < 0.01 or ***P < 0.001. (Ctrl, control; ET, endotoxin; IL-6, interleukin-6). -ET (white square); +ET (black square).

To check if the anti-inflammatory effect previously observed with I.2 was due to the Y_{2+3} subfraction, the ability of the latter to inhibit ET-induced IL-6 was evaluated. SCp2 cells were pretreated with different Y_{2+3} concentrations, not exceeding 30 µg/ml, using two modes of treatment. Short-term treatment at 5, 10, 15 or 20 µg/ml resulted in a concentration-dependent downregulation of ET-induced IL-6 levels (Figure 3B). This reduction was significant at all the tested concentrations and exceeded 50% inhibition at the highest Y_{2+3} concentration (20 µg/ml). Long-term treatment at 5 µg/ml significantly downregulated ET-induced IL-6 levels by more than 50% (Figure 3C).

3.3.2 POTENCY OF Y_{2+3} VERSUS ITS PRESUMED FATTY ACID COMPONENTS, FISH OIL OR CONJUGATED LINOLEIC ACID IN REGULATING ENDOTOXIN-INDUCED INTERLEUKIN-6 LEVELS IN SCP2 CELLS

The effect of Y_{2+3} in inhibiting ET-induced IL-6 was compared to that of short- or long-term treatment with each of the individual FA constituents, i.e. palmitic and stearic acid and the two most common C18:2 and C18:1 isomers: linoleic (cis-9, cis-12-octadecadienoic acid) and oleic (cis-9-octadecenoic acid) acid, respectively, at concentrations similar to those previously used with Y_{2+3}. It was noted that Y_{2+3} significantly reduced ET-induced IL-6 levels upon both short- and long-term treatment of SCp2 cells (Figure 4A and 4B). However, none of the individual FAs could reduce IL-6 levels at concentrations ranging from 5-20 µg/ml following short-term treatment (Figure 4A) or at a concentration of 5 µg/ml following long-term treatment (Figure 4B). Furthermore, neither short-term treatment at 5-20 µg/ml, nor long-term treatment at 5 µg/ml with a synthetic mix of palmitic, linoleic (cis-9, cis-12-octadecadienoic acid), oleic (cis-9-octadecenoic acid) and stearic acid in the same proportion as in Y_{2+3} could reduce ET-induced IL-6 levels (Figure 4A and 4B). In fact, in both modes of treatment the mix induced higher levels of IL-6 than those induced by ET alone, similarly for linoleate in short-term treatment and stearate and palmitate in long-term treatment. Noteworthy is that linoleate was cytotoxic to cells in long-term treatment mode.

n-3 FAs and CLA are notoriously associated with anti-inflammatory properties and are available in many forms as over-the-counter supplements. The ability of fish oil, containing the n-3 FAs EPA and DHA (1:0.76 ratio), to reduce ET-induced IL-6 levels was compared to that noted with Y_{2+3}. SCp2 cells were exposed to short- or long-term treatment with fish oil at concentrations similar to those used with Y_{2+3}. In contrast to Y_{2+3}, short-term fish oil treatment did not reduce IL-6 levels induced by ET, but rather enhanced such levels by at least 40% (Figure 5A). However, long-term treatment significantly reduced IL-6 to approximately 25% of the control levels (Figure 5B). Worth mentioning is the fact that fish oil reduced IL-6 levels more than Y_{2+3} at similar concentrations upon long-term treatment.

The ability of short- or long-term CLA treatment to reduce ET-induced IL-6 levels in SCp2 cells was also compared to that of Y_{2+3}. At noncytotoxic concentrations (0.1, 0.5, 1 and 3 µg/ml), short-term CLA treatment did not reduce IL-6 levels, except for a marginal, but significant, reduction at 3 µg/ml (Figure 5C). This reduction was less than that observed with Y_{2+3} at 10 µg/ml. Following long-term treatment, CLA (0.1, 0.5 or 1 µg/ml) significantly reduced IL-6 levels more so than that noted for Y_{2+3} at the 0.5 and 1 µg/ml level (Figure 5D). Concentrations of CLA at 3 and 5 µg/ml were cytotoxic to cells upon long- and short-term treatment, respectively.

3.3.3 EFFECT OF Y_{2+3} ON INTERLEUKIN-1-INDUCED CYCLOOXYGENASE-2 EXPRESSION IN MODE-K CELLS

The effect of Y_{2+3} on COX-2 protein levels in Mode-K cells was assessed by pretreating the cells with Y_{2+3} at 10 µg/ml for 8 or 12 hr prior to 6-hr treatment with 10 ng/ml of IL-1 or cotreating cells with Y_{2+3} and IL-1 for 8 hr. Y_{2+3} caused a significant decrease in IL-1-induced COX-2 levels at 12-hr pretreatment as well as 8-hr cotreatment with IL-1 (Figure 6A). As with SCp2 cells, the effect of the synthetic mixture of FA components of Y_{2+3} on COX-2 protein levels in IL-1-treated Mode-K cells was tested. At 10 µg/ml, a similar concentration to Y_{2+3}, the synthetic mix did not reverse the IL-1-induced COX-2 levels in Mode-K cells (Figure 6B, left panel). The synthetic mix failed to reverse these levels even at a higher concentration of 60 µg/ml (Figure 6B, right panel).

A

B

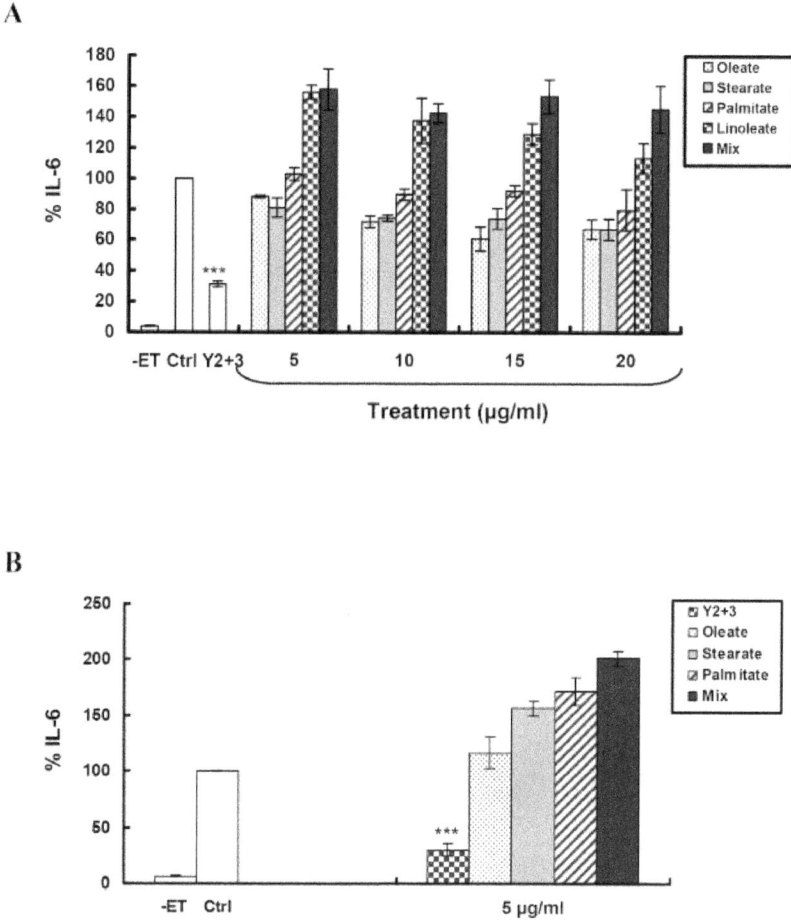

FIGURE 4: Exposure of SCp2 cells to individual FA components of Y_{2+3} or a synthetic FA mix does not reduce ET-induced IL-6 levels. SCp2 cells were treated (A) on day 3 of culture 30 min before ET (short-term exposure) or (B) for 3 days (long-term exposure), as of day 1 of culture, with EtOH (Ctrl), Y_{2+3}[a], palmitate, linoleate[b], oleate, stearate or a synthetic FA mix at different concentrations. Cells were treated on day 3 with ET at 10 μg/ml in DM supplemented with 1% FBS and their media collected 9 hr post-ET. The values depicted are the means (± S.D.) of a triplicate treatment. Statistical significance of the difference from Ctrl+ET is with ***P < 0.001. (Ctrl, control; -ET, untreated cells; IL-6, interleukin-6). [a]For short-term exposure (A), cells were treated with Y_{2+3} at 10 μg/ml. [b]Long-term exposure (B) to linoleate at 5 μg/ml was cytotoxic to cells.

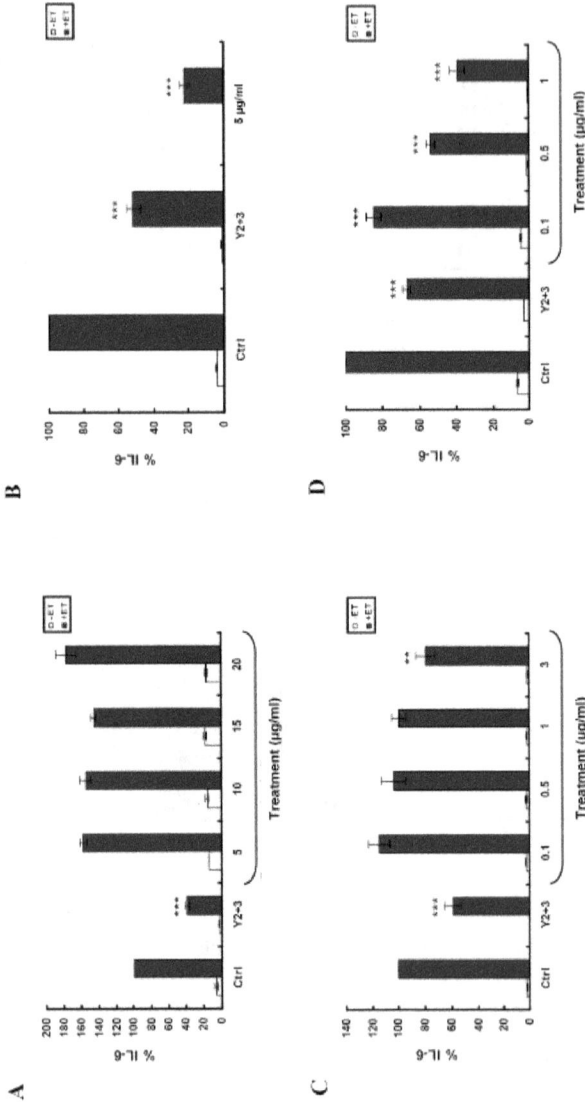

FIGURE 5: Exposure of SCp2 cells to Y$_{2+3}$ reduces ET-induced IL-6 levels more potently than fish oil and CLA. SCp2 cells were treated (A and C) on day 3 of culture 30 min before ET (short-term exposure) or (B and D) for 3 days (long-term exposure), as of day 1 of culture, with EtOH (Ctrl), Y$_{2+3}$[a] fish oil (A and B) or CLA[b] (C and D) at different concentrations. Cells were treated on day 3 with ET at 10 μg/ml in DM supplemented with 1% FBS and their media collected 9 hr post-ET. The values depicted are the means (± S.D.) of a triplicate treatment. Statistical significance of the difference from Ctrl+ET is with **P < 0.01 or ***P < 0.001. (Ctrl, control; ET, endotoxin; IL-6, interleukin-6). [a]Cells were treated with Y$_{2+3}$ at 5 or 10 μg/ml for long- (B and D) and short-term (A and C) exposure, respectively. [b]Short- and long-term exposures to CLA at 5 and 3 μg/ml, respectively, were cytotoxic to cells. -ET (white square); +ET (black square).

A

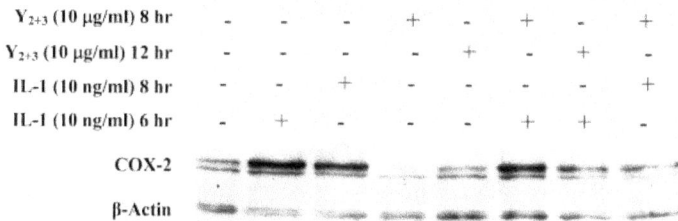

Y₂₊₃ (10 µg/ml) 8 hr	-	-	-	+	-	+	-	+
Y₂₊₃ (10 µg/ml) 12 hr	-	-	-	-	+	-	+	-
IL-1 (10 ng/ml) 8 hr	-	-	+	-	-	-	-	+
IL-1 (10 ng/ml) 6 hr	-	+	-	-	-	+	+	-

COX-2

β-Actin

B

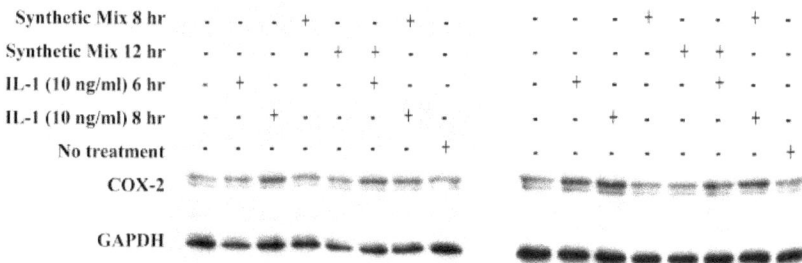

Synthetic Mix 8 hr

Synthetic Mix 12 hr

IL-1 (10 ng/ml) 6 hr

IL-1 (10 ng/ml) 8 hr

No treatment

COX-2

GAPDH

FIGURE 6. Exposure of Mode-K cells to Y_{2+3}, but not to a synthetic FA mix, reduces IL-1-induced COX-2 protein levels. Mode-K cells were treated on day 2 of culture 8 or 12 hr before IL-1 (pretreatment) or on day 3 (cotreatment) with (A) Y_{2+3} at 10 µg/ml or (B) a synthetic FA mix at different concentrations (Left: 10 µg/ml; Right: 60 µg/ml) in FBS-free medium. Cells were treated on day 3 with IL-1 at 10 ng/ml in the absence of FBS and their proteins extracted 6 or 8 hr post-IL-1 for western blot analysis. β-actin or GAPDH was used to demonstrate equal loading. (COX-2, cyclooxygenase-2; IL-1, interleukin-1).

3.4 DISCUSSION

In this study, we report the existence of anti-inflammatory activities in *R. constantinopolitanus* (Arabic name: Hawdhan fa'ri), commonly used in Eastern Mediterranean folk medicine, using in-vitro models of inflammation. Previous work in our laboratory established an in-vitro model of inflammation [26]. In this model, treatment of mouse mammary cells with ET at 10 µg/ml, a noncytotoxic concentration, enhanced nuclear factor (NF)-κB DNA-binding activity, suppressed β-casein expression and up-regulated pro-inflammatory mediators, including gelatinases (MMP-2 and MMP-9) and cytokines (IL-6 and TNF-α). Consequently, SCp2 mouse mammary epithelial cell strain was utilized to assess potential in-vitro anti-inflammatory activities in *R. constantinopolitanus*. In reviewing the literature, we highlighted the role phenols, flavonoids and terpenoids play in treating inflammation [27]. Accordingly, I.2, the chloroform fraction derived from the crude MeOH extract of the plant and presumably rich in these compounds, was assessed for its anti-inflammatory effects in ET-treated SCp2 cells. Due to its importance in the transition from the acute to the chronic phase of inflammation [28], IL-6 has been chosen as an inflammation marker to be monitored in our study. I.2 significantly reduced ET-induced IL-6 levels without altering cell viability or morphology. From there, I.2 was further fractionated and purified to yield a FA mix, Y_{2+3}. Short- and long-term exposure to Y_{2+3} generated an IL-6 inhibitory profile similar to that of I.2 without causing cytotoxicity, but at relatively lower concentrations, indicating that the inhibitory effect noted in I.2 was possibly due to Y_{2+3}.

Numerous reports have shown the occurrence of FAs in members of the Ranunculaceae family [29-31]. Chemical investigation demonstrated the presence of palmitic acid, C18:2 and C18:1 isomers and stearic acid (1:5:8:1 ratio) in Y_{2+3}. In a similar study, these FAs, along with others, were reported to exist in *Ranunculus* ternatus [30], a Chinese medicinal plant used as an analgesic for headache and toothache and for treating congestion, corneal pterygium and malaria.

The comparison between the anti-inflammatory activity of Y_{2+3} and other commonly known biologically active FAs suggested that the higher potency of Y_{2+3} was not due to its presumed FAs, i.e. palmitic and stearic acid and at least not the two most common isomers of C18:2 and C18:1: linoleic and oleic acid, respectively. Even when tested at concentrations exceeding the ones normally present in Y_{2+3} mix, none of the FAs reduced ET-induced IL-6 levels. Furthermore, the synthetic FA mix, containing these FAs in the same ratio as in Y_{2+3}, did not reduce IL-6 levels in SCp2 cells. Y_{2+3} has demonstrated comparable anti-inflammatory effects in IL-1-stimulated mouse intestinal epithelial Mode-K cells. Y_{2+3} effectively downregulated COX-2 expression in these cells, an activity not noted in its synthetic FA mix. Nevertheless, the above observations do not exclude potential combinatorial effects for these FAs. This suggestion is supported by a study that demonstrated antifertility activities in *Azadirachta indica* seed extract and in one of its fractions (containing palmitate, linoleate, oleate and stearate, in addition to methyl palmitate and methyl oleate), which were reduced upon further fractionation. In the same study, regrouping the obtained subfractions to reconstitute the original mixture in a similar proportion did not regenerate the original biological activity [32]. This was attributed to the synergism of the constituents of the mixture as they existed in the seed. Although this could be the case in our study, however, our results can be explained also by possible occurrence of CLA and/or its precursor vaccenic acid as the C18:2 and C18:1 isomers, respectively. Knowing that the anti-inflammatory role of CLA, unlike oleate, palmitate and stearate, was highlighted by different studies [9,14], we opted to investigate the effect of CLA on IL-6 production by SCp2 cells.

In addition, various reports demonstrated the efficacy of CLA, EPA and DHA in reversing inflammation [2,33-36]. Our comparative studies denote similar or more potent effects for Y_{2+3} in SCp2 cell culture model that could be noticed within a shorter exposure time or with less cytotoxic effects. Compared to fish oil, Y_{2+3} was able to reduce IL-6 levels within a shorter period of time; however, at longer exposures, fish oil was more potent than Y_{2+3}. Similarly, CLA was less effective than Y_{2+3}, even at the maximum noncytotoxic concentration for short durations, but exhibited more potent effect after long-term exposure. This suggests the presence of biologically active CLA isomer(s) in Y_{2+3} that could be synergized by the other FA constituents of Y_{2+3}. Worth noting is the presence of a marketable formula of CLA that contains, in addition, palmitic, linoleic, oleic and stearic acid (Tonalin CLA, WeightLossGuide, Sarasota, FL, USA).

Studies have confirmed that dietary PUFA supplementation is capable of ameliorating IBD [37,38]. For instance, using a pig model of dextran sodium sulfate (DSS)-induced colitis, both n-3 PUFA- and CLA-rich diets were shown to exert anti-inflammatory effects [39]. In a related preliminary study, Y_{2+3} synergized the anti-inflammatory activities in salograviolide A (SA), a sesquiterpene lactone purified from Centaurea ainetensis [24,40], whereby intraperitoneal (i.p.) administration of Y_{2+3}:SA mix reduced pro-inflammatory cytokine levels in colons of iodoacetamide-induced ulcerative colitis (UC) rats (Data not shown).

3.5 CONCLUSION

Y_{2+3}, the naturally occurring FA combination derived from *R. constantinopolitanus*, reduces ET-induced IL-6 levels and IL-1-induced COX-2 expression in-vitro more efficiently than the highly reputable CLA and fish oil and within a shorter period of time. Our preliminary studies demonstrate similar effects for Y_{2+3} in an in-vivo model of IBD, making it a promising plant-derived anti-inflammatory FA mix. The mechanism of action of this mixture and the nature of its C18:1 and C18:2 isomers have not been fully elucidated. Finally, a better understanding of the specific cellular targets of Y_{2+3} could prove invaluable in determining the role played by FAs in inflammation prevention and resolution.

REFERENCES

1.   Bendyk A, Marino V, Zilm PS, Howe P, Bartold PM: Effect of dietary omega-3 polyunsaturated fatty acids on experimental periodontitis in the mouse. J Periodontal Res 2009, 44:211-216.
2.   Changhua L, Jindong Y, Defa L, Lidan Z, Shiyan Q, Jianjun X: Conjugated linoleic acid attenuates the production and gene expression of proinflammatory cytokines in weaned pigs challenged with lipopolysaccharide. J Nutr 2005, 135:239-244.
3.   Du C, Fujii Y, Ito M, Harada M, Moriyama E, Shimada R, Ikemoto A, Okuyama H: Dietary polyunsaturated fatty acids suppress acute hepatitis, alter gene expression

and prolong survival of female Long-Evans Cinnamon rats, a model of Wilson disease. J Nutr Biochem 2004, 15:273-280.

4. Jaudszus A, Krokowski M, Möckel P, Darcan Y, Avagyan A, Matricardi P, Jahreis G, Hamelmann E: Cis-9,trans-11-conjugated linoleic acid inhibits allergic sensitization and airway inflammation via a PPARgamma-related mechanism in mice. J Nutr 2008, 138:1336-1342.

5. Sadeghi S, Wallace FA, Calder PC: Dietary lipids modify the cytokine response to bacterial lipopolysaccharide in mice. Immunology 1999, 96:404-410.

6. Sane S, Baba M, Kusano C, Shirao K, Andoh T, Kamada T, Aikou T: Eicosapentaenoic acid reduces pulmonary edema in endotoxemic rats. J Surg Res 2000, 93:21-27.

7. Calder PC: Polyunsaturated fatty acids and inflammation. Biochem Soc Trans 2005, 33:423-427.

8. Calder PC: Polyunsaturated fatty acids, inflammatory processes and inflammatory bowel diseases. Mol Nutr Food Res 2008, 52:885-897.

9. O'Shea M, Bassaganya-Riera J, Mohede IC: Immunomodulatory properties of conjugated linoleic acid. Am J Clin Nutr 2004, 79(Suppl 6):1199-1206.

10. Zainal Z, Longman AJ, Hurst S, Duggan K, Caterson B, Hughes CE, Harwood JL: Relative efficacies of omega-3 polyunsaturated fatty acids in reducing expression of key proteins in a model system for studying osteoarthritis. Osteoarthr Cartilage 2009, 17:882-891.

11. Gil A: Polyunsaturated fatty acids and inflammatory diseases. Biomed Pharmacother 2002, 56:388-396.

12. Nies LK, Cymbala AA, Kasten SL, Lamprecht DG, Olson KL: Complementary and alternative therapies for the management of dyslipidemia. Ann Pharmacother 2006, 40:1984-1992.

13. Pariza MW, Park Y, Cook ME: The biologically active isomers of conjugated linoleic acid. Prog Lipid Res 2001, 40:283-298.

14. Zulet MA, Marti A, Parra MD, Martinez JA: Inflammation and conjugated linoleic acid: mechanisms of action and implications for human health. J Physiol Biochem 2005, 61:483-494.

15. Barbour EK, Al Sharif M, Sagherian VK, Habre AN, Talhouk RS, Talhouk SN: Screening of selected indigenous plants of Lebanon for antimicrobial activity. J Ethnopharmacol 2004, 93:1-7.

16. Cao BJ, Meng QY, Ji N: Analgesic and anti-inflammatory effects of *Ranunculus japonicus* extract. Planta Med 1992, 58:496-498.

17. Li H, Zhou C, Pan Y, Gao X, Wu X, Bai H, Zhou L, Chen Z, Zhang S, Shi S, Luo J, Xu J, Chen L, Zheng X, Zhao Y: Evaluation of antiviral activity of compounds isolated from *Ranunculus* sieboldii and *Ranunculus* sceleratus. Planta Med 2005, 71:1128-1133.

18. Mares D: Antimicrobial activity of protoanemonin, a lactone from ranunculaceous plants. Mycopathologia 1987, 98:133-140.

19. Prieto JM, Recio MC, Giner RM, Máñez S, Ríos JL: Pharmacological approach to the pro- and anti-inflammatory effects of *Ranunculus* sceleratus L. J Ethnopharmacol 2003, 89:131-137.

20. Schinella GR, Tournier HA, Prieto JM, Rios JL, Buschiazzo H, Zaidenberg A: In-hibition of Trypanosoma cruzi growth by medical plant extracts. Fitoterapia 2002, 73:569-575.

21. Duan H, Zhang Y, Xu J, Qiao J, Suo Z, Hu G, Mu X: Effect of anemonin on NO, ET-1 and ICAM-1 production in rat intestinal microvascular endothelial cells. J Eth-nopharmacol 2006, 104:362-366.

22. Lee TH, Huang NK, Lai TC, Yang AT, Wang GJ: Anemonin, from Clematis crassifo-lia, potent and selective inducible nitric oxide synthase inhibitor. J Ethnopharmacol 2008, 116:518-527.

23. Martin ML, Ortíz de Urbina AV, Montero MJ, Carrón R, San Román L: Pharmaco-logic effects of lactones isolated from Pulsatilla alpina subsp. apiifolia. J Ethnophar-macol 1988, 24:185-191.

24. Saliba NA, Dakdouki S, Homeidan F, Kogan J, Bouhadir K, Talhouk S, Talhouk R: Bio-guided identification of an anti-inflammatory guaianolide from Centaurea ainetensis. Pharm Biol 2009, 47:701-707.

25. Homaidan FR, Chakroun I, El-Sabban ME: Regulation of nuclear factor-kappaB in intestinal epithelial cells in a cell model of inflammation. Mediators Inflamm 2003, 12:277-283.

26. Safieh-Garabedian B, Mouneimne GM, El-Jouni W, Khattar M, Talhouk R: The ef-fect of endotoxin on functional parameters of mammary CID-9 cells. Reproduction 2004, 127:397-406.

27. Talhouk RS, Karam C, Fostok S, El-Jouni W, Barbour EK: Anti-inflammatory bio-activities in plant extracts. J Med Food 2007, 10:1-10.

28. Gabay C: Interleukin-6 and chronic inflammation. Arthritis Res Ther 2006, 8(Suppl 2):3.

29. Aitzetmuller K: An unusual fatty acid pattern in Eranthis seed oil. Lipids 1996, 31:201-205.

30. Chen J, Yao C, Xia LM, Ouyang PK: [Determination of fatty acids and organic acids in *Ranunculus* ternatus Thunb using GC-MS]. Guang Pu Xue Yu Guang Pu Fen Xi 2006, 26:1550-1552.

31. Spencer GF, Kleiman R, Earle FR, Wolff IA: Unusual olefinic fatty acids in seed oils from two genera in the Ranunculaceae. Lipids 1970, 5:277-278.

32. Garg S, Talwar GP, Upadhyay SN: Immunocontraceptive activity guided fraction-ation and characterization of active constituents of neem (Azadirachta indica) seed extracts. J Ethnopharmacol 1998, 60:235-246.

33. Lo CJ, Chiu KC, Fu M, Lo R, Helton S: Fish oil decreases macrophage tumor ne-crosis factor gene transcription by altering the NF kappa B activity. J Surg Res 1999, 82:216-221.

34. Puglia C, Tropea S, Rizza L, Santagati NA, Bonina F: *In vitro* percutaneous absorp-tion studies and in vivo evaluation of anti-inflammatory activity of essential fatty acids (EFA) from fish oil extracts. Int J Pharm 2005, 299:41-48.

35. Shen CL, Dunn DM, Henry JH, Li Y, Watkins BA: Decreased production of inflam-matory mediators in human osteoarthritic chondrocytes by conjugated linoleic acids. Lipids 2004, 39:161-166.

36. Tappia PS, Grimble RF: Complex modulation of cytokine induction by endotoxin and tumour necrosis factor from peritoneal macrophages of rats by diets containing

fats of different saturated, monounsaturated and polyunsaturated fatty acid composition. Clin Sci (Lond) 1994, 87:173-178.

37. Belluzzi A: Polyunsaturated fatty acids (n-3 PUFAs) and inflammatory bowel disease (IBD): pathogenesis and treatment. Eur Rev Med Pharmacol Sci 2004, 8:225-229.

38. Wild GE, Drozdowski L, Tartaglia C, Clandinin MT, Thomson AB: Nutritional modulation of the inflammatory response in inflammatory bowel disease--from the molecular to the integrative to the clinical. World J Gastroenterol 2007, 13:1-7.

39. Bassaganya-Riera J, Hontecillas R: CLA and n-3 PUFA differentially modulate clinical activity and colonic PPAR-responsive gene expression in a pig model of experimental IBD. Clin Nutr 2006, 25:454-465.

40. Al-Saghir J, Al-Ashi R, Salloum R, Saliba NA, Talhouk RS, Homaidan FR: Anti-inflammatory properties of Salograviolide A purified from Lebanese plant Centaurea ainetensis. BMC Complement Altern Med 9:36.

41. Post GE: The plants. In Flora of Syria, Palestine and Sinai. Volume 1. 2nd edition. Edited by Dinsmore JE. Beirut: American Press; 1932::14.

CHAPTER 4

AN EXTRACT OF THE MEDICINAL MUSHROOM *AGARICUS BLAZEI* MURILL CAN PROTECT AGAINST ALLERGY

LINDA K. ELLERTSEN AND GEIR HETLAND

4.1 BACKGROUND

Agaricus blazei Murill (AbM) of the family *Basidiomycetes* is a popular edible medicinal mushroom, originally native to a small village, Piedade, in the highland areas of Atlantic forest near São Paulo, Brazil. It has traditionally been used for the prevention of a range of diseases, including cancer, hepatitis, atherosclerosis, hypercholesterolemia, diabetes and dermatitis [1,2]. Because of its alleged health effects, the mushroom was brought to Japan in the mid-1960s and subjected to biomedical research. AbM was found to be rich in immuno-modulating substances such as β-glucans [3,4] and proteoglycans [5], and it had anti-infection [6,7] and anti-tumor [4,5] effects in mice.

Anti-tumor and anti-infection immunity are both due to Th1 responses, which also do promote autoimmune disease when overshooting. On the other hand, anti-helminth and anti-rejection immunity are due to Th2 responses, which may also induce IgE-mediated allergy, whereas delayed-

This chapter was originally published under the Creative Commons Attribution License. Ellertsen LK and Hetland G. An extract of the medicinal mushroom Agaricus blazei *Murill can protect against allergy.* Clinical and Molecular Allergy *7,6 (2009). doi:10.1186/1476-7961-7-6.*

type hypersensitivity is believed to involve Th1 cells. Since, according to the original Th1/Th2 dichotomy [8] there is an inverse relationship between Th1 and Th2 responses, we set out to look for substances that increased Th1 responses and thus, presumably, would reduce allergy. Moreover, we looked for substances with broad immunogenic specificity and hence a broad range of possible therapeutical activity. This criterion fits substances containing so-called pathogen-associated molecular patterns, which stimulate innate immunity via binding to a few different receptors with broad specificities like Toll-like receptors and dectin-1.

In order to test putative functional Th1-stimulating substances, a mouse model for systemic bacterial infection was chosen rather than a tumor model, because of the more rapid outcome of an anti-bacterial than an anti-tumor response. We tested different β-glucans, which are known stimulators of innate immunity with anti-tumor [9] and anti-infection [10] activities. We found that one β-1,3-glucan from *Sclerotinia sclerotiorum* was highly protective against sepsis in a mouse model for systemic *S. pneumoniae*, although only when given i.p. and not p.o. [11]. However, surprisingly, we detected that s.c. administration of both this β-glucan and other β-glucans from barley and baker's yeast, in addition to moulds per se, also increased specific IgE levels in a mouse model for allergy [12,13]. This is in agreement with the finding of increased allergic responses of mold-derived β-1,3-glucan in an airway inhalation model in the mouse [14]. Since AbM is another more recently discovered source of strong innate stimulatory properties [15,16], with a high content of β-glucan and anti-tumor properties in the mouse [3], we tested whether extracts of AbM from different producers had anti-infection effects in the said mouse model for pneumococcal sepsis. We found that the current extract, AndoSan™, containing approximately 80% of AbM and 20% of two other *Basidiomycetes* mushrooms; *Hericium erinaceum* and *Grifola frondosa*, was the most effective: It was the only extract that decreased bacteremia statistically significantly and increased the survival rate of the exposed animals [17]. Moreover, it had more profound anti-infection effect even when given p.o. via a gastric catheter than did any of the above β-glucans given i.p..

There are anecdotes about persons who have used AbM for other purposes than allergy, and who have experienced less allergic symptoms when ingesting the remedy. To our knowledge the very few papers on AbM or other *Basidiomycetes* mushrooms and allergy in English scientific literature rather report on induction of allergy; cheilitis and increased delayed-type sensitivity due to AbM [18,19], hypersensitivity pneumonitis caused by *Grifola frondosa* [20], and allergic contact dermatitis from *Hericeum erinaceum* exposure [21]. Based on preliminary anti-infection and anti-allergy results in our laboratory with the current extract of mainly AbM (AndoSan™), a patent application was filed in 2004 [22]. There are other publications on beneficial effects of the mushrooms in the patent literature, foremost of Japanese origin: One patent (A61K 35/84, 05.08.2002) claims that an essence extracted from mycelium of *Basidiomycetes*, including *Hericium erinaceum*, can prevent and cure allergic symptoms, especially atopic dermatitis. Another (WO 02/15917) claims the use of AbM in treatment of autoimmune and skin diseases, due to down-regulation of immune function. Yet another (WO 93/207923) describes the isolation from *Agaricus hortensis* of anti-allergic components, especially for dermatological usage. Extracts of AbM have also been found to have anti-allergic effect based on inhibition of basophilic leukocytes (US2003/0104006). Finally, EP0413053 describes a process for producing an anti-allergic substance from *Basidiomycetes* mycelium, including that of AbM and *Grifola frondosa*.

The aim of the present study was to examine whether the extract that was most effective against systemic pneumococcal infection, also could protect against allergy development when given to a mouse model for allergy. For this purpose the model allergen ovalbumin (OVA) was injected s.c. and AbM extract as adjuvant was given orally, and levels of specific IgE and IgG2a antibodies were determined in serum. In addition, Th1, Th2 and Treg cytokines were measured in supernatants of cultured spleen cells from the mice.

4.2 METHODS

4.2.1 MICE

These were inbred, female, pathogen-free, 6–8 weeks old NIH/OlaHsd, C57Bl/6 and Balb/c obtained from Gl. Bomholt gård Ltd (Ry, Denmark) and rested for 1 week after arrival. They were housed 8 animals per cage, individually earmarked, and given water and egg-free feed ad libitum. Experiments were performed according to law and regulations for animal experiments in Norway, which are in agreement with the Helsinki declaration, and they were approved by the local Animal Board under the minister of Agriculture in Norway.

4.2.2 REAGENTS

An aqueous extract of mycelium of AbM (82%), containing additionally *Hericium erinaceum* (15%) and *Grifola frondosa* (3%) (AndoSan™), grown commercially, was given by ACE Co., Ltd., Gifu, Japan. It was stored at 4°C in dark bottles and kept sterile until being instilled intragastrically in the mice. The AbM mixed powder contains per 100 g the following constituents: moisture 5.8 g, protein 2.6 g, fat 0.3 g, carbohydrates 89.4 g of which β-glucan constitutes 2.8 g, and ash 1.9 g, and its final concentration was 340 g/l. The amount per liter of the extract for sodium was 11 mg, phosphorus 254 mg, calcium 35 mg, potassium 483 mg, magnesium 99 mg and zinc 60 mg. The LPS content of AndoSan™ was found, using the *Limulus* amebocyte lysate test (COAMATIC Chromo-LAL; Chromogenix, Falmouth, MA, USA) with detection limit 0.005 EU/ml (1 EU = 0.1 ng/ml), to be a miniscule concentration of <0.5 pg/ml. The results from tests for heavy metals were conformable with strict Japanese regulations for health foods. AndoSan™ had been heat-sterilized (124°C for 1 h) by the producer. Since this mushroom extract is a commercial product, the method for its production is a business secret. Ovalbumin (OVA) (Sigma, St. Louis, MO, USA; cat.no. A7641) and Al(OH)$_3$ were dissolved in PBS of pH 7.3, and each animal was immunized with 10 μg of OVA and 2 mg of Al(OH)$_3$ in a total volume of 0.5 ml in the tail base.

4.2.3 EXPERIMENTAL DESIGN

Groups of 8 mice were given either 200 μl (according to their assumed maximal ventricular volume) of the AbM extract, AndoSan™, or PBS orally via a gastric tube and injected a day later with OVA $+Al(OH)_3$ s.c. in the tail base or injected first with OVA $+Al(OH)_3$ s.c. and given AndoSan™ or PBS p.o. on day 19. With Balb/c mice both OVA and 20 µl of AndoSan™ or PBS were injected s.c. in one hind foot pad (for Balb/c mice). Then both groups were boosted with OVA s.c. on day 20, before sacrifice and exanguination and removal of the spleen or the foot pad-draining popliteal lymph nodes (PLN) (for Balb/c mice), on day 26. Some mice (C57Bl/6) were given additional AbM or PBS treatment on both day -1 and day 19 before the OVA boosting. The scheme in Table 1 shows the different set-ups.

TABLE 1: Scheme for experimental design in murine allergy model

Exp #	# Mice, strain	Treatment before and/or after OVA immunization		Harvest
1	16 NIH/OlaHsd	AndoSan™ or PBS p.o.* (200 µl) ↓		serum, spleen ↑
2	16 NIH/OlaHsd		AndoSan™/PBS p.o. ↓	serum, spleen ↑
3	8 C57Bl/6	AndoSan™/PBS p.o. and/or ↓	AndoSan™/PBS p.o. ↓	serum, spleen ↑
4	8 Balb/c	AndoSan™/PBS s.c. in foot pad (20 µl)** ↓		serum, PLN ↑
Day	-1	0	19, 20	26
Immuniza-tion		↑ OVA (10 µg) + Al(OH)₃ s.c. in tail-base or foot pad +	↑ OVA s.c	↑ Sacrifice

*200 µl of AndoSan™ or PBS was given p.o. via a gastric catheter. ** OVA and Al(OH)3 (2 mg) was dissolved in AndoSan™ or PBS before s.c. injection in foot pad.

4.2.4 SPLEEN CELL CULTURES

The spleen was removed from each sacrificed mouse and put in a tube containing Hank's Balanced Salt Solution (HBSS; Gibco BRL, Paisley, Scotland). A single cell suspension was prepared under sterile condition by placing the spleen on top of a wire-net in a Petri dish containing 2 ml HBSS. The spleen was punctured by a canula (BD Microlance™ 3 needle,

Becton Dickinson AB, Sweden) and thereafter a bended glass staff was used to rub the cells from the spleen capsule through the wire net to make a single cell suspension. The cell suspensions were washed in HBSS and re-suspended in RPMI (RPMI 1640 culture medium with 20 mM L-glutamine (Gibco)), containing 10% FCS, 100 U penicillin G and 0.1 mg/ml strep-tomycin (PAA Laboratories GmbH). The cell concentration was measured with a Coulter Counter ZI (Beckman Coulter Inc., FL, USA). The spleen cells were seeded into a 24-well culture plates (Costar Inc., NY, USA) to a final concentration of 5×10^6 cells/ml. OVA or Con A were added to a final concentration of 1 mg/ml and 6 μg/ml, respectively, except for unstimulated controls. The cells were cultured at 37°C and in 5% CO_2 for 48 or 72 hours. Thereafter the plates were centrifuged at 1200 rpm for 5 minutes, and super-natants were collected and stored at -80C until analysis.

4.2.5 ASSAYS

Mouse IgE anti-OVA and IgG2a anti-OVA antibodies were measured in serum, and levels of cytokines IFNγ, IL-2 (Th1 response), IL-4, IL-5 (Th2 response) and IL-10 (Treg cytokine) in cell culture supernatants by ELISAs. Whereas the former Ig ELISAs were in-house (sandwich anti-OVA IgE and simple an-ti-OVA IgG2a [13]) and the cut-off set to give negative results in serum from naïve mice, the ones for the cytokines were from R&D Systems, Minneapolis, MN, USA. The excised PLN from both injected and non-injected hind limb were weighed and compared as a parameter for local inflammation.

4.2.6 STATISTICS

Sigma Stat (Systat Software, Inc., 1735 Technology Drive Suite 430 San Jose, CA) statistical and graphics package was used. When the data were normally distributed parametric assays were used, otherwise non-paramet-ric assays. Student's t-test was used for comparing two groups. One-way ANOVA was used for single repeated measurements, and two-ways ANO-VA for two experiments with repeated measurements. P values below 0.05 were considered statistically significant.

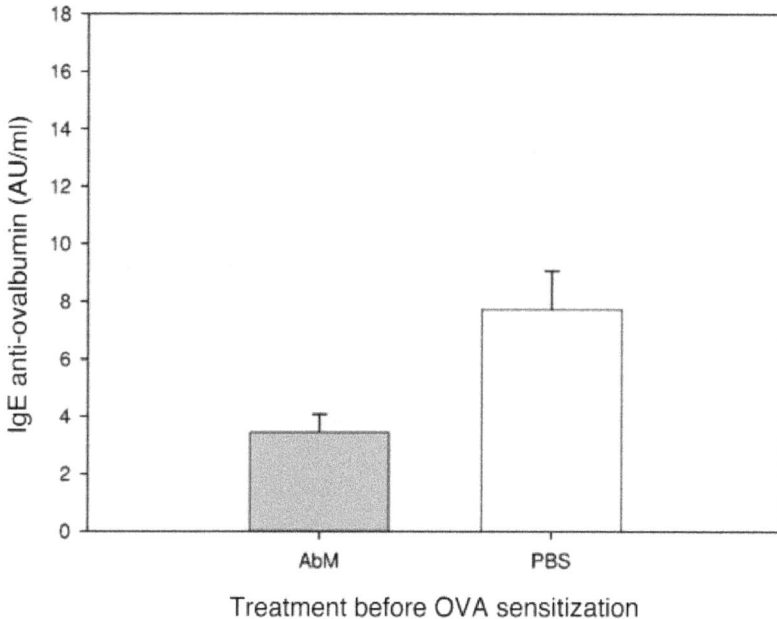

FIGURE 1: Levels of OVA-specific IgE measured in mouse serum on day 26 after OVA-pretreatment with AbM. Mice were given 200 μl of AndoSan™ extract or PBS intragastrically on day -1 and injected with 10 μg of OVA s.c. in the tail base on day 0 and again on day 20, before exsanguination for serum on day 26. Values are given in arbitrary units (AU)/ml and means + 1 s.e.m. for groups of 16 mice (groups of 8 per each of 2 experiments). Anti-OVA IgE levels were lower in AbM (AndoSan™) than in PBS treated groups ($p = 0.002$, two-way ANOVA).

4.3 RESULTS

4.3.1 SERUM ANTI-OVA IGE AND IGG2A ANTIBODIES

We used a mouse model for allergy to examine whether the medicinal mushroom AbM could protect against this disease. Experiments were conducted in three mouse strains with OVA as model allergen and a mushroom extract, AndoSan™, mainly containing AbM, or PBS control as adjuvant. In two experiments with NIH/Ola mice, AbM treatment prior to OVA immunization reduced the levels of serum anti-OVA IgE antibodies significantly (p = 0.002, two-way ANOVA) compared with similar PBS pre-OVA treatment (Figure 1) when the animals were sacrificed about 4 weeks after OVA immunization. The levels of serum anti-OVA IgG2a tended to be higher in the AbM group (Figure 2), but were not statistically significantly different from the PBS control. Furthermore, when AbM, as compared with PBS, was given near 3 weeks after the allergen immunization of such mice, this treatment also significantly reduced the levels of anti-OVA IgE (p = 0.048, two-way ANOVA) (Figure 3). In these two experiments the levels of anti-OVA IgG2a in the AbM group, relative to PBS, seemed to be even higher (Figure 4) than observed above, but were due to large variation not statistically different from the control.

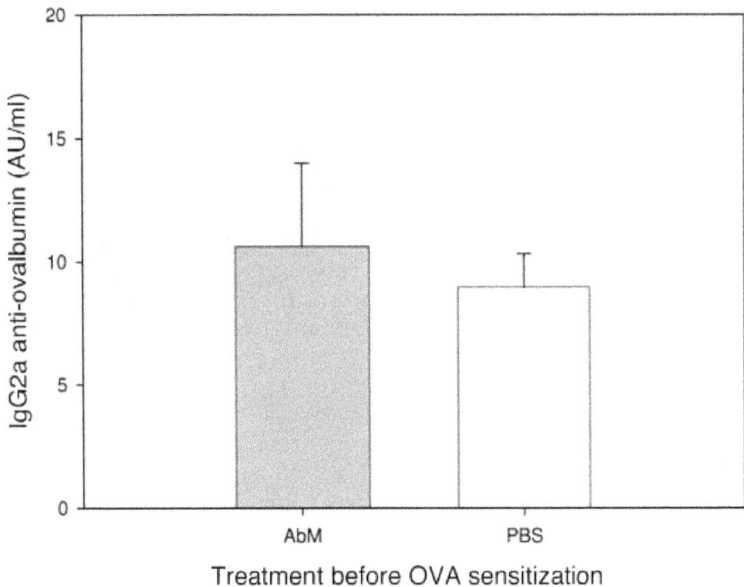

FIGURE 2: Levels of IgG2a measured in mouse serum on day 26 after OVA-pretreatment with AbM. Mice were given 200 μl of AndoSan™ extract or PBS intragastrically on day -1 and injected with 10 μg of OVA s.c. in the tail base on day 0 and again on day 20, before exsanguination for serum on day 26. Values are given in arbitrary units (AU)/ml and means + 1 s.e.m. for groups of 16 mice (groups of 8 per each of 2 experiments).

The next set-up was similar to the ones above, but with C57Bl/6 mice and included groups that were treated with AbM or PBS either before or after OVA immunization, or both before and after the immunization. Figure 5 shows a tendency towards lower anti-OVA IgE levels in the AbM compared with PBS treated groups (p = 0.064, one way ANOVA), albeit the levels of specific IgE of the PBS-OVA-PBS control (last column in Figure 5) was relatively far lower than the two other PBS controls. The IgG2a levels were all-over below the detection limit of the assay and thus too low for data analysis. In a third set-up with Balb/c mice, a similar but statistically not significant trend of AbM-induced lower IgE and higher serum anti-OVA IgG2a levels was still found when using the foot pad of the mice for s.c. injection of both OVA and a 1/10 volume of AndoSan™ (data not shown).

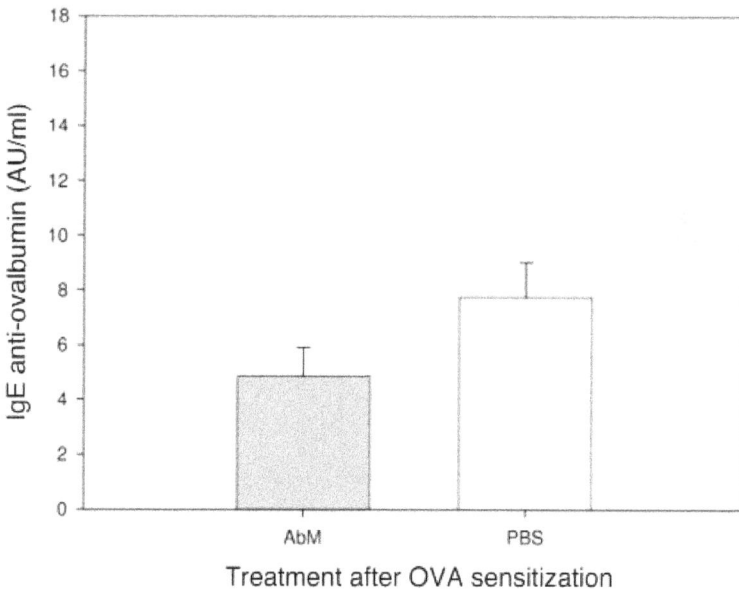

FIGURE 3: Levels of OVA-specific IgE measured in mouse serum on day 26 after OVA-post treatment with AbM. Mice were injected with 10 µg of OVA on day 0 and given 200 µl of AndoSan™ extract or PBS intragastrically on day 19, before OVA booster on day 20 and sacrifice on day 26. Values are given in AU/ml and means + 1 s.e.m. for groups of 16 mice (groups of 8 per each of 2 experiments). Anti-OVA IgE levels were lower in AbM (AndoSan™) than PBS treated groups (p = 0.048, two-way ANOVA).

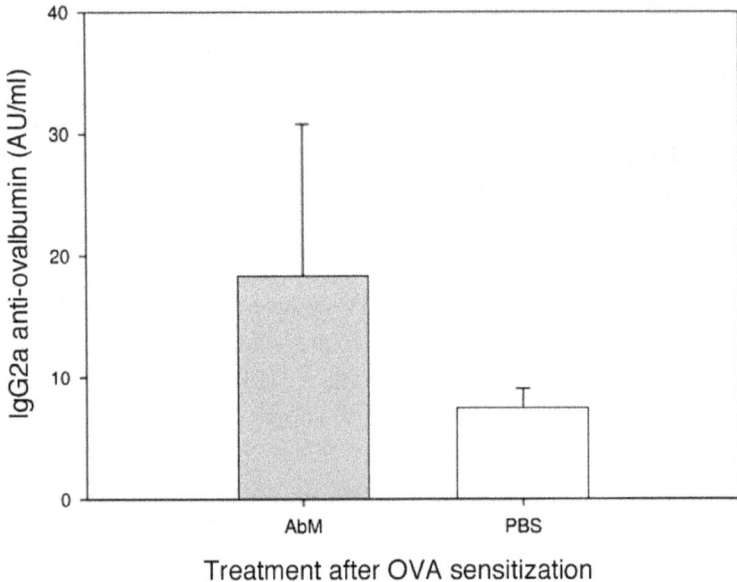

FIGURE 4: Levels of IgG2a measured in mouse serum on day 26 after OVA-post treatment with AbM. Mice were injected with 10 µg of OVA on day 0 and given 200 µl of AndoSan™ extract or PBS intragastrically on day 19, before OVA booster on day 20 and sacrifice on day 26. Values are given in AU/ml and means + 1 s.e.m. for groups of 16 mice (groups of 8 per each of 2 experiments).

4.3.2 CYTOKINES IN SPLEEN CELL CULTURES AND WEIGHT OF PLN

Occasionally, there were in single experiments reduced levels (p < 0.05), except increased levels once for IL-2, and otherwise no significant differences in all the five cytokines measured; IFNγ, IL-2, IL-4, IL-5 and IL-10, in spleen cell culture supernatants from animals treated with AbM relative to PBS control, either before or after OVA immunization. Table 2 gives cytokine levels as indices of those for AbM-treated relative to those for PBS treated controls. For each experiment the highest read-outs above the detection limit of each assay was used, for set-up with either OVA or Con A *in vitro* stimulated cell cultures. When all indices for all groups of

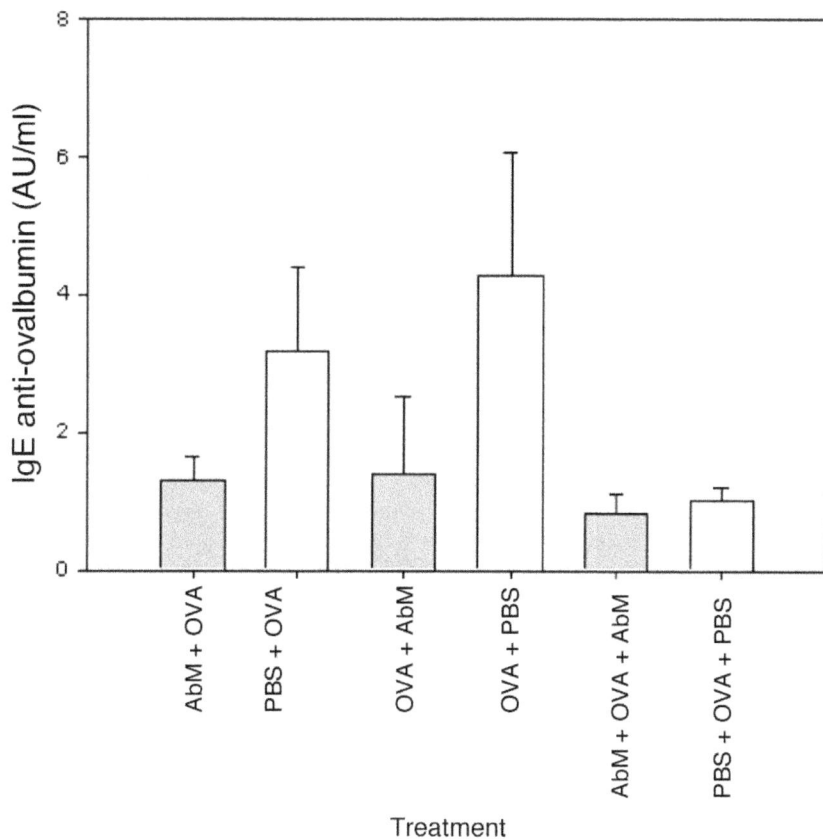

FIGURE 5: Levels of OVA-specific IgE measured in mouse serum on day 26 after either pre- or post-OVA treatment with AbM. Mice were either given 200 μl of AndoSan™ extract or PBS intragastrically on day -1 and injected with 10 μg of OVA s.c. in the tail base on day 0, or injected with OVA on day 0 and given AndoSan™ extract or PBS intragastrically on day 19, or given AndoSan™ extract or PBS both before (day -1) and after (day 19) OVA injection (day 0). All groups were OVA boosted on day 20 and sacrificed on day 26. Values are given in AU/ml and means + 1 s.e.m. for groups of 8 mice (p = 0.064, one-way ANOVA for difference between the groups).

Th2 cytokines (mean index: 0.87 ± 0.05) were compared with all indices of Th1 cytokines (mean index: 1.07 ± 0.05), Th2 cytokines were significantly lower ($p = 0.026$). Hence, there seemed to be a tendency of reduced Th2 relative to Th1 cytokine levels in the AbM groups. There were similar weights of the excised PLN from the AbM and PBS groups, suggesting no local inflammatory response to the mushroom extract.

TABLE 2: Cytokines in supernatants of cultured spleen cells from mice treated with AndoSan™ or PBS p.o. before or after sensitization against OVA s.c..

Cytokine	Pre-OVA treatment	Post-OVA treatment
	AndoSan™/PBS index	AndoSan™/PBS index
IFNγ	$1.13^* \pm 0.06$	$0.90^* \pm 0.11$
IL-2	$1.06^{*, **} \pm 0.13$	1.07 ± 0.00
IL-4	0.95 ± 0.15	$0.82^* \pm 0.10$
IL-5	0.83 ± 0.08	0.78 ± 0.05
IL-10	$0.88^* \pm 0.08$	0.89 ± 0.01

*The indices are given as mean $\pm$ s.e.m. of 2–5 experiments in duplicates, each comprising 8 mice per group, of the highest read-out data of either OVA or Con A stimulated cultures for either 48 h or 72 h is given for each experiment. *In one of the experiments cytokine levels in supernatants of cell cultures from AndoSan™ treated mice were lower than from PBS treated mice ($p < 0.05$). **In one of the experiments cytokine levels in supernatants of cell cultures from AndoSan™ treated mice were higher than from PBS treated mice ($p < 0.05$). All over, indices for Th2 cytokines were lower than indices for Th1 cytokines ($p = 0.026$). The lack of data from some experiments is due to values below detection limit of assay.*

4.4 DISCUSSION

Our results are strengthened by the similar findings, observed in two different mouse strains after s.c. injection of OVA in the tail base, and in a third mouse strain (Balb/c) after s.c. injection of both mushroom extract and OVA in the foot pad. In the latter Th2-prone mice the so-called PLN assay was used, which was originally employed for toxicological screening of substances that would inflame the foot pad-draining PLN, but which is also convenient for examining systemic IgE response in serum to an allergen given with adjuvant [23]. The lacking increase in PLN weight in mice injected AbM extract relative to PBS in the foot pad, agrees with the assumed anti-inflammatory anti-allergic effect of the AbM as seen from the tendency of generally lowering of Th2 cytokine levels in spleen cell cultures ex vivo.

Increased specific IgE levels are not equivalent with allergic disease, but a prerequisite for IgE-mediated allergy. Hence, our findings of decreased anti-OVA IgE levels secondary to AbM intake in animals that were otherwise sensitized to OVA, strongly indicates a protective effect of AbM against IgE-mediated allergy. We did not examine allergy signs in the mice. These would have been similar to egg allergy, as in food allergy. Possible skin rashes would have been difficult to assess in the mice, and nude mice could not have been used because they lack normal lymphocytes, which are a prerequisite for an allergic immune response. In possible follow-up studies, the allergen should be given via the natural route; e.g. p.o. if using ovalbumin, although this would be costly. Instead, a common food allergen like peanut could have been used, or if one wished to examine airways allergy in the case of aeroallergens, another cheap aeroallergen like birch pollen, although with novel ELISAs for these antigens. The finding of relatively far lower anti-OVA IgE levels in the repeated PBS controls in Figure 5, may be due to the stress invoked by such repeated intragastric procedure. In preliminary experiments, in which repeated pre-OVA treatment of mice with the mushroom extract or PBS was delivered intragastrically by the highly trained technicians to increase the dose, all mice looked sick and one animal died, presumably from stress, which is known to impair immunity.

Previously, we have used pure β-glucans from yeast and fungi together with ovalbumin s.c. in the very same PLN model and, contrary to the present observation, found increased specific anti-OVA IgE levels in serum [12,13]. Hence, either the administration route is critical, or the particular β-glucans of the current mushroom extract does either promote a different outcome than the other β-glucans, or other stronger anti-allergic immunomodulating substances in the mushroom extract do overcome a possible general "pro-allergic" effect of β-glucans. If the latter is true, we assume that the anti-allergy effects of the AbM extract in vivo is mediated via immunomodulating substances in the extract that are smaller and more readily absorbable than β-glucans.

As to possible side effects, there are conflicting reports regarding the effect of AbM on liver function. Whereas one report suggests that use of

AbM for several weeks may have induced severe hepatic dysfunction in three cancer patients [24], another says that AbM extract normalized liver function in patients with chronic hepatitis B virus infection [25]. Moreover, our studies on patients with chronic hepatitis C virus infection [26] and on AbM intake in healthy volunteers [27], revealed no pathological effect whatsoever on hematological parameters including those for liver-, pancreatic- and renal function, even when volumes equivalent by body weight to that given to the mice, were taken.

The generally observed AbM-induced all-over reduction in Th2 cytokines IL-4 and IL-5 relative to Th1 cytokines IFNγ and IL-2 production ex vivo in our present cultures of spleen cells, agrees with the original Th1/Th2 dichotomy [8]. However, this theory has been modified towards suggesting that T regulatory cells are crucial for fine-tuning both Th1 and Th2 responses by the regulatory cytokines IL-10 and TGF-β. However, our measurement of suggestive reduced levels of the Treg cytokine IL-10 in the AbM groups, is difficult to interpret. In contrast, when the extract was given *in vitro* to cell cultures there was an increase in proinflammatory cytokines [15]. This apparent discrepancy must be due to the fact that whereas cells *in vitro* are subjected to all substances in the extract including β-glucans with large m.w., which are abundant in AbM [3], mainly smaller substances are taken up from the digestive tract in humans and are active in the blood in vivo. Although, β-glucans in the intestines could stimulate Peyer's patches in jejunum, we have in fact observed that the genes in leukocytes predominantly affected by AbM *in vitro* and in vivo were quite different [26,28]. Whereas genes related to proinflammatory cytokines were strongly induced *in vitro*—presumably by β-glucan, genes involved in cell signalling and cycling and transcriptional regulation and thus foremost related to anti-tumor defence, were upregulated in vivo [26]. Thus, the microarray analyses agree with the assumption that AbM extract especially promotes a Th1 anti-tumor and anti-infection response in the body and hence reciprocally inhibits a Th2 response. This is supported by the reported immuno-modulatory effects of AbM in mice [19].

β-glucans may stimulate macrophages and other cells of innate immunity after binding to cellular receptors like CD11b/18, Toll-like receptor and dectin-1 [reviewed in [17]]. Stimulation by AbM of peripheral blood leukocytes resulted both in an upregulation of such receptors [26,28,29], activation of NFKB via TLR2 stimulation [30], and mediation via them of increased release of proinflammatory cytokines [15] and Th1 cytokines IFNγ, IL-12, and IL-23α [16,28,31]. Although one report of reduced release of Th2 cytokine IL-4 after AbM stimulation *in vitro* also found reduced IL-2 and IFNγ levels [32], IL-12- and IFNγ-mediated NK cell activation by AbM p.o. has been documented in mice [16]. Even though the present AbM extract should occasionally give reduced IFNγ levels, the increased expression of the IFN receptor gene after AbM extract intake in humans [26], may overcome a reduction in the concentration of the ligand and result in an increased Th1 response. When measuring different cytokines in serum from humans after 12 days intake of the current AndoSan™ extract mainly containing AbM, there was a significant reduction in both pro-inflammatory, Th1 and Th2 cytokines [31]. This indicates a general anti-inflammatory effect of AndoSan™ in vivo, which agrees with its current anti-allergic effect.

For intragastric delivery of AbM extract a volume of 200 μl was chosen because this is, according to our veterinary, the maximal ventricular volume in a 5–6 weeks old mouse. In an initial experiment, we tried to give the AbM extract repeatedly on subsequent days via a gastric catheter in order to possibly inhibit the specific IgE response completely. However, this procedure was dropped because it was too stressful for the mice even in hands of our well-trained technicians. The unexpected result in the last two columns of Figure 5 may in fact reflect this concern. Also, we did not use a higher concentration of this extract than what was sold on the health food market. If translated to human intake, the equivalent of 200 μl to a 25 g mouse would be 560 ml to a 70 kg individual. In fact, a daily low intake in healthy volunteers of 60 ml AndoSan™ for 12 days gave a significant 50% reduction in levels of the allergy-promoting cytokine IL-4 in blood and left the other allergy-related cytokines IL-5, IL-7 and IL-13 at negligible levels [27]. Addition of AbM extract to drink water for the mice in our set-up would have been more natural, but the intake of AbM is impossible to monitor as accurately as with intragastric delivery. In the current allergy model we did not test other extracts of AbM from other manufacturers that did not have a significant effect against pneumococcal infection in mice [17]. Therefore, the question is not fully answered as to whether there is an absolute link between the anti-bacterial infection and anti-allergy effect of a substance or an extract like AndoSan™. Moreover, even though we have seen that Agaricus bM is the main TLR2 stimulating mushroom of AndoSan™ [30], it is likely that the former anti-bacterial and current anti-allergic effect of this mixed mushroom product may be partly due to possible synergistic effects of the other mushrooms, *Hericium erinaceum* and *Grifola frondosa*, and components thereof contained in the extract. The mouse model of allergic airways disease should be used in a follow-up study with OVA and the mushroom extract in order to confirm that also allergic symptoms like development of airways hyper responsiveness are reduced by AndoSan™ intake. Whether the AbM extract is effective against allergy in the human setting must be tested in a clinical trial, e.g. in persons with aeroallergy during the pollen season taking 60 ml a day for a few weeks.

4.5 CONCLUSION

From our results with mice we conclude that a mushroom extract, mainly containing AbM, may prevent the development of IgE-mediated allergy when given before allergen immunization. Even more interesting, the extract seemed to have a therapeutic effect when given together with or as late as 3 weeks after the allergen immunization. Three weeks in the mouse equals several months in a human, suggesting that also established allergy in patients can be reverted.

REFERENCES

1.   Wasser SP, Weis AL: Therapeutic effects of substances occurring in higher *basidiomycetes* mushrooms: a modern perspective. Crit Rev Immunol 1999, 19:65-96.
2.   Huang N: Brazilian mushroom (Gee Song Rong). In Cultivation of eight rare and precious gourmet mushrooms. Edited by Huang. Chinese Agriculture University Press; 1997::95-101.
3.   Ohno N, Furukawa M, Miura NN, Adachi Y, Motoi M, Yadomae T: Antitumor beta glucan from the cultured fruit body of *Agaricus blazei*. Biol Pharm Bull 2001, 24:820-828.

4. Firenzuoli F, Gori L, Lombardo G: The medicinal mushroom *Agaricus blazei* Murill: Review of literature and pharmaco-toxicological problems. Evid Based Complement Alternat Med 2008, 5:3-15.

5. Itoh H, Ito H, Amano H, Noda H: Inhibitory action of a (1-->6)-beta-D-glucan-protein complex (F III-2-b) isolated from *Agaricus blazei* Murill ("himematsutake") on Meth A fibrosarcoma-bearing mice and its antitumor mechanism. Jpn J Pharmacol 1994, 66:265-271.

6. Bernardshaw S, Johnson E, Hetland G: An extract of the mushroom *Agaricus blazei* Murill administered orally protects against systemic Streptococcus pneumoniae infection in mice. Scand J Immunol 2005, 62:393-398.

7. Bernardshaw S, Hetland G, Grinde B, Johnson E: An extract of the mushroom *Agaricus blazei* Murill protects against lethal septicemia in a mouse model for fecal peritonitis. Shock 2006, 25:420-425.

8. Romagnani S: The Th1/Th2 paradigm. Immunol Today 1997, 18:263-266.

9. Seljelid R: A water-soluble aminated beta-1-3D-glucan derivative causes regression of solid tumores in mice. Biosci Rep 1986, 6:845-851.

10. Reynolds JA, Kastello MD, Harrington DG, Crabbs CL, Peters CJ, Jemski JV, Scott GH, Di Luzio NR: Glucan-induced enhancement of host resistance to selected infectious diseases. Infect Immun 1980, 30:51-57.

11. Hetland G, Ohno N, Aaberge IS, Løvik M: Protective effect of β-glucan against systemic Streptococcus pneumoniae infection in mice. FEMS Immunology and Medical Microbiology 2000, 27:111-116.

12. Ormstad H, Groeng EC, Løvik M, Hetland G: The fungal cell wall component β-1,3-glucan has an adjuvant effect on the allergic response to ovalbumin in mice. J Toxicol Environ Health Part A 2000, 61:55-67.

13. Instanes C, Ormstad H, Rydjord B, Wiker HG, Hetland G: Mould extracts increase the allergic response to ovalbumin in mice. Clin Exp Allergy 2004, 34:1634-1641.

14. Wan GH, Li CS, Guo SP, Rylander R, Lin RH: An airborne mold-derived product, beta-1,3-D-glucan potentiates airway allergic responses. Eur J Immunol 1999, 29:2491-2497.

15. Bernardshaw S, Hetland G, Ellertsen LK, Aaland Tryggestad AM, Johnson E: An extract of the medicinal mushroom *Agaricus blazei* Murill differentially stimulates production of pro-inflammatory cytokines in human monocytes and human vein endothelial cells *in vitro*. Inflammation 2005, 29:147-153.

16. Yuminamochi E, Koike T, Takeda K, Horiuchi I, Okumura K: Interleukin-12- and interferon-gamma-mediated natural killer cell activation by *Agaricus blazei* Murill. Immunology 2007, 121:197-206.

17. Hetland G, Johnson E, Lyberg T, Bernardshaw S, Tryggestad AMA, Grinde B: Effects of the medicinal mushroom *Agaricus blazei* Murill on immunity, infection and cancer. Scand J Immunol 2008, 68:363-370.

18. Suehiro M, Kishimoto S: Cheilitis due to *Agaricus blazei* Murill mushroom extract. Contact Derm 2007, 56:293-294.

19. Chan Y, Chang T, Chan CH, Yeh YC, Chen CW, Shieh B, Li C: Immunomodulatory effect of *Agaricus blazei* Murill in Balb/cByJ mice. J Microbiol Immunol Infect 2007, 40:201-208.

20. Tanaka H, Tsunematsu K, Makamura N, Suzuki K, Tanaka N, Takeya I, Saikai T, Abe S: Successful treatment of hyper-sensitivity pneumonitis caused by *Grifola frondosa* (Maitake) mushroom using a HFA-BDP extra-fine aerosol. Intern Med 2004, 43:737-740.

21. Maes MF, van Baar HM, van Ginkel CJ: Occupational allergic contact dermatitis from the mushroom White Pom Pom (Hericeum erinaceum). Contact Derm 1999, 40:289-290.

22. Hetland G: Applicant/Inventor: Use of the mushroom *Agaricus blazei* Murill for the production of medicaments suitable for treating infections and allergies. WO 2005/065063 (Priority; Jan 2004)

23. Løvik M, Hogseth AK, Gaarder PI, Hagemann R, Eide I: Diesel exhaust particles and carbon black have adjuvant activity on the local lymph node response and systemic IgE production to ovalbumin. Toxicology 1997, 121:165-178.

24. Mukai H, Watanabe T, Ando M, Katsumata N: An alternative medicine, *Agaricus blazei*, may have induced severe hepatic dysfunction in cancer patients. Jpn J Clin Oncol 2006, 36:808-810.

25. Hsu CH, Hwanq KC, Chiang YH, Chou P: The mushroom *Agaricus blazei* Murill extract normalizes liver function in patients with chronic hepatitis B. J Altern Complement Med 2008, 14:299-301.

26. Grinde B, Hetland G, Johnson E: Effects on gene expression and viral load of a medicinal extract from *Agaricus blazei* in patients with chronic hepatitis C infection. Int Immunopharmacol 2006, 6:1311-1314.

27. Johnson E, Førland DT, Sætre L, Bernardshaw SV, Lyberg T, Hetland G: Effect of an extract based on the medicinal mushroom *Agaricus blazei* Murill on release of cytokines, chemokines and leukocyte growth factors in human blood ex vivo and in vivo. Scand J Immunol 2009, 69:242-250.

28. Ellertsen LK, Hetland G, Johnson E, Grinde B: Effect of a medicinal extract from *Agaricus blazei* Murill on gene expression in a human monocyte cell line as examined by microarrays and immuno assays. Int Immunopharmacol 2006, 6:133-143.

29. Bernardshaw S, Lyberg T, Hetland G, Johnson E: Effect of an extract of the medicinal mushroom *Agaricus blazei* Murill on expression of adhesion molecules and production of reactive oxygen species in monocytes and granulocytes in human whole blood ex vivo. APMIS 2007, 1157:19-25.

30. Tryggestad AMA, Espevik T, Førland DT, Ryan L, Hetland G: The medicinal mushroom *Agaricus blazei* Murill activates NF-KB via TLR2. 13th Int. Congress of Immunology, Rio de Janerio, 2007:P2.23 INI-02 Signalling pathways of innate immune receptors; abstract P1193

31. Kasai H, He LM, Kawamura M, Yang PT, Deng XW, Munkanta M, Yamashita A, Terunuma H, Hirama M, Horiuchi I, Natori T, Koga T, Amano Y, Yamaguchi N, Ito M: IL-12 Production Induced by *Agaricus blazei* Fraction H (ABH) Involves Toll-like Receptor (TLR). Evid Based Complement Alternat Med 2004, 1:259-267.

32. Kuo YC, Huang YL, Chen CC, Lin YS, Chuang KA, Tsai WJ: Cell cycle progression and cytokine gene expression of human peripheral blood mononuclear cells modulated by *Agaricus blazei*. J Lab Clin Med 2002, 140:176-187.

CHAPTER 5

ANTI-OXIDATIVE EFFECTS OF THE BIENNIAL FLOWER OF *PANAX NOTOGINSENG* AGAINST H_2O_2-INDUCED CYTOTOXICITY IN CULTURED PC12 CELLS

ROY CHI-YAN CHOI, ZHIYONG JIANG, HEIDI QUN XIE, ANNA WING-HAN CHEUNG, DAVID TAI-WAI LAU, QIANG FU, TINA TINGXIA DONG, JIJUN CHEN, ZHENGTAO WANG, AND KARL WAH-KEUNG TSIM

5.1 BACKGROUND

Radix Notoginseng (*Sanqi*, the root of *Panax notoginseng*) is a Chinese herbal medicine used in China to promote blood circulation, remove blood stasis, induce blood clotting, relieve swelling and alleviate pain [1,2]. Moreover, *Panax notoginseng* is beneficial for coronary heart disease, cerebral vascular disease as well as learning and memory improvement [3-7]. These therapeutic effects are attributed to its active ingredients, namely saponins [8,9], flavonoids [10] and polysaccharides [11,12].

This chapter was originally published under the Creative Commons Attribution License. Choi RC-Y, Jiang Z, Xie HQ, Cheung AW-H, Lau DT-W, Fu Q, Dong TT, Chen J, Wang Z, and Tsim KW-K. Anti-oxidative Effects of the Biennial Flower of Panax notoginseng Against H₂O₂-induced Cytotoxicity in Cultured PC12 Cells. Chinese Medicine 5,38 (2010). doi:10.1186/1749-8546-5-38.

Saponins isolated from *Radix notoginseng* increase the blood flow of coronary arteries [13], prevent platelet aggregation [14], decrease oxygen consumption by heart muscles [15], restore learning impairment induced by chronic morphine administration [16] and protect neuronal cell death against oxidative stress [17]. Flavonoids increase the coronary flow, reduce myocardial oxygen consumption and lower arterial pressure [10]. A flavonol glycoside called quercetin 3-O-β-D-xylopyranosyl-β-D-galactopyranoside (RNFG) from the root and rhizome of *Panax notoginseng* is promising in treating Alzheimer's disease through inhibiting amyloid-β aggregation and amyloid-β-induced cytotoxicity in cortical neuron cultures. Such neuroprotection effect was mediated by the suppression of apoptosis triggered by amyloid-β [18]. Moreover, polysaccharide extracted from the root-rhizome of *Panax notoginseng* is also considered to be an active constituent with immuno-stimulating activities *in vitro* [11,12,19].

While the therapeutic effects of the root of *Panax notoginseng* have been demonstrated, the pharmacological effects of other parts of *Panax notoginseng* are largely unknown. The present study examines the anti-oxidation effects of other parts of *Panax notoginseng*.

5.2 METHODS

5.2.1 PLANT MATERIALS AND PREPARATION

Fresh *Panax notoginseng* from Wenshan in Yunnan Province (China) was identified morphologically during harvest. Voucher specimen (number 03-6-8) of *Panax Notoginseng* was confirmed by genetic analysis [20] and deposited at the Department of Biology, Hong Kong University of Science and Technology. For water extraction, the biennial flower, stem and leaf, root-rhizome, fiber root and/or sideslip (10 g) were boiled in 80 ml of water for two hours twice. The extract was then dried by lyophilization with an extraction efficiency of 15-18%. For ethanol extraction, biennial flower (10 g) was sonicated in 100 ml of 30%, 50%, 70% and 90% ethanol for 30 minutes twice. The extract was dried by rota-evaporation at 60°C with an extraction efficiency of 5-8%. The water and ethanol extracts were re-dissolved in water to 100 mg/ml stock concentration.

5.2.2 CELL CULTURE

Rat pheochromatocytoma PC12 cell line was obtained from ATCC (CRL-1721; USA). The cells were maintained in Dulbecco's modified Eagles medium (DMEM) supplemented with 6% fetal bovine serum and 6% horse serum at 37°C in a water-saturated 7.5% CO_2 incubator. Reagents for cell cultures were purchased from Invitrogen Technologies (USA).

5.2.3 IN VITRO XANTHINE OXIDASE ACTIVITY

Xanthine oxidase activity assay was described previously [21]. In brief, the herbal extracts (0.1 mg/ml) were pre-mixed with 0.05U/ml xanthine oxidase for 20 minutes. Then 0.4 mM xanthine and 0.24 mM hydroxyl amine were incubated for 20 minutes at 37°C. Reactions were stopped by adding 0.1% SDS to the mixture and measured at 550 nm absorbance. Vitamin C at various concentrations (0, 17.6, 35.2, 52.8 and 88 μg/ml) served as the positive control of anti-oxidation. All the chemicals were purchased from Sigma (USA).

5.2.4 CELL VIABILITY TEST

Cultured PC12 cells in 96-well-plate (5000 cells/well) were pre-treated with various extracts (1 mg/ml) for 24 hours. After washed with PBS and replaced by fresh culture medium, the cultures were treated with 13.6 μg/ml hydrogen peroxide (H_2O_2) for 24 hours. Cell viability test was performed with the addition of thiazolyl blue tetrazolium bromide (MTT) (Sigma, USA) in PBS at a final concentration of 5 mg/ml for four hours. After the solution was removed, the purple precipitate inside the cells was re-suspended in DMSO and then measured at 570 nm absorbance [22].

H_2O_2 at various concentrations (0, 1.7, 3.4, 6.8 and 13.6 µg/ml) served as a control for the cytotoxicity test.

5.2.5 DETERMINATION OF ROS FORMATION

The reactive oxygen species (ROS) level in cell cultures was determined according to the method by Zhu et al. [22]. Cultured PC12 cells in 96-well-plate were pre-treated with the water and ethanol extracts of biennial flower (1 mg/ml) for 24 hours, and then the cells were labeled by 100M dichlorofluorescin diacetate (DCFH-DA, Sigma, USA) in HBSS for one hour at 25°C. Cultures were treated with 13.6 µg/ml H_2O_2 for one hour. The amount of intracellular H_2O_2-induced ROS was detected by fluorometric measurement with excitation at 485 nm and emission at 530 nm (SPECTRA max® GEMINI XS, Molecular Devices Corporation, USA).

5.2.6 STATISTICAL ANALYSIS

Individual data were expressed as mean ± standard deviation (SD). A post-hoc Dunnett's test was used to obtain corrected P values in group comparisons. Statistical analyses were performed with one-way ANOVA (version 13.0, SPSS, USA). Data were considered as significant when $P < 0.05$ and highly significant when $P < 0.001$.

5.3 RESULTS

5.3.1 ANTI-OXIDATIVE EFFECTS OF PANAX NOTOGINSENG'S BIENNIAL FLOWER

To reveal the anti-oxidative effects of *Panax notoginseng*, we carried out an *in vitro* assay of xanthine oxidase effects. The abnormality of the xanthine oxidase causes pathological disorders [23-25]; thus, the enzyme is a

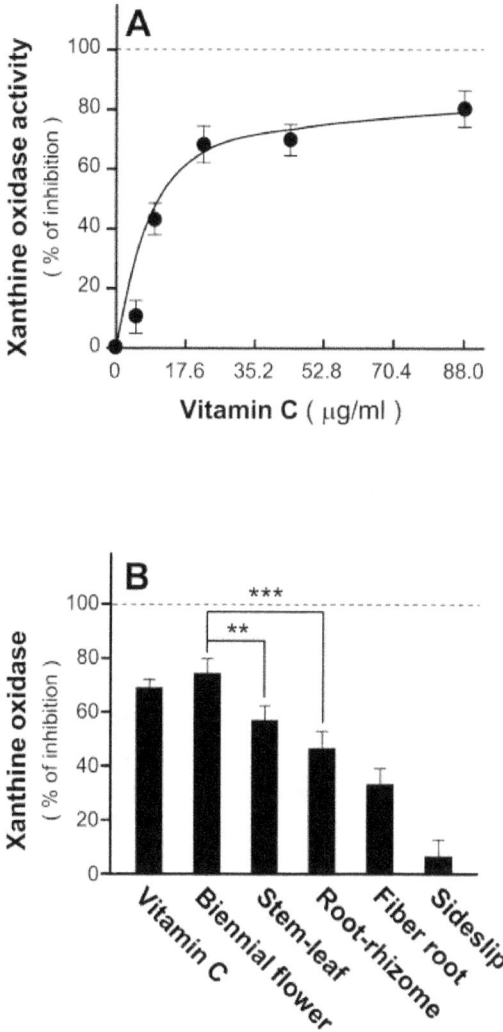

FIGURE 1: *In vitro* anti-oxidative effects of extracts from various parts of *Panax notoginseng*. A: Vitamin C at various concentrations (0, 17.6, 35.2, 52.8 and 88 μg/ml) was pre-incubated with xanthine oxidase before the addition of the xanthine substrate. The xanthine oxidase activity was measured at 550 nm absorbance. B: Extracts (0.1 mg/ml) from the biennial flower, stem-leaf, rhizome and fiber root of *Panax notoginseng* were assayed for their anti-xanthine oxidase activity as in [A]. Vitamin C (35.2 μg/ml) served as positive control. Data were expressed as% of inhibition where all the values were normalized by the control (no drug treatment), Mean ± SD, n = 6. Statistical significance is indicated as ** P = 0.00876 for biennial flower vs stem-leaf; and *** P = 0.000586 for biennial flower vs root-rhizome.

biological marker for anti-oxidative effects. In the presence of vitamin C at various concentrations (0, 17.6, 35.2, 52.8 and 88 μg/ml), xanthine oxidase effects were suppressed in a dose-dependent manner, with maximum inhibition of 80% as compared with the control (Figure 1A), validating this anti-oxidation assay. Different parts of *Panax notoginseng* including the biennial flower, stem-leaf, root-rhizome, fiber root and sideslip were separated from the whole plant (Figure 2) and subjected to water extraction. Individual extract was tested on its anti-oxidation effects against xanthine oxidase. Water extract (0.1 mg/ml) from the biennial flower possessed the strongest anti-oxidative effects (about 80% of enzyme inhibition) among various parts of *Panax notoginseng* while the extract from sideslip showed the least effects (Figure 1B). Vitamin C (35.2 μg/ml) served as a positive control with an inhibition rate of about 70%. These results suggested that different parts of *Panax notoginseng* all possessed anti-oxidative effects with varying degrees.

The above *in vitro* anti-oxidative effects of *Panax notoginseng* could be mediated by a direct interaction between the herb-derived active ingredient(s) and xanthine oxidase. However, we speculate that such interaction may not be allowed inside the cell because the cell permeability and cellular absorption of the active ingredients are unknown. For this reason, a cell-based assay using neuronal PC12 cell was employed. PC12 cell is a popular study model in analyzing the neuroprotective effects against oxidation and other insults [22,26,27]. To inducing oxidative stress, we treated the cultures with various concentrations of H_2O_2 (0-13.6 μg/ml) and assayed for their cell viability. The neuronal cytotoxicity of PC12 cells induced by H_2O_2 was demonstrated by a dose-dependent decrease of cell viability (Figure 3A). At 13.6 μg/ml concentration of H_2O_2, about 50% cells survived. Under such cytotoxic condition, pre-treatment of the extracts from the biennial flower, stem-leaf and rhizome (1 mg/ml) protected PC12 cells against H_2O_2 insult (Figure 3B). Among all the tested extracts, the neuroprotective effects of the biennial flower were more robust than those of stem-leaf and rhizome. On the other hand, the extract of fiber root did not show any significant response while the sideslip was not included due to its negative effects in anti-oxidation. Pre-treatment of vitamin C was performed in control. These results showed that the water extract of the biennial flower of *Panax notoginseng* exhibited significant anti-oxidative effects.

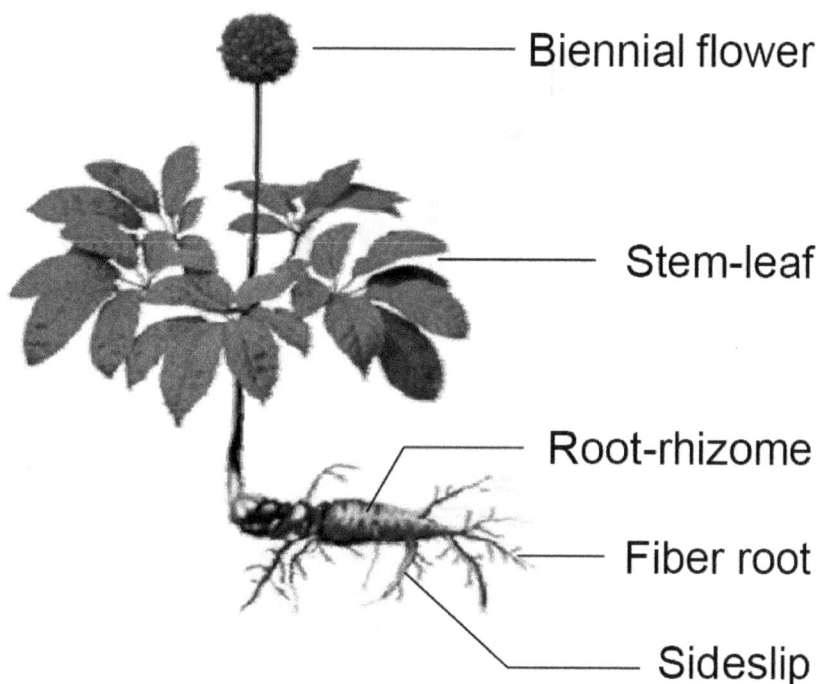

FIGURE 2: A schematic diagram to illustrate various parts of Panax notoginseng.

5.3.2 COMPARISON OF ANTI-OXIDATIVE EFFECTS BY WATER AND ETHANOL EXTRACTS

To reveal the importance of solvent selection, we used various concentrations of ethanol (30%, 50%, 70% and 90%) in the extraction of the biennial flower. The anti-oxidative effects of the ethanol extracts (0.1 mg/ml) were compared with those of water extraction. The ethanol extracts of the biennial flower showed lesser anti-oxidative effects (Figure 4); both 30% and 90% ethanol extracts exerted about 18% inhibition whereas 50% ethanol extract did not show inhibition at all. Vitamin C served as positive control. Moreover, the neuroprotective effects of the ethanol extracts were tested in cultured PC12 cells. Pre-treatments of 50%, 70% and 90% ethanol extracts did not protect the neuronal cultures against H_2O_2-induced cell

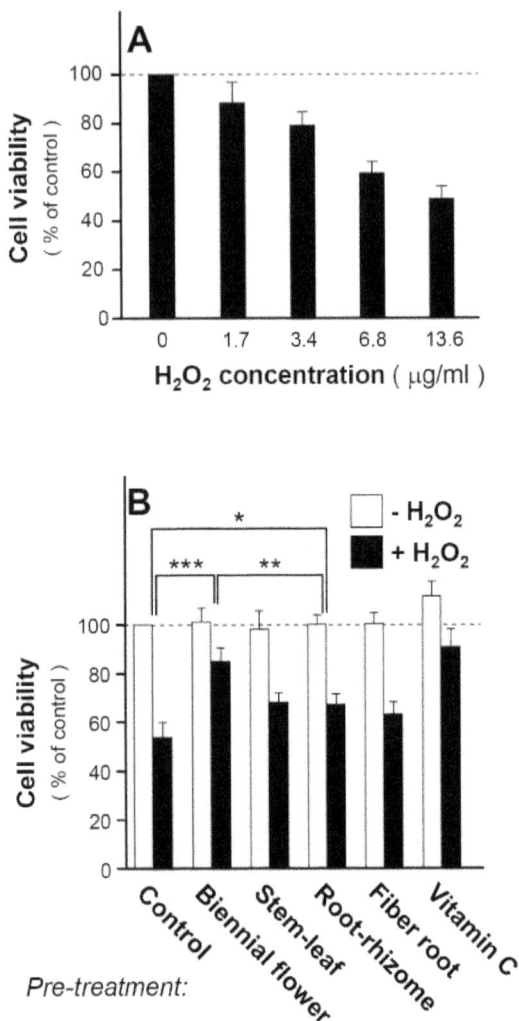

FIGURE 3: Anti-oxidative effects by the extract of the biennial flower of *Panax notoginseng* against H_2O_2-induced cytotoxicity in PC12 cells. A: Various concentrations of H_2O_2 (0, 1.7, 3.4, 6.8 and 13.6 μg/ml) were added onto cultured PC12 cells, incubated for 24 hours and determined with cell viability assay. B: Extracts (1 mg/ml) from biennial flower, stem-leaf, rhizome and fiber root of *Panax notoginseng* were pre-treated with PC12 cells for 24 hours before the addition of H_2O_2 (13.6 μg/ml) for cytotoxicity test as in [A]. Vitamin C (35.2 μg/ml) served as a positive control. Data were expressed as% of control where the value of untreated culture was set as 100%, Mean ± SD, n = 4. Statistical significance is indicated as * P = 0.0412 for root-rhizome vs control); ** P = 0.00826 for biennial flower vs root-rhizome and *** P = 0.000215 for biennial flower vs control.

death (Figure 5A) while 30% ethanol extract slightly exerted neuroprotective effects. The water extract performed the best. To further confirm the anti-oxidative effects of the water extract in PC12 cells, we pre-treated the cultures with various water extracts (0.01-10 mg/ml) and then with H_2O_2 and performed cell viability assay. The survival rate of PC12 cells under H_2O_2 insult was improved in a dose-dependent manner (Figure 5B). The saturation dose was at about 1 mg/ml. Therefore, water extracts of the biennial flower showed stronger anti-oxidative effects than ethanol extracts.

To elucidate the anti-oxidative mechanism of the biennial flower, we chose reactive oxygen species (ROS) for the investigation because ROS promote the oxidation of lipid, protein and DNA, thereby affecting the normal cell physiology, leading to neuronal demise [28,29]. Cultured PC12 cells were pre-labeled with an ROS indicator and then treated with various concentrations of H2O2 (0-400 µM). Upon the addition of H_2O_2, ROS formation increased in a dose-dependent manner (Figure 6A). Such elevation of ROS in cultured PC12 cells was reduced by the pre-treatment of water extract of the biennial flower, with about 30% ROS inhibition (Figure 6B). By contrast, 30% ethanol extract slightly reduced the amount of H_2O_2-induced ROS whereas 50%, 70% and 90% of ethanol extracts did not show any effects.

5.4 DISCUSSION

The present study, for the first time, demonstrated the anti-oxidative effects possessed by the water extract of the biennial flower of *Panax notoginseng* through the suppression of H_2O_2-induced ROS formation and neuroprotection against H_2O_2 insult. More importantly, it was the biennial flower instead of the root-rhizome that showed the strongest effects. These results support the multi-functional roles of *Panax notoginseng* and warrant further studies to explore other pharmacological effects of the plant. In terms of identifying the possible active ingredient(s) from the biennial flower, the anti-oxidation effects of different ethanol extracts were shown to be significantly less potent than that of the water extract, suggesting that the majority of active compounds might be preferentially water soluble. However, a continuous work of activity-guided fractionation is required

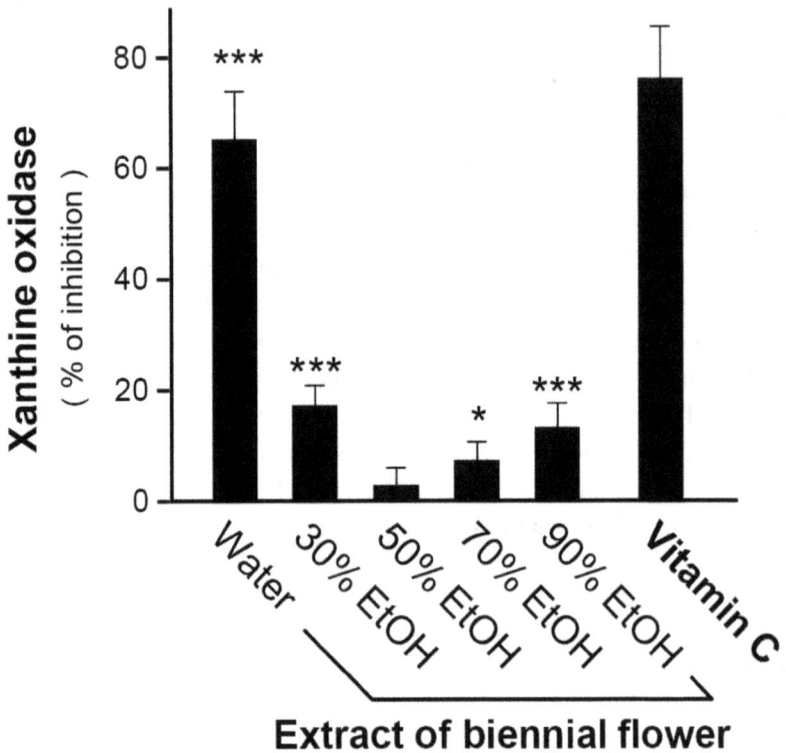

FIGURE 4: Comparison of anti-xanthine oxidase effects between the water- and ethanol-extracts of the biennial flower. Biennial flower of *Panax notoginseng* was extracted by water or various concentrations of ethanol (30, 50 70 and 90%). Extracts (0.1 mg/ml) were tested for their anti-oxidative effects against xanthine oxidase as in Figure 1. Vitamin C (35.2 µg/ml) served as positive control. Data were expressed as% of inhibition where all the values were normalized by the control (no drug treatment), Mean ± SD, n = 6. Statistical significance is indicated as * P = 0.0419 for control (without extract) vs 70% EtOH and *** P = 0.0000852 for control (without extract) vs water, P = 0.000725 for control (without extract) vs 30% EtOH and P = 0.000897 for control (without extract) vs 90% EtOH.

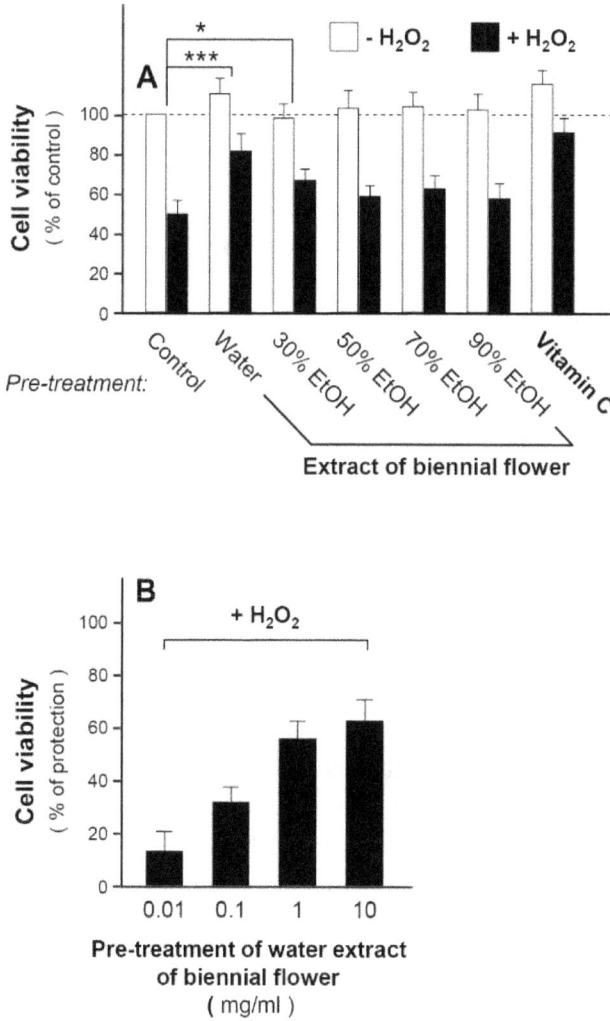

FIGURE 5: Dose-dependent effects of the water extract of the biennial flower against H2O2-induced cytotoxicity in PC12 cells. A: Extracts (1 mg/ml) of biennial flower by water and ethanol extractions were pre-treated with PC12 cells for 24 hours before the addition of H_2O_2 (13.6 μg/ml) for cytotoxicity test as in Figure 2. Vitamin C (35.2 μg/ml) served as positive control. B: Dose-dependent response was performed by pre-treating the culture with various concentrations of the water extract of the biennial flower (0.01-10 mg/ml). Data were expressed as% of control where the value of untreated culture was set as 100%, Mean ± SD, n = 4. Statistical significance is indicated as * P = 0.00471 for control (without extract) vs 30% EtOH and *** P = 0.000693 for control (without extract) vs water.

to purify and identify the candidates from the water extract of biennial flower. In this case, the high solubility of those active compounds in water will facilitate the preparation of health food supplements and drinks that could be developed from the biennial flower. Indeed, this new application will increase the economic value of *Panax notoginseng*.

Neuronal action of *Panax notoginseng* on the brain possesses various aspects. Saponins derived from the herb have been shown to prevent the neuronal cell death against hypoxia condition. The mechanism was related to the improvement of energy metabolism [30]. The therapeutic effect of saponins derived from *Panax notoginseng* was further supported by promoting the absorption of hematoma in hemorrhagic apoplexy at super-early stage in rat [31], and protecting the neuron against insults and promoting functional rehabilitation in patients after cerebral hemorrhage [32]. In addition, the co-treatment of icariin and sponins derived from *Panax notoginseng* exerted significant prophylactic and therapeutic effects in rat models of Alzheimer's disease *in vivo* [33], as well as ameliorated the learning and memory deficit and blood viscosity by protecting neurons from oxidative stress in ischemic brain [34]. For neurotrophic effects, the phosphorylated neurofilament- and MAP2-expressing neurites could be extended in SK-N-SH cells by the treatment of saponins and *Panax notoginseng* extracts, suggesting the possible axonal and dendritic formation activity [35]. Therefore, the multi-functional effects of saponins from *Panax notoginseng* might be a good candidate in mediating the anti-oxidation activities because of the high extractability of saponins by water. This speculation was in accordance to our previous finding that the amounts of four active constituents, notoginsenoside R1, ginsenoside Rg1, Rb1 and Rd, by water extraction were higher than that of 30% and 70% ethanol extractions [36]. In addition to saponins, a flavonol glycoside, named RNFG, isolated from *Panax notoginseng* also possesses the neuroprotective effect against amyloid-β-induced apoptosis and cytotoxicity at cellular level, and which improves the learning and memory process in rats [18]. Interestingly, this compound also exerts a significant anti-oxidative activity by lowering the amount of reactive oxygen species (ROS) induced by H_2O_2 in cultured PC12 cells. Based on the above findings, it should be very interesting to know if the biennial flower contains RNFG, and which could have neuroprotective effect in cell cultures and in animal study. Therefore,

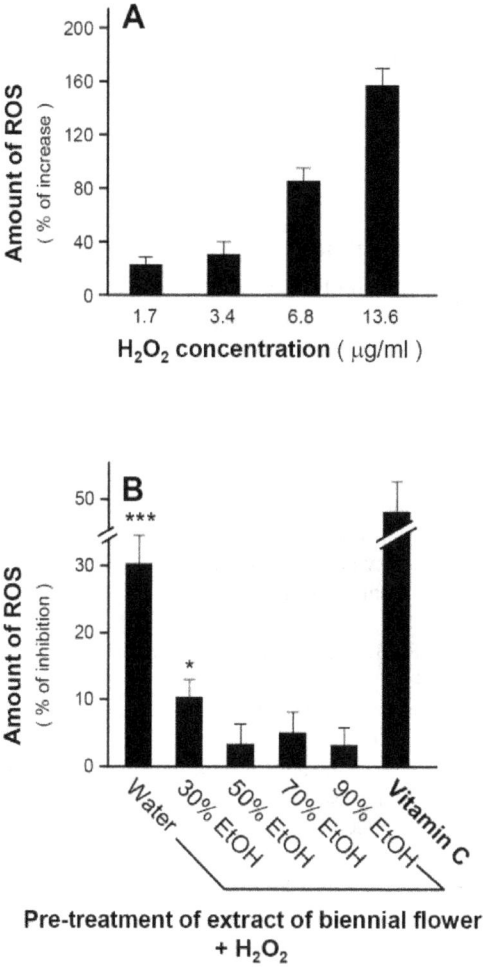

FIGURE 6. Suppression of the formation of H_2O_2-induced ROS formation in PC12 cells by water extracts of the biennial flower. A: Cultured PC12 cells were pre-labeled DCFH-DA for one hour before the addition of various concentrations of H_2O_2 (0, 1.7, 3.4, 6.8 and 13.6 μg/ml) for another hour. The amount of ROS was fluorometrically measured with excitation at 485 nm and emission at 530 nm. B: Water and ethanol extracts of the biennial flower (1 mg/ml) were pre-treated with the PC12 cells for 24 hours. H_2O_2 (13.6 μg/ml) was used in the ROS formation assay as in A. Vitamin C (35.2 μg/ml) served as positive control. Data were expressed as% of inhibition where all the values were normalized by the control (no drug treatment), Mean ± SD, n = 4. Statistical significance is indicated as * P = 0.00419 for control (without extract) vs 30% EtOH and *** P = 0.000269 for control (without extract) vs water.

the identification and isolation of the possible active ingredients (saponins, flavonoids, flavonol glycoside or others) will be essential to extend and support the multi-functional usages of *Radix notoginseng* in future.

5.5 CONCLUSION

The present study demonstrates the biennial flower of *Panax notoginseng* to have neuroprotection effect on cultured neurons and the underlying protection mechanism may involve anti-oxidation.

REFERENCES

1. Lei XL, Chiou GC: Cardiovascular pharmacology of *Panax notoginseng* (Burk) F.H. Chen and Salvia miltiorrhiza. Am J Chin Med 1986, 14:145-152.
2. Cicero AF, Vitale G, Savino G, Arlett R: *Panax notoginseng* (Burk.) effects on fibrinogen and lipid plasma level in rat fed on a high-fat diet. Phytother Res 2003, 17:174-178.
3. Zheng GZ, Yang CR: Biology of *Panax Notoginseng* and Its Application. Beijing: Science Press; 1994.
4. Zheng XY, (ed.): Pharmacopoeia of the People's Republic of China. Beijing: Chemistry Industry Press; 2000.
5. Chan P, Thomas GN, Tromlinson B: Protective effects of trilinolein extracted from *Panax notoginseng* against cardiovascular disease. Planta Med 2002, 68:1024-1028.
6. Kim HC, Shin EJ, Jang CG, Lee MK, Eun JS, Hong JT, Oh KW: Pharmacological action of Panax ginseng on the behavioral toxicities induced by psychotropic agents. Arch Pharm Res 2005, 28:995-1001.
7. Chuang CM, Hsieh CL, Lin HY, Lin JG: *Panax notoginseng* Burk attenuates impairment of learning and memory functions and increases ED1, BDNF and beta-secretase immunoreactive cells in chronic stage ischemia-reperfusion injured rats. Am J Chin Med (Gard City N Y) 2008, 36:685-693.
8. Wu W, Zhang XM, Liu PM, Li JM, Wang JF: Effects of *Panax notoginseng* saponin Rg1 on cardiac electrophysiological properties and ventricular fibrillation threshold in dogs. Acta Pharm Sin 1995, 16:459-463.
9. Chen JC, Chen LD, Tsauer W, Tsai CC, Chen BC, Chen YJ: Effects of Ginsenoside Rb2 and Rc on inferior human sperm motility *in vitro*. Am J Chin Med (Gard City N Y) 2001, 29:155-160.
10. Wei JX, Wang JF, Chang LY, Du YC: Chemical studies of san-chi *Panax notoginseng* I: Studies on the constituents of San-Chi root hairs. Acta Pharm Sin 1980, 15:359-364.

11. Gao H, Wang F, Lien EJ, Trousdale MD: Immunostimulating polysaccharides from Panax notoginseng. Pharm Res 1996, 13:1196-1200.

12. Wu Y, Wang D: Structural characterization and DPPH radical scavenging activity of an arabinoglucogalactan from *Panax notoginseng* root. J Nat Prod 2008, 71:241-245.

13. Huang YS, Yang ZC, Yan BG, Hu XC, Li AN, Crowther RS: Improvement of early postburn cardiac function by use of *Panax notoginseng* and immediate total eschar excision in one operation. Burns 1999, 25:35-41.

14. Wang J, Xu J, Zhong JB: Effect of Radix Notoginseng saponins on platelet activating molecule expression and aggregation in patients with blood hyperviscosity syndrome. Zhongguo Zhong Xi Yi Jie He Za Zhi 2004, 24:312-316.

15. Chen ZH, Wang DC, Li HL, Wei JX, Wang JF, Du YC: Hemodynamic effects of san chi (Panax notoginseng) root, leaf, flower and saponins on anesthetized dogs. Acta Pharm Sin 1983, 18:818-822.

16. Qi D, Zhu Y, Wen L, Liu Q, Qiao H: Ginsenoside Rg1 restores the impairment of learning induced by chronic morphine administration in rats. J Psychopharmacol 2009, 231:74-83.

17. Bao HY, Zhang J, Yeo SJ, Myung CS, Kim HM, Kim JM, Park JH, Cho J, Kang JS: Memory enhancing and neuroprotective effects of selected ginsenosides. Arch Pharm Res 2005, 28:335-342.

18. Choi RC, Zhu JT, Leung KW, Chu GK, Xie HQ, Chen VP, Zheng KY, Lau DT, Dong TT, Chow PC, Han YF, Wang ZT, Tsim KW: A flavonol glycoside, isolated from roots of Panax notoginseng, reduces amyloid-beta-induced neurotoxicity in cultured neurons: signaling transduction and drug development for Alzheimer's disease. J Alzheimers Dis 2010, 19:795-811.

19. Ohtani K, Mizutani K, Hatono S, Kasai R, Sumino R, Shiota T, Ushijima M, Zhou J, Fuwa T, Tanaka O: Sanchinan-A, a reticuloendothelial system activating arabinogalactan from sanchi-ginseng (roots of Panax notoginseng). Planta Med 1987, 53:166-169.

20. Cui XM, Lo CK, Yip KL, Dong TT, Tsim KW: Authentication of *Panax notoginseng* by 5S-rRNA spacer domain and random amplified polymorphic DNA (RAPD) analysis. Planta Med 2003, 69:584-586.

21. Li SP, Zhao KJ, Ji ZN, Song ZH, Dong TT, Lo CK, Cheung JK, Zhu SQ, Tsim KW: A polysaccharide isolated from Cordyceps sinensis, a traditional Chinese medicine, protects PC12 cells against hydrogen peroxide-induced injury. Life Sci 2003, 73:2503-2513.

22. Zhu JT, Choi RCY, Chu GK, Cheung AW, Gao QT, Li J, Jiang ZY, Dong TT, Tsim KW: Flavonoids possess neuroprotective effects on cultured pheochromocytoma PC12 cells: a comparison of different flavonoids in activating estrogenic effect and in preventing beta-amyloid-induced cell death. J Agric Food Chem 2007, 55:2438-2445.

23. Aruoma OI, Bahorun T, Jen LS: Neuroprotection by bioactive components in medicinal and food plant extracts. Mutat Res 2003, 544:203-215.

24. Bonomini F, Tengattini S, Fabiano A, Bianchi R, Rezzani R: Atherosclerosis and oxidative stress. Histol Histopathol 2008, 23:381-390.

25. Förstermann U: Oxidative stress in vascular disease: causes, defense mechanisms and potential therapies. Nat Clin Pract Cardiovasc Med 2008, 5:338-349.

26. Tabakman R, Jiang H, Shahar I, Arien-Zakay H, Levine RA, Lazarovici P: Neuroprotection by NGF in the PC12 *in vitro* OGD model: involvement of mitogen-activated protein kinases and gene expression. Ann N Y Acad Sci 2005, 1053:84-96.

27. Li SP, Zhang GH, Zeng Q, Huang ZG, Wang YT, Dong TT, Tsim KW: Hypoglycemic activity of polysaccharide, with antioxidation, isolated from cultured Cordyceps mycelia. Phytomedicine 2006, 13:428-433.

28. Behl C, Moosmann B: Antioxidant neuroprotection in Alzheimer's disease as preventive and therapeutic approach. Free Radic Biol Med 2002, 33:182-191.

29. Perez-Pinzon MA, Dave KR, Raval AP: Role of reactive oxygen species and protein kinase C in ischemic tolerance in the brain. Antioxid Redox Signal 2005, 7:1150-1157.

30. Jiang KY, Qian ZN: Effects of *Panax notoginseng* saponins on posthypoxic cell damage of neurons *in vitro*. Zhongguo Yao Li Xue Bao 1995, 16:399-402.

31. Nie YX, Wang D, Zhang X: Effect of *panax notoginseng* saponins injection on brain edema in intracerebral hemorrhage rats. Zhongguo Zhong Xi Yi Jie He Za Zhi 2006, 26:922-925.

32. Wei SG, Meng LQ, Huang RY: Effect of *Panax notoginseng* saponins on serum neuronal specific enolase and rehabilitation in patients with cerebral hemorrhage. Zhongguo Zhong Xi Yi Jie He Za Zhi 2007, 27:159-162.

33. Xiao XF, Zheng M, Qu LH, Lou YJ: Effects of icariin combined with the *Panax notoginseng* saponins on behavior and acetylcholinesterase activity induced by β-amyloid peptide 25-35 lateral ventricle injection in rats. Chin J MAP 2005, 22:178-181.

34. Zheng M, Qu L, Lou Y: Effects of icariin combined with *Panax notoginseng* saponins on ischemia reperfusion-induced cognitive impairments related with oxidative stress and CA1 of hippocampal neurons in rat. Phytother Res 2008, 22:597-604.

35. Tohda C, Matsumoto N, Zou K, Meselhy MR, Komatsu K: Axonal and dendritic extension by protopanaxadiol-type saponins from ginseng drugs in SK-N-SH cells. Jpn J Pharmacol 2002, 90:254-262.

36. Dong TT, Zhao KJ, Huang WZ, Leung KW, Tsim KW: Orthogonal array design in optimizing the extraction efficiency of active constituents from roots of Panax notoginseng. Phytother Res 2005, 19:684-688.

CHAPTER 6

CYTOTOXIC ACTIVITY OF PROTEINS ISOLATED FROM EXTRACTS OF *CORYDALIS CAVA* TUBERS IN HUMAN CERVICAL CARCINOMA HELA CELLS

ROBERT NAWROT, MARIA WOLUN-CHOLEWA, WOJCIECH BIALAS, DANUTA WYRZYKOWSKA, STANISLAW BALCERKIEWICZ, AND ANNA GOZDZICKA-JOZEFIAK

6.1 BACKGROUND

Plants from the family Papaveraceae are frequently used in traditional medicine as a remedy for treatment of several diseases. Such plants include *Corydalis cava* Schweigg. & Koerte; syn. *Corydalis bulbosa* (L.) Pers. non (L.) DC. and *Chelidonium majus* L. studied earlier by our group (Greater Celandine). The two species are closely related and belong to order Papaverales [1,2]. Milky sap as well as extracts of the whole *Chelidonium majus* plant has been used to treat papillae, warts, condylomae, which are a visible effect of human papilloma virus (HPV) infection. It has

This chapter was originally published under the Creative Commons Attribution License. Nawrot R, Wolun-Cholewa M, Bialas W, Wyrzykowska D, Balcerkiewicz S and Gozdzicka-Jozefiak A. Cytotoxic Activity of Proteins Isolated from Extracts of Corydalis cava *Tubers in Human Cervical Carcinoma HeLa Cells.* BMC Complementary and Alternative Medicine *10,78 (2010). doi:10.1186/1472-6882-10-78.*

also been found that they have antimicrobial, antitumor, anti-inflammato-ry, antifungal, and fungistatic properties [3]. The tuber of *Corydalis sp.* contains isoquinoline alkaloids of apomorphine type, e.g. bulbocapnine, corydaline, which manifest analgetic, sedating and narcotic effects [4-7]. The plant has been used for the treatment of severe neurological disorders and mental diseases. It was also used in cases of asomnia, tension and anxiety conditions [7]. Some species of *Corydalis* are used in East Asia as analgetic drugs: in the traditional Chinese medicine, the species of *Corydalis yanhusho* was used to alleviate post-traumatic, colic, abdominal and menstrual pains [7]. Moreover, extracts of the same species showed anti-cancerous metastasis effect *in vitro* [8]. Anti-tumour activity of *Corydalis* species was also reported for Korean *Corydalis turtschaninovii*, which is effective for the treatment of inflammatory, allergic diseases and tumours [9]. Isoquinoline alkaloids contained in alcohol extracts of tubers in many species of *Corydalis*, affect metabolism of neurotransmitters [10]. Active compounds in such extracts include alkaloids, such as bulbocapnine, co-rydaline and corydine [11]. The similar curing properties of *Chelidonium majus* milky sap were attributed mainly to alkaloids, such as chelidonine, sanguinarine, berberine, coptosine, chelerythrine, and also several flavo-noids and phenolic acids [12]. However, different findings show that all of them may be potentially toxic for human either alone or in combination [13,14].

Our earlier studies have shown that biological activity of *Chelidonium majus* milky sap may be related to its protein content. The majority of the identified proteins can be linked to direct and indirect stress and defense reactions, e.g. against different pathogens [15-17]. We have recently dis-covered that purified plant proteins from *Chelidonium majus* milky sap with nucleolytic activity, which probably belong to pathogenesis-related (PR) protein family, are capable of inducing apoptosis in human cervical cancer HeLa cells [17].

Therefore, the objective of our study was to evaluate the effect of puri-fied proteins from extracts of *Corydalis cava* tubers with nucleolytic ac-tivity on HeLa tumour cells and to identify the protein content of such purified fractions using tandem mass spectrometry.

6.2 METHODS

6.2.1 PLANT MATERIAL

Corydalis cava plants were collected during 2007 and 2008 in the neighbourhood of Poznań, Poland, during flowering, in April. A voucher specimen was deposited at the Department of Molecular Virology, Faculty of Biology, Adam Mickiewicz University in Poznan, Poland.

6.2.2 PROTEIN EXTRACT

The protein extract was prepared from tubers, dissolved in 0.1 M Tris-Cl buffer, pH 8.0, containing 10% glycerol (extract : buffer ratio was 1:1). The tuber extract (50% v/v) samples were separated into a supernatant, and a pellet fraction, by centrifugation at 12000 rpm for 20 min at 4°C as described in the protocol [16], with modifications. Supernatants were stored at -20°C for further analysis. Protein concentration was determined according to Lowry et al. [18].

6.2.3 ISOLATION AND PURIFICATION OF PROTEINS

For isolation and purification of proteins, crude extracts from *C. cava* tubers collected in April were used. About 0.5-µg protein was loaded on HT Heparin column (GE Healthcare) (0.7 × 2.5 cm) equilibrated with 0.1 M Tris-HCl, pH 8.0, 10% glycerol. The column was eluted with a linear gradient of 0 to 2 M NaCl in the same buffer. The absorbance at 280 nm and DNase activity of all fractions (volume 1 ml) were determined.

6.2.4 ANALYSIS BY SDS-PAGE

In order to verify the protein composition of chromatographic fractions, sodium dodecyl sulfate polyacrylamide gel electrophoresis (SDS-PAGE) was carried out in a slab mini-gel apparatus according to Laemmli 1970 [19], using 10% polyacrylamide as the separating gel and 5% polyacrylamide as the stacking gel. The proteins were reduced by heating them at 100°C in the presence of 2-mercaptoethanol for 5 min. After SDS-PAGE, the gels were fixed and stained with silver according to Shevchenko et al. [20].

6.2.5 IN-GEL NUCLEASE ASSAY

An in-gel DNase assay was performed according to Thelen and Northcote [21], with modifications [22]. For in-gel DNase assay, *C. cava* tuber extracts or fractions after purification were dissolved in SDS-PAGE sample buffer without a reducing agent, incubated at 37°C for 10 min, and subjected to SDS-PAGE in 10% polyacrylamide gel containing denatured calf thymus DNA (40 µg/ml). After the electrophoresis and removal of SDS, the gels were washed with reaction buffer (10 mM Tris-HCl, pH 8.0, containing 10 mM $CaCl2$). DNase activity was visualized by staining the gel with ethidium bromide.

6.2.6 CELL CULTURE AND VIABILITY ASSAY

HeLa cells were cultured in RPMI 1640 supplemented with 5% FCS, 2 mmol/l L-glutamine, 100 µg/ml streptomycin and 100 U/ml penicillin. Viability of cell cultures was appraised using XTT colorimetric test, based on a dynamics of XTT (tetrazoline 2,3-bis(2-methoxy-4-nitro-5-sulfofenylo)-2H-5-carboxyanilide) stain reduction by viable cells with the formation of a colored product. Intensity of the fluorescence was measured at the wavelength of 450 nm. Percentage of mitochondrial metabolism activity inhibition was calculated according to the following equation: 100-(OD drug treated cells - OD medium alone/OD untreated cells-OD medium alone*100). Each experiment was conducted independently in 8 cultures and in each culture at least 200 cells were scored. Statistical analysis of the results involved the t-test for unpaired data using the STATISTICA ver.6.1 software. P value < 0.05 was considered to represent threshold of significance.

6.2.7 LC-ESI-MS/MS ANALYSIS

Stained protein bands were excised from the gel and analyzed by liquid chromatography coupled to mass spectrometer in the Laboratory of Mass Spectrometry, Institute of Biochemistry and Biophysics, Polish Academy of Sciences, Warsaw, Poland. Samples were concentrated and desalted on RP-C18 precolumn (LC Packings, UK) and further peptide separation was achieved in a nano-HPLC RP-C18 column (LC Packings, 75 mM i.d.) of a UltiMate nano-HPLC system, using a 50-min linear acetonitrile gradient. Column outlet was directly coupled to Finningan Nanospray ion source of LTQ-FT (Thermo, USA) mass spectrometer working in the regime of data dependent MS to MS/MS switch. An electrospray voltage of 1500 V and a cone voltage of 30 V were used.

6.2.8 MS/MS DATA ANALYSIS

The data were analysed automatically by database matching against the NCBInr protein database (NCBI, Bethesda, USA) with a Viridiplantae filter, using the MASCOT database search engine (Matrix science, London, UK; http://www.matrixscience.com webcite) [23].

6.3 RESULTS

6.3.1 ISOLATION AND PURIFICATION OF PROTEINS FROM CORYDALIS CAVA TUBER EXTRACTS ON A HEPARIN COLUMN

In order to evaluate if biological activity of *Corydalis* tuber extracts is related to the proteins contained in them, the proteins of nucleolytic activity were isolated from the tubers by purification on a HT Heparin column (Figure 1A) using ÄKTA Explorer™ chromatographic system (Amersham Biosciences). Following the application of the extract to the column (0.7 × 2.5 cm), molecules which did not bind to the column were eluted using elution buffer (buffer A: 100 mM Tris, pH 8.0, 10% glycerol). The first eight fractions of 1.5 ml each represented the flow-through fractions. The subsequent fractions were eluted using a linear gradient of NaCl (from 0 to 2 M) (19 fractions of 1 ml each). In all the fractions, absorbance was measured at 280 nm (Figure 1A), indicating the presence of purified proteins in fractions 16-18. Protein fractions purified on heparin column were tested for DNase activity using in-gel DNase assay (Figure 1B) according to Thelen and Northcote [21]. Nucleolytic activity was demonstrated in fraction numbers 16, 17 and 18. All the fractions were also separated in SDS-containing polyacrylamide gel (SDS-PAGE), which was stained with silver according to Shevchenko et al. [20] (Figure 1C). Fraction numbers 16 and 17 each contained five protein bands of molecular weights (MW) approx. 30, 32, 35, 38 and 68 kDa, while the fraction number 18 contained an additional fraction of MW around 140 kDa.

6.3.2 ANALYSIS OF MITOCHONDRIAL ACTIVITY OF HELA CELLS

All the fractions with nuclease activity were tested for cytotoxic activity in human cervical carcinoma HeLa cells. For the analysis, proteins contained in fraction numbers 16, 17, 18 and 19 were used, from three different rounds of purification. The buffer used for tuber extract isolation (0.1 M Tris, 10% glycerol), at the concentration of 26.7 µl/ml served as a negative control. For each fraction, 48 h cultures of HeLa cells were conducted in the presence of three protein concentrations: 42, 83 and 167 ng/ml from three purification rounds. HeLa cells on the plates were subjected to the action of XTT/PBS solution (1 mg XTT/ml in PBS + 1.53 mg PMS/ml in PBS) in order to estimate cell viability. Following incubation, the results were recorded using a small plate ELISA reader (Labsystems Multiskan MCC/340) with readout at 450 nm. The results are presented in Table 1.

TABLE 1: Mitochondrial activity inhibition in neoplastic HeLa cells under the effect of purified protein fractions from extracts of *C. cava* tubers.

Fraction no.	Protein concentration [ng/ml]	Mean value of HeLa cells inhibition [%]	Standard deviation [%]
16	42	4.55	3.53
16	83	15.57	2.42
16	167	35.31	4.32
17	42	8.66	5.19
17	83	22.35	2.40
17	167	39.15	3.34
18	42	12.59	5.37
18	83	32.42	3.13
18	167	43.45	3.06
19	42	5.90	5.43
19	83	15.18	7.10
19	167	21.78	6.06

Proteins from three rounds of purification were administered at concentrations of 42; 83; and 167 ng/ml. The data was analyzed using STATISTICA (version 6.1) software. [%] - inhibition of mitochondrial activity of HeLa cells under effect of examined proteins as compared to the control.

The cytotoxic effect of studied proteins in relation to HeLa cell line was clearly marked and it depended on the applied dose of protein: the most pronounced effect was obtained with protein fractions administered at the highest concentration (167 ng/ml), while at the intermediate concentration (83 ng/ml), the effect was appropriately lower compared to the highest concentration. Fraction 18 exerted the highest cytotoxic effect at the concentration of 167 ng/ml: 43.45 ± 3% cells underwent mitochondrial activity inhibition (Table 1). Protein fractions at the lowest protein concentration (42 ng/ml) manifested the least pronounced cytotoxic effect (e.g., fraction 16: 4.55 ± 3.5%, table 1). In the experiments, the control was provided by the pure elution buffer (0.1 M Tris, 10% glycerol), added to HeLa cells at the concentration of 26.7 μl/ml, which did not exert any effect on mitochondrial activity of HeLa cells.

TABLE 2: Defense-related proteins identified in fractions after purification of nucleases from extracts of *Corydalis cava* tubers using LC-ESI-MS/MS.

No. of protein band[a]	Identified protein[b]	Accesion No.[c]	Matched peptides[d]	Score[e]	Mol. mass (Da)[f]	pI[g]	Sequence coverage (%)[h]
1, 2, 3, 4,	peroxidase [*Nicotiana tabacum*] (PR-9)	gi|14031049	16	560	39495	5.99	13
5, 6	heat shock protein 70 [*Chlorella zofingiensis*]	gi|18482472	4	180	70112	8.29	8
1	pectinesterase [*Phaseolus vulgaris*]	gi|21060	2	112	23967	9.52	4
2	SODP_PETHY Superoxide dismutase (ISS) [*Ostreococcus tauri*]	gi|116056311	2	74	42244	11.68	4
4	GRP-like protein 2 [*Gossypium hirsutum*]	gi|110559491	3	69	41333	6.01	8
5	disease resistance protein (TIR-NBS-LRR class), putative [*Arabidopsis thaliana*]	gi|15229962	1	64	117364	7.49	0
3	ribosomal protein S12 [*Mesostigma viride*]	gi|11466414	1	55	13815	11.32	9
1	DNA-binding protein [*Zea mays*]	gi|195658581	1	54	27597	6.49	4
4	chloroplast nucleoid DNA-binding protein-related [*Arabidopsis thaliana*]	gi|18391062	1	53	48429	7.48	2
4	RPP13-like protein [*Arabidopsis arenosa*]	gi|46410122	1	52	70976	5.51	2

a) Assigned numbers of protein bands as indicated in Fig. 1C.
b) Identified homologous proteins and organism from which it proceeds.
c) Database accession numbers according to: NCBInr (nr); trEMBL (trm).
d) Number of matched peptides with Mascot Search data (http://www.matrixscience.com webcite).
e) Mascot Search Probability Based Mowse Score. Ions score is -10*Log(P), where P is the probability that the observed match is a random event. Individual ions scores > 48 indicate identity or extensive homology (p < 0.05).
f) Theoretical mass (kDa) of identified proteins. The values were retrieved from the protein database.
g) Theoretical pI of identified proteins. The values were retrieved from the protein database.
h) Amino acid sequence coverage for the identified proteins.

6.3.3 IDENTIFICATION OF PROTEINS IN PURIFIED FRACTIONS BY MASS SPECTROMETRY

The protein bands were numbered 1 to 6 (Figure 1C), excised from the gel stained with silver [20] and sent for identification by mass spectrometry (LC-ESI-MS/MS) at the Laboratory of Mass Spectrometry, Institute of Biochemistry and Biophysics, Polish Academy of Sciences (IBB PAN) in Warsaw, Poland. The data was analyzed using MASCOT (http://www. matrixscience.com webcite).

Results of protein identification using tandem mass spectrometry analysis (LC-ESI-MS/MS) are presented in Table 2. It contains a list of identified proteins from fractions of *Corydalis cava* tuber extracts. Results of the identification show that proteins contained in bands of fraction numbers 16-18 belong to plant pathogenesis- (PR) and defense-related proteins. Most of the identified proteins is directly or indirectly involved in defense reactions of the plant against various stresses, e.g. against attack of a pathogen (Table 2).

Analysis of DNase activity has demonstrated the presence of a band with nucleolytic activity in fractions 16, 17 and 18 of molecular weight around 30 kDa (Figure 1B). Comparison of SDS-PAGE gel following the separation of the same fractions and staining with the silver method (Figure 1C), demonstrates an analogous band of around 30 kDa molecular weight (No. 1) identified as DNA-binding protein from Zea mays with a very similar molecular weight of 27.6 kDa (Table 2). Thus, the studied fraction contains a number of proteins with defense and metabolic significance for the plant.

Table 2 lists identified defense-related proteins with plant species in which the proteins were detected as well as protein scores and sequence coverages. The number of compatible peptides for individual results ranged between 1 and 43, sequence coverage in a single case reached the maximum value of 26%. In the Table 2, numbers of protein bands were indicated in which particular proteins were identified (Figure 1C).

6.4 DISCUSSION

Plants that belong to family Papaveraceae, like Greater Celandine (*Chelidonium majus* L.) and *Corydalis cava* Schweigg. & Koerte, are a rich

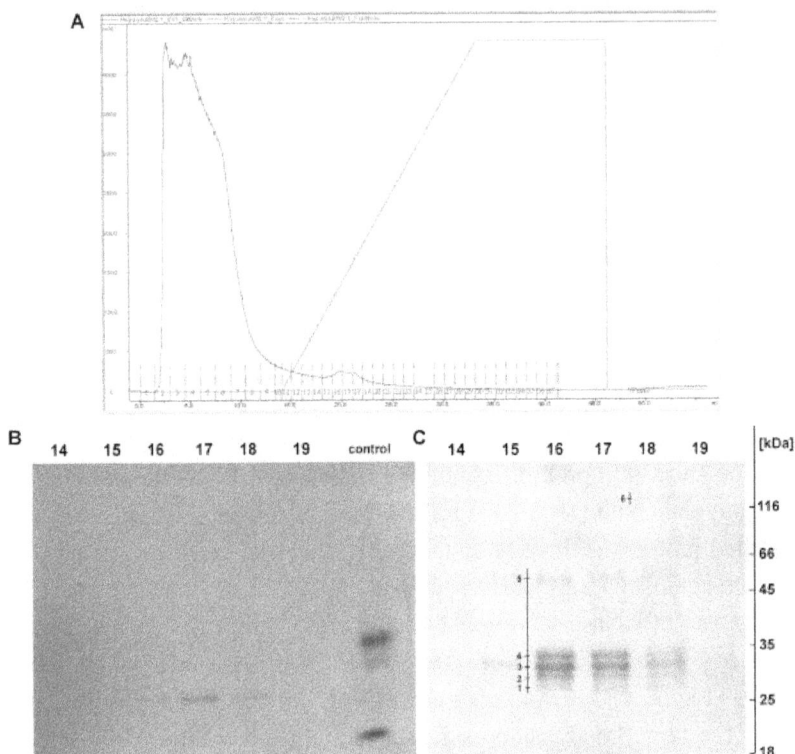

FIGURE 1: Protein purification and electrophoretic analysis. (A) Chromatographic profile of protein purification from *C. cava* tuber extracts in HT Heparin column (GE Healthcare). Fractions 1 to 9 represented flow-through fractions, 10 to 27 were eluted with a linear NaCl gradient (from 0 to 2 M). The absorbance of all fractions was measured at 280 nm and their DNase activity was estimated using in-gel assay. Proteins present in fractions 16, 17 and 18 were identified using LC-ESI-MS/MS. Fractions 16-19 following three rounds of purification were used in tests on HeLa tumour cell line. (B) In-gel DNase pattern of the gel in which DNase activity of protein fractions originating from *C. cava* tuber extracts was estimated. ssDNA containing 10% SDS-PAGE, following electrophoresis and incubation (12 h) in 10 mM Ca^{2+} buffer, pH 8.0, was stained with ethidium bromide and viewed under UV light. Nucleolytic activity was noted in fractions Nos.16, 17 and 18 of MW around 30 kDa. Control: purified nucleases from *Chelidonium majus* milky sap served as positive control. (C) 10% SDS-PAGE following electrophoresis of fraction-contained proteins and silver staining according to Shevchenko et al. [20]. The separated fractions were identical to those in the gel in Fig. 1B. Fractions nos. 16 and 17 each contained 5 protein bands of MW around 30, 32, 35, 38 and 68 kDa, while fraction no. 18 contained an additional band of MW around 140 kDa. The protein bands were numbered 1-6, excised from the gel and sent for identification by mass spectrometry (LC-ESI-MS/MS). M - Protein Molecular Weight Marker (Fermentas).

source of various biologically active substances with strong pharmaco-logical activity. The mechanism of this activity is still unknown, but very important compounds are the proteins contained in the plants. Our earlier studies showed that biological activity of *Chelidonium majus* milky sap may be related to its protein content. The protein fractions which con-tained two nucleases induced apoptosis in human cervical cancer HeLa cells [17].

Most probably, the present study represents the first investigations on the effect of purified PR proteins from tuber extracts of a pharmacologi-cally active plant on cell lines. The cytotoxic effect of studied proteins toward HeLa cell line cells has been evident and dependent on increasing dose of the protein.

Results of protein identification in fractions from purification of *C. cava* tuber extracts using LC-ESI-MS/MS analysis have shown that proteins contained in bands of fractions 16-18 belong to plant pathogenesis- and defense-related proteins, indirectly or directly involved in plant defense reactions against stresses of various kind. Many of them belong to the PR protein family involved in plant defense against the pathogen attack. The family includes 17 protein classes of variable activities [24]. *C. cava* tubers are exposed to the attack of fungal, viral, bacterial and other patho-gens during the entire vegetation season as well as during winter time [25]. Accumulation of high number and variability of defense proteins in tubers together with several secondary metabolites, such as isoquinoline alkaloids, provides an effective and long-time protection against attack of pathogens. Moreover, defense-related proteins contained in *C. cava* tubers resemble 21 proteins identified earlier by our group in *Chelidonium majus* milky sap [15].

The studies represent preliminary demonstration of the effect exerted by tuber proteins from a plant of pharmacological significance on cells of a tumour cell line. The investigated protein fractions comprise a mixture of plant defense-related proteins. In subsequent studies, an effort will be made to isolate the individual proteins and examine their effect on tu-mour cells individually and in combinations as well. Nevertheless, the synergistic action of all the compounds present in plant protein extracts is very important for their activity. Many effective and extensively studied compounds of plant origin are, in fact, crude protein mixtures, such as phytotherapeutical drug bromelain, which is crude, aqueous extract from the stems and immature fruits of pineapples (Ananas comosus from the family Bromeliaceae), constituting a complex mixture of different thiol-endopeptidases and other components such as phosphatases, glucosidases, peroxidases, cellulases, glycoproteins, carbohydrates and several proteinase inhibitors [26]. Also, *Viscum album* L. extracts (VAE, European mistletoe) are composed of pharmacologically relevant compounds like: mistletoe lectins (ML I, II and III), viscotoxins and other low molecular proteins, VisalbCBA (*Viscum album* chitin-binding agglutinin), oligo- and polysaccharides, flavonoids, vesicles, triterpene acids, and others. Whole VAE as well as several of the compounds are cytotoxic and the mistletoe lectins have strong apoptosis-inducing effects [27].

Although the mechanism of presented activity of *C. cava* proteins is unknown, their defensive role for the plant could be very important. Many plant defense-related proteins belong to small (14-40 amino acids), linear, cationic peptides. These peptides have membrane lytic properties and potent activity against a broad spectrum of microorganisms. They organize into ordered secondary structures (α-helix and β-sheet) in the membrane [28]. Above a threshold concentration, peptides disturb the cell membrane and cause cell death due to membrane disintegration [29].

6.5 CONCLUSIONS

Presented studies confirm that biological activity of *C. cava* extracts may also be related to proteins contained in the extracts. For possible further applications, the biologically active plant proteins should be separated from alkaloids and other secondary metabolites, which in higher doses might be toxic [14]. The studies represent preliminary demonstration of the effect exerted by tuber proteins from a plant of pharmacological significance on cells of a tumour cell line. In the subsequent studies, an effort will be made to isolate the individual proteins and examine their effect on tumour cells individually and in combinations.

REFERENCES

1. Cronquist A: An Integrated System of Classification of Flowering Plants. New York, Columbia University Press; 1981.
2. Reveal JL: System of Classification. PBIO 250 Lecture Notes: Plant Taxonomy. Department of Plant Biology, University of Maryland; 1999.
3. Colombo ML, Bosisio E: Pharmacological activities of *Chelidonium majus* L. (Papaveraceae). Pharm Res 1996, 33:127-134.
4. Rueffer M, Bauer W, Zenk MH: The formation of corydaline and related alkaloids in *Corydalis cava* in vivo and *in vitro*. Can J Chem 1994, 72:170-175.
5. Hänsel R, Sticher O: Pharmakognosie-Phytopharmazie. Heidelberg, Springer Verlag; 2004.
6. Freudenreich O: Ocular side effects associated with dietary supplements and herbal medicines. Drugs Today 2005, 41:537.
7. Cheng ZH, Guo Y-L, Wang H-Y, Chen G-Q: Qualitative and quantitative analysis of quaternary ammonium alkaloids from Rhizoma *Corydalis* by matrix-assisted laser desorption/ionization Fourier transform mass spectrometry coupled with a selective precipitation reaction using Reinecke salt. Anal Chim Acta 2006, 555:269-277.
8. Gao JL, Shi JM, He K, Zhang QW, Li SP, Lee SM, Wang YT: Yanhusuo extract inhibits metastasis of breast cancer cells by modulating mitogen-activated protein kinase signaling pathways. Oncol Rep 2008, 20:819-824.
9. An HJ, Rim HK, Chung HS, Choi IY, Kim NH, Kim SJ, Moon PD, Myung NY, Jeong HJ, Jeong CH, Chung SH, Um JY, Hong SH, Kim HM: Expression of inducible nitric oxide synthase by *Corydalis turtschaninovii* on interferon-gamma stimulated macrophages. J Ethnopharmacol 2009, 122:573-578.
10. Schäfer HL, Schäfer H, Schneider W, Elstner EF: Sedative action of extract combinations of Eschscholtzia californica and *Corydalis cava*. Arzneimittelforschung 1995, 45:124-126.
11. Adsersen A, Kjølbye A, Dall O, Jäger AK: Acetylcholinesterase and butyrylcholinesterase inhibitory compounds from *Corydalis cava* Schweigg. & Kort. J Ethnopharmacol 2007, 113:179-182.
12. Tome F, Colombo ML: Distribution of alkaloids in *Chelidonium majus* and factors affecting their accumulation. Phytochemistry 1995, 40:37-39.
13. Benninger J, Schneider HT, Schuppan D, Kirchner T, Hahn EG: Acute hepatitis induced by greater celandine (*Chelidonium majus*). Gastroenterology 1999, 117:1234-1237.
14. Stickel F, Pöschl G, Seitz HK, Waldherr R, Hahn EG, Schuppan D: Acute hepatitis induced by Greater Celandine (*Chelidonium majus*). Scand J Gastroenterol 2003, 38:565-568.
15. Nawrot R, Kalinowski A, Gozdzicka-Jozefiak A: Proteomic analysis of *Chelidonium majus* milky sap using two-dimensional gel electrophoresis and tandem mass spectrometry. Phytochemistry 2007, 68:1612-1622.

16. Nawrot R, Lesniewicz K, Pienkowska J, Gozdzicka-Jozefiak A: A novel extracellular peroxidase and nucleases from a milky sap of *Chelidonium majus* L. Fitoterapia 2007, 78:496-501.
17. Nawrot R, Wołuń-Cholewa M, Goździcka-Józefiak A: Nucleases isolated from *Chelidonium majus* L. milky sap can induce apoptosis in human cervical carcinoma HeLa cells but not in Chinese Hamster Ovary CHO cells. Folia Histochem Cytobiol 2008, 46:79-83.
18. Lowry OH, Rosebrough NJ, Farr AL, Randall RJ: Protein measurement with the Folin phenol reagent. J Biol Chem 1951, 193:265-275.
19. Laemmli UK: Cleavage of structural proteins during the assembly of the head of bacteriophage T4. Nature 1970, 227:680-685.
20. Shevchenko A, Wilm M, Vorm O, Mann M: Mass spectrometric sequencing of proteins silver-stained polyacrylamide gels. Anal Chem 1996, 68:850-858.
21. Thelen MP, Northcote DH: Identification and purification of a nuclease from Zinnia elegans L.: a potential molecular marker for xylogenesis. Planta 1989, 179:181-195.
22. Ito J, Fukuda H: ZEN1 is a key enzyme in the degradation of nuclear DNA during programmed cell death of tracheary elements. Plant Cell 2002, 14:3201-3211.
23. Perkins DN, Pappin DJ, Creasy DM, Cottrell JS: Probability-based protein identification by searching sequence databases using mass spectrometry data. Electrophoresis 1999, 20:3551-3567.
24. Sels J, Mathys J, De Coninck BM, Cammue BP, De Bolle MF: Plant pathogenesis-related (PR) proteins: a focus on PR peptides. Plant Physiol Biochem 2008, 46:941-950.
25. Olesen JM, Ehlers BK: Age determination of individuals of *Corydalis* species and other perennial herbs. Nord J Bot 2008, 21:187-194.
26. Maurer HR: Bromelain: biochemistry, pharmacology and medical use. Cell Mol Life Sci 2001, 58:1234-1245.
27. Kienle GS, Glockmann A, Schink M, Kiene H: Viscum album L. extracts in breast and gynaecological cancers: a systematic review of clinical and preclinical research. J Exp Clin Cancer Res 2009, 28:79.
28. Zhong J, Chau Y: Antitumor activity of a membrane lytic peptide cyclized with a linker sensitive to membrane type 1-matrix metalloproteinase. Mol Cancer Ther 2008, 7:2933-2940.
29. Shai Y: Mode of action of membrane active antimicrobial peptides. Biopolymers 2002, 66:236-248.

CHAPTER 7

ARCTIGENIN FROM *ARCTIUM LAPPA* INHIBITS INTERLEUKIN-2 AND INTERFERON GENE EXPRESSION IN PRIMARY HUMAN T LYMPHOCYTES

WEI-JERN TSAI, CHU-TING CHANG, GUEI-JANE WANG, TZONG-HUEI LEE, SHWU-FEN CHANG, SHAO-CHUN LU, AND YUH-CHI KUO

7.1 BACKGROUND

The central event in the generation of immune responses is the activation and clonal expansion of T cells. Interaction of T cells with antigens initiates a cascade of biochemical events and gene expression that induces the resting T cells to activate and proliferate [1]. Activation of nuclear factor of activated T cells (NF-AT) and a series of genes such as interleukin-2 (IL-2) and interferon-γ (IFN-γ) are pivotal in the growth of T lymphocytes induced by antigens [2,3]. Thus, growth modulators or other external events affecting T cell proliferation are likely to act by controlling the expression or function of the products of these genes [4]. The immune responses to invasive organisms, if inappropriately intense or prolonged, may paradoxically aggravate the injury or even cause death. The use of immunomodulatory medications must therefore be discreet. Regulation of

This chapter was originally published under the Creative Commons Attribution License. Tsai W-J, Chang C-T, Wang G-J, Lee T-H, Chang S-F, Lu S-C, and Kuo Y-C. Arctigenin from Arctium lappa *Inhibits Interleukin-2 and Interferon Gene Expression in Primary Human T Lymphocytes.* Chinese Medicine *6,12 (2011). doi:10.1186/1749-8546-6-12.*

T lymphocyte activation and proliferation and cytokine production is one of the action mechanisms [5,6].

Chinese medicinal herbs are now widely acknowledged for their immunomodulatory activities [1]. A member of the Compositae family, *Arctium lappa* (Niubang) is regarded as an effective Chinese medicine for alleviation of rheumatic pain and fever [7]. Arctigenin (AC), a bioactive component of *A. lappa*, has various biological activities including: (1) inhibition of nitric oxide, interlukin-6 and tumor necrosis factor-α production in macrophages [8,9]; (2) anti-proliferative activity against leukemia cells [10]; and (3) protective effects on hepatocytes from CCl_4 injury [11]. Definitive evidence for its effects on T cell-mediated immune responses has been scarce.

The present study aims to elucidate the effects of AC on T lymphocytes proliferation, production and gene expression of IL-2 and IFN-γ in T lymphocytes induced by anti-CD3/CD28 antibodies (Ab) and NF-AT activation.

7.2 METHODS

7.2.1 PREPARATION OF ARCTIGENIN (AC)

AC was isolated from dried ground of *A. lappa* L. by using reported methods [12]. Briefly, ground *A. lappa* (1 kg) was extracted with ethanol (2L × 3) at room temperature. The solvent was removed under reduced pressure and the residue was partitioned between H_2O and ethyl acetate (EtOAc). The concentrated EtOAc extracts (60 mg) were subjected to chromatography over silica gel and eluted with n-hexane/EtOAc (4:1), n-hexane/EtOAc (1:1) and EtOAc successively. AC (4.5 mg; $C_{21}H_{24}O_6$; MW 372; Figure 1) was purified from EtOAC fraction with bioassay-guided separation. Mass and NMR spectral data for this compound were identical with those previously reported [12]. AC, with the purity above 98%, was dissolved in dimethylsulfoxide (DMSO) to a concentration of 100 mM and then stored at 4°C until use.

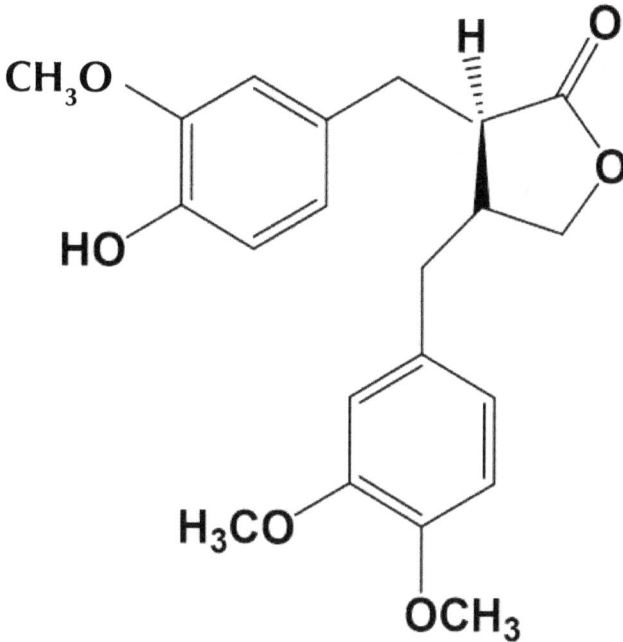

FIGURE 1: Chemical structure of AC.

7.2.2 PARTICIPANTS

Ten healthy male participants aged between 20 and 32 years (mean 26) were selected for this study. The experimental protocol were reviewed and approved by the institutional human experimentation committee of Fu-Jen University. Written informed consent was obtained from all participants.

7.2.3 PREPARATION OF PRIMARY HUMAN T LYMPHOCYTES

Heparinized human peripheral bloods (80 ml) were obtained from healthy donors. The peripheral blood was centrifuged at 850 × g (Sorvall Legend RT, Kendro, Germany) at 4°C for ten minutes to remove the plasma. The blood cells were diluted with phosphate buffered saline (PBS) and then centrifuged in a Ficoll-Hypaque discontinuous gradient (specific gravity 1.077) at $420 \times g$ (Sorvall Legend RT, Kendro, Germany) for 30 minutes. The peripheral blood mononuclear cell (PBMC) layers were collected and washed with cold distilled water and 10× Hanks' buffer saline solution (HBSS) to remove red blood cells. T lymphocytes were separated from PBMC by nylon wool columns (Wako Chemicals, USA). Purified T lymphocytes had >87% CD3+ cells and <0.5% CD14+ or CD19+ cells. The cells were re-suspended to a concentration of 2×10^6 cells/ml in RPMI-1640 medium supplemented with 2% fetal calf serum (FCS), 100 U/ml penicillin and 100 µg/ml streptomycin [4].

7.2.4 LYMPHOPROLIFERATION TEST

The lymphoproliferation test was modified from a previously described method [13]. Briefly, the density of T lymphocytes was adjusted to 2×10^6 cells/ml before use. Cell suspension (100 µl) was applied into each well of a 96-well flat-bottomed plate (Nunc 167008, Nunclon, Denmark) with or without anti-CD3 (1 µg/ml)/CD28 (3 µg/ml) antibody (eBioscience, USA). Cyclosporin A (CsA, 2.5 µM), an immuno-suppressor, was used as a reference drug [14]. AC was added to the cells at various concentrations (6.25, 12.5 and 25 µM). The plates were incubated in 5% CO_2-air humidified atmosphere at 37°C for three days. Subsequently, tritiated thymidine (1 µCi/well, New England Nuclear, USA) was added into each well. After incubated for 16 hours, the cells were harvested on glass fiber filters by an automatic harvester (Dynatech, Multimash 2000, UK). Radioactivity (counting per minute, CPM) in the filters was measured by a scintillation counter (LS 6000IC, Beckman Instruments Inc., USA). The inhibitory activity of AC on T lymphocytes proliferation was calculated according to the following formula:

Inhibitory activity (%) = [Control group (CPM) - Experiment group (CPM)]/ Control group (CPM) × 100%

7.2.5 DETERMINATION OF IL-2 AND IFN-γ PRODUCTION

Primary human T lymphocytes (2×10^5 cells/well) were cultured with anti-CD3/CD28 Ab alone or in combination with cyclosporin A (CsA) or various concentrations of AC for three days. The cell supernatants were then collected and assayed for IL-2 and IFN-γ concentrations by enzyme immunoassays (EIAs; R&D systems, USA).

7.2.6 DETERMINATION OF CELL VIABILITY

Resting or anti-CD3/CD28 Ab-activated T lymphocytes were cultured in a medium, namely DMSO (0.1%), or various concentrations of AC (6.25, 12.5 and 25 μM) for four days. After stained by trypan blue, total, viable and non-viable cell numbers were counted with a hemocytometer under microscope. The percentage of viable cells was calculated according to the following formula:

Viability (%) = (Viable Cell Number/Total Cell Number) × 100%

7.2.7 EXTRACTION OF TOTAL CELLULAR RNA

T lymphocytes (5×10^6) were activated with or without anti-CD3/CD28 Ab and co-cultured with 6.25, 12.5 or 25 μM of AC for 18 hours. T lymphocytes were collected and lysed by RNA-Bee™ (Tel-Test, USA). After centrifugation with $12000 \times g$ (Sigma 2K15, B Braun, Germany) at 4°C for 15 min, the supernatants were extracted with a phenol-chloroform mixture. The extracted RNA was precipitated with 100% cold ethanol. The total cellular RNA was pelleted by centrifugation and re-dissolved in diethyl pyrocarbonate (DEPC)-treated water. The concentration of RNA was calculated according to its optical density at 260 nm.

7.2.8 REVERSE TRANSCRIPTION-POLYMERASE CHAIN REACTION (RT-PCR)

RT-PCR was carried out according to a previously described method [15]. Briefly, RNA (1 μg) was reverse-transcribed to cDNA by the Advantage™ RT-for-PCR kit (Clontech, USA) according to the manufacturer's instructions. Briefly, 10 μl of cDNA was mixed with 0.75 μM primers, four units of Taq polymerase, 10 μl of reaction buffer consisting of 2 mM Tris-HCl (pH8.0), 0.01 mM ethylenediaminetetraacetate (EDTA), 0.1 mM dithiothreitol (DTT), 0.1% Triton X-100, 5% glycerol and 1.5 mM $MgCl_2$, and 25 μl of water making up a total volume of 50 μl. All primer pairs for the glyceraldehyde-3-phosphate dehydrogenase (GAPDH), IL-2, and IFN-γ were designed according to the published human cDNA sequence data (Table 1). Settings of the PCR thermocycler were as follows: denaturing at 94°C for 1 minute, annealing at 60°C for 1 minute and elongation at 72°C for 80 seconds for the first 35 cycles and finally elongation at 72°C for 10 minutes. After the reaction, the amplified products were run on 1.8% agarose gel for electrophoresis.

TABLE 1: Oligonucleotide sequences of the primers used for amplification of IL-2, IFN-γ and GAPDH mRNA in primary human T lymphocytes

Cytokine	Sequence	Predicted size (bp)
IL-2	5'-GTC ACA AAC AGT GCA CCT AC-3' 5'-GAA AGT GAA TTC TGG GTC CC-3'	262
IFN-γ	5'-GCA GAG CCA AAT TGT CTC CT-3' 5'-ATG CTC TTC GAC CTC GAA AC-3'	320
GAPDH	5': TGA AGG TCG GAG TCA ACG GAT TTG GT 3': CAT GTG GGC CAT GAG GTC CAC CAC	983

7.2.9 LUCIFERASE ASSAY

Jurkat cells (5×10^4) were transfected by pGL4.30 (luc2P/NFAT-RE/Hygro) with Lipofectamin™ 2000 (Invitrogen, USA) for 24 hours according to the manufacturer's instructions. Then, the cells were cultured with anti-CD3 (1 μg/ml)/CD28 (3 μg/ml) Ab in the presence or absence of AC (6.25,

12.5 and 25 μM) or CsA (2.5 μM) for four hours. Total cell lysates were extracted with 1× reporter lysis buffer (Promega, USA). Total cell lysates (10 μg) were used to determine luciferase activity by the Luciferase Assay System (Promega, USA).

7.2.10 STATISTICAL ANALYSIS

Data were presented as mean ± standard deviation (SD). The differences between groups were assessed with student's t test and corrected with the Bonferroni test. Correlations between AC concentration and activity parameters were calculated with Pearson product-moment correlation test. P < 0.05 was considered statistically significant.

7.3 RESULTS

7.3.1 EFFECTS OF AC ON PRIMARY HUMAN T LYMPHOCYTES PROLIFERATION

Using indicated concentrations of AC isolated from *A. lappa*, we treated resting cells or cells activated with anti-CD3/CD28 Ab. Cell proliferation was determined by tritiated thymidine uptake. As shown in Figure 2A, treatment with anti-CD3/CD28 Ab for three days increased cell proliferation by about 11-fold (P = 0.002). Neither the resting or the activated cells was affected by DMSO treatment in terms of the tritiated thymidine uptake. While AC had little effect on tritiated thymidine uptake in resting T lymphocytes, the enhanced uptake observed in the activated cells was significantly suppressed by 6.25, 12.5 and 25 μM AC (P = 0.006, P = 0.007 and P = 0.002 respectively). The inhibition of AC on the activated cells were in a dose-dependent manner (r = -0.963, P = 0.0374). At 6.25 μM, the inhibitory percentage of AC was 37.0 ± 5.0% on T lymphocytes proliferation activated by anti-CD3/CD28 Ab. The corresponding degree of inhibition for 12.5 μM was 52.1 ± 2.9% whereas that for 100 μM was

78.0 ± 4.0%. The IC50 of AC on activated primary human T lymphocytes proliferation was 15.7 ± 3.2 µM.

7.3.2 VIABILITY OF PRIMARY HUMAN T LYMPHOCYTES TREATED WITH VARIOUS CONCENTRATIONS OF AC

We examined the viabilities of resting or anti-CD3/CD28 activated T lymphocytes treated with 6.25, 12.5 and 25 µM respectively for four days. AC had no cytotoxicity, ie the viabilities of resting or activated cells were not significantly decreased after treatment with various concentrations of AC for four days (Figure 2B). In comparison with the medium-treated group, neither the viability of the resting T lymphocytes nor that of the anti-CD3/CD28-activated T lymphocytes was reduced by DMSO, indicating that decreased T lymphocytes proliferation by AC was not related to direct cytotoxicity.

7.3.3 EFFECTS OF AC ON IL-2 AND IFN-γ PRODUCTION IN PRIMARY HUMAN T LYMPHOCYTES

Production of IL-2 and IFN-γ is a hallmark of activated T lymphocytes [16]. To investigate whether AC affected IL-2 and IFN-γ productions in T lymphocytes, we stimulated the cells with anti-CD3/CD28 Ab in the presence or absence of various concentrations of AC (6.25, 12.5 and 25 µM) for three days. Supernatants were then collected and the productions of IL-2 and IFN-γ were determined with EIA. Treatment with anti-CD3/CD28 Ab for three days stimulated IL-2 and IFN-γ productions in primary human T lymphocytes by about 29-fold ($P = 0.004$) and 23-fold ($P = 0.006$) respectively (Figure 3). By contrast, the stimulated production of IL-2 and IFN-γ in activated primary human T lymphocytes was significantly suppressed by 6.25, 12.5 and 25 µM AC (IL-2: $P = 0.001$, $P = 0.001$ and $P = 0.001$ respectively; IFN-γ: $P = 0.001$, $P = 0.001$ and $P = 0.005$ respectively). The inhibitory activity of AC was in a dose-dependent manner (IL-2: $r=-0.972$, $P = 0.0278$; IFN-γ: $r = -0.936$, $P = 0.0642$). AC impaired IL-2 and IFN-γ productions in primary human T lymphoctyes induced by anti-CD3/CD28 Ab.

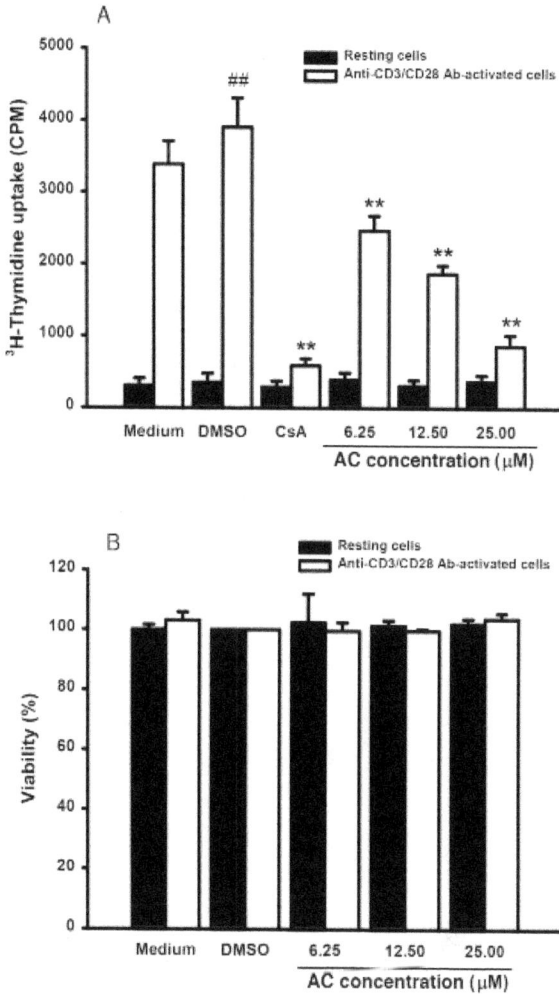

FIGURE 2: Effects of AC on cell proliferation and cell viability in primary human T lymphocytes. Primary human T lymphocytes (2 × 105/well) were stimulated with or without anti-CD3 (1 μg/ml)/CD28 (3 μg/ml) Ab and treated with medium, 0.1%DMSO, or the indicated concentration of AC, or CsA (2.5 μM). (A) After incubated for 72 hours, the proliferation of T lymphocytes was detected by tritiated thymidine uptake (1 μCi/well). After incubated for 16 hours, the cells were harvested by an automatic harvester, then radioactivity was measured by liquid scintillation counting. (B) After 96 hr incubation, T cells were harvested and numbers of total, viable, and nonviable cells were counted after trypan blue staining. Each bar represents the mean ± SD of three independent experiments. ## $P < 0.01$: vs. the cells treated with DMSO. ** $P < 0.01$: vs. the cells treated with DMSO and anti-CD3/CD28 Ab.

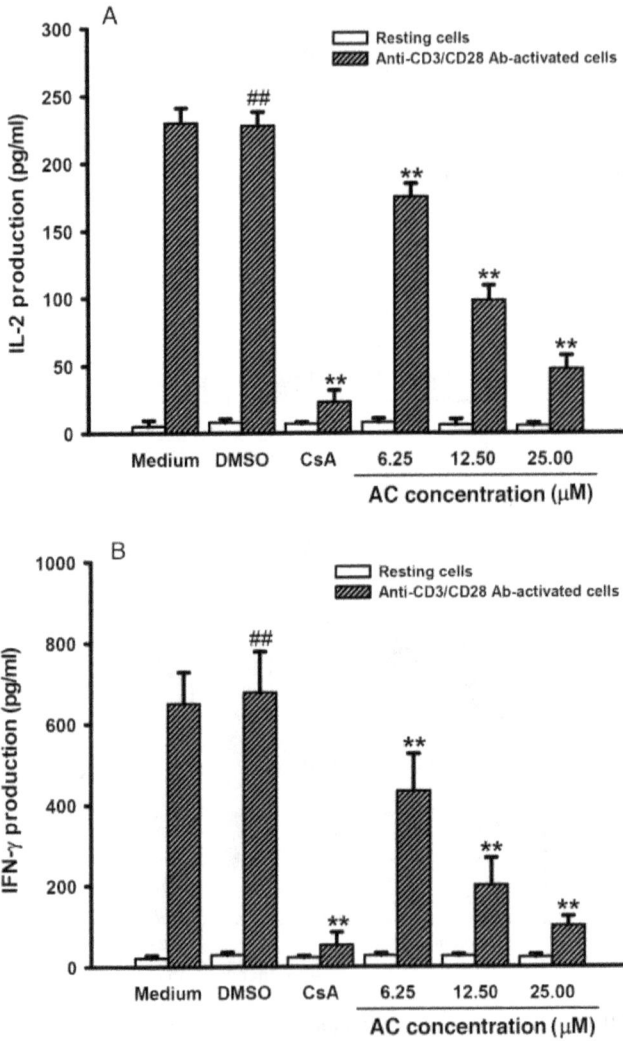

FIGURE 3: IL-2 and IFN-γ production in primary human T lymphocytes treated with AC. Primary human T lymphocytes C (2×10^5/well) were treated by 0, 6.25, 12.5 and 25 μM of AC or CsA (2.5 μM) with or without anti-CD3 (1 μg/ml)/CD28 (3 μg/ml) Ab for three days. Then the cell supernatants were collected and IL-2 and IFN-γ concentrations were determined by EIA, respectively. Each bar is the mean ± SD of three independent experiments. ## $P < 0.01$: vs. the cells treated with DMSO. ** $P < 0.01$: vs. the cells treated with DMSO and anti-CD3/CD28 Ab.

7.3.4 INHIBITORY EFFECTS OF AC ON IL-2 AND IFN-γ GENE EXPRESSION IN PRIMARY HUMAN T LYMPHOCYTES

To determine whether AC reduced IL-2 and IFN-γ production was related to gene expression, we extracted total cellular RNA from activated primary human T lymphocytes in the presence or absence of AC for 18 hours, ready for RT-PCR. The results of RT-PCR are in Figure 4. The mRNA for GAPDH was detectable in the samples treated with medium (Lane 1), DMSO (0.1%; Lane 2), AC (6.25, 12.5 and 25 μM; Lanes 3 to 5), anti-CD3/CD28 Ab (Lane 6), DMSO and anti-CD3/CD28 Ab (Lane 7), and AC and anti-CD3/CD28 Ab (Lanes 8 to 10) respectively (Figure 4A and 4B). The results indicated that the levels of IL-2 (P = 0.003) and IFN-γ (P = 0.001) mRNA in T lymphocytes were significantly induced by anti-CD3/CD28 Ab. By contrast, PCR products for both cytokines amplified from activated T lymphocytes RNA preparations were reduced by AC. The laser densitometry analysis demonstrated that the ratio of IL-2 to GAPDH mRNAs in anti-CD3/CD28 Ab-activated T lymphocytes were significantly decreased by 6.25, 12.5 and 25 μM AC (P = 0.001, P = 0.001 and P = 0.001 respectively). AC (25 μM) also significantly ameliorated the ratio of IFN-γ to GAPDH mRNAs in activated T lymphocytes (P = 0.001). Thus, AC inhibited IL-2 and IFN-γ production.

7.3.5 INHIBITORY EFFECTS OF AC ON NF-AT ACTIVATION

We used the luciferase assay to determine effects of AC on one major transcription factor, NF-AT, induced by CD3/CD28 signaling and involved in IL-2 and IFN-γ gene regulation [17]. The reporter cells, Jurkat cells transfected with pGL4.30 (luc2P/NFAT-RE/Hygro), were cultured in the presence of AC (6.25, 12.5 and 25 μM) for four hours. The cellular proteins were then extracted from the cells and subjected to the luciferase activity assay. As shown in Figure 5, anti-CD3/CD28 Ab induced a 4.6-fold increase in luciferase activity (P = 0.001) whereas the vehicle (0.1% DMSO) did not affect this induction. CsA significantly interrupted the luciferase activity in activated T cells (P = 0.001). However, treatment with 6.25, 12.5 and 25 μM of AC significantly decreased the luciferase activity of anti-CD3/CD28 Ab-activated cells in a dose-dependent manner (r = -0.958, P = 0.0418). Thus, AC modulated NF-AT activation.

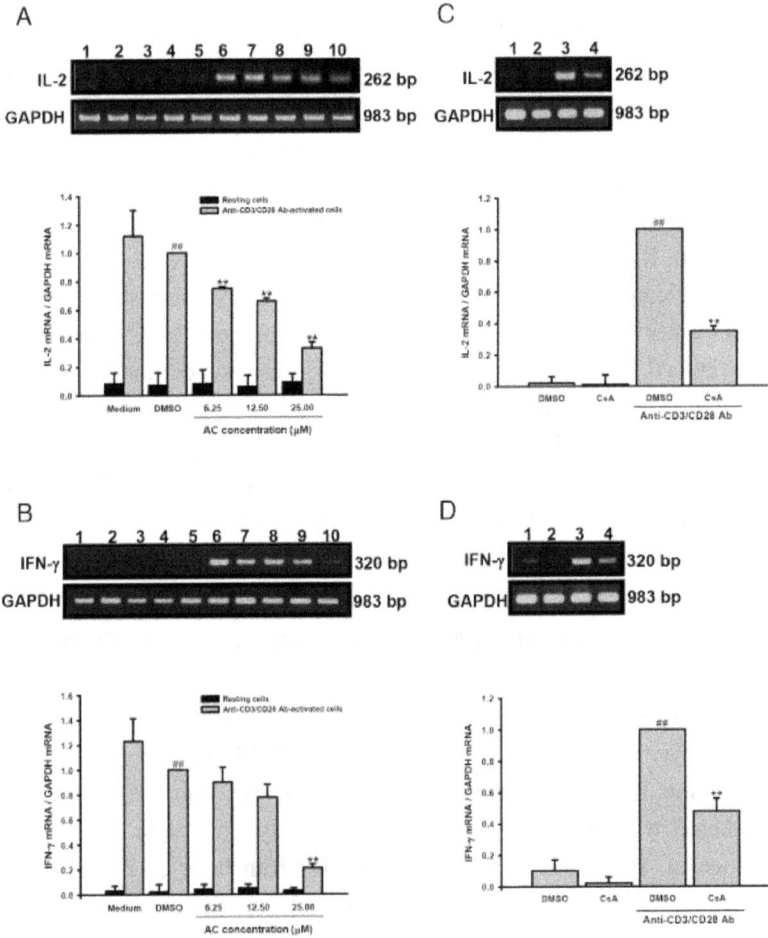

FIGURE 4: Effects of AC on IL-2 and IFN-γ transcripts in primary human T lymphocytes induced by anti-CD3/CD28 Ab. Primary human T lymphocytes (5×10^6) activated with or without anti-CD3 (1 μg/ml)/CD28 (3 μg/ml) Ab in the presence or absence of 6.25, 12.5 or 25 μM AC or CsA (2.5 μM) for 18 hr. The total cellular RNA was isolated from T lymphocytes and aliquots of 1 μg of RNA were reverse-transcribed for synthesis of cDNA. Briefly, 10 μl of cDNA was applied for the PCR test. The PCR was done as described in Materials and Methods. After the reaction, the amplified product was taken out of the tubes and run on 2% agarose gel. (A) and (B): Lane 1 - medium, Lane 2 - 0.1% DMSO, Lanes 3 to 5 - 6.25, 12.5 and 25 μM AC, Lane 6 - anti-CD3/CD28 Ab, Lane 7 - DMSO and anti-CD3/CD28 Ab, Lanes 8 to 10 - 6.25, 12.5 or 25 μM AC and anti-CD3/CD28 Ab. (C) and (D): Lane 1 - 0.1% DMSO, Lane 2 - CsA, Lane 3 - DMSO and anti-CD3/CD28 Ab, Lane 4 - CsA and anti-CD3/CD28 Ab. Graphical representation of laser densitometry of IL-2 and IFN-γ mRNA expression in resting or anti-CD3/CD28 Ab-stimulated PBMC in the presence or absence of AC or CsA. Each band was quantitated using laser-scanning densitometer SLR-2D/1D (Biomed Instruments, USA). The ratio of each cytokine mRNA to GAPDH mRNA was calculated. Each bar is the mean ± SD of three independent experiments. ## $P < 0.01$: vs. the cells treated with DMSO. ** $P < 0.01$: vs. the cells treated with DMSO and anti-CD3/CD28 Ab.

7.3.6 EFFECTS OF CSA ON IL-2, IFN-γ AND CELL PROLIFERATION IN T LYMPHOCYTES ACTIVATED WITH ANTI-CD3/CD28 AB

To determine whether AC decreased NF-AT activation, gene expression of IL-2 and IFN-γ and cell proliferation in T lymphocytes, we added CsA (2.5 μM), an NF-AT inhibitor, into T lymphocytes and analyzed gene expression of IL-2 and IFN-γ as well as cell proliferation. While IL-2 ($P = 0.001$) and IFN-γ mRNA ($P = 0.002$) were significantly induced in anti-CD3/CD28 Ab-activated T lymphocytes, CsA signigicantly blocked IL-2 ($P = 0.001$) and IFN-γ ($P = 0.008$) expression in the cells (Figures 4C and 4D). CsA also significantly reduced IL-2 ($P = 0.001$) and IFN-γ ($P = 0.003$) production in the activated cells (Figures 3A and 3B). Furthermore, the T lymphocyte proliferation stimulated by anti-CD3/CD28 Ab was significantly suppressed by CsA (Figure 2A; $P = 0.003$).

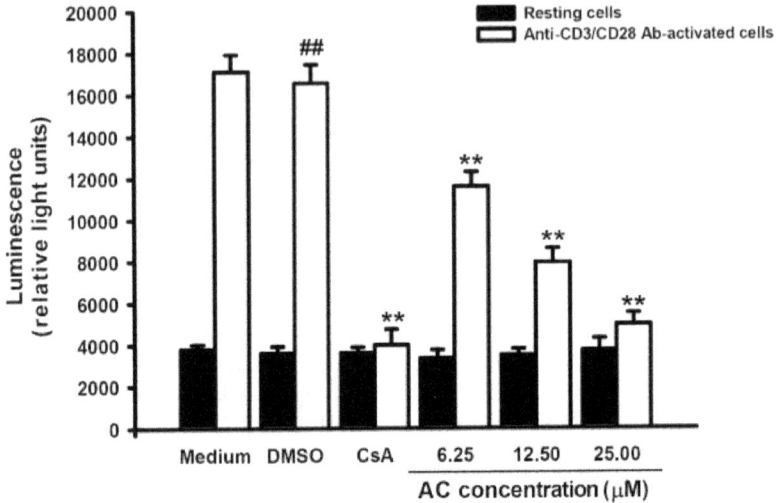

FIGURE 5: Effects of AC on NF-AT activation. Jurkat cells (5×10^4) were transfected with pGL4.30 (luc2P/NFAT-RE/Hygro) by Lipofectamin™ 2000 (Invitrogen, USA) for 24 hours according to the manufacturer's instructions. Then, the cells were cultured with anti-CD3 (1 μg/ml)/CD28 (3 μg/ml) Ab in the presence or absence of AC (6.25, 12.5 and 25 μM) or CsA (2.5 μM) for four hours. Total cell lysates were extracted with 1× reporter lysis buffer (Promega, USA), then 10 μg of total cell lysates were used to determine luciferase activity by the Luciferase Assay System (Promega, USA). Each bar is the mean ± SD of three independent experiments. ## $P < 0.01$: vs. the cells treated with DMSO. ** $P < 0.01$: vs. the cells treated with DMSO and anti-CD3/CD28 Ab.

7.4 DISCUSSION

Several pharmacological effects were identified in *A. lappa* such as antibacterial infection, scavenging free radicals [18], binding platelet-activating factors [19] and inhibiting acute ear swelling [20]. This study showed that AC from *A. lappa* had a profound inhibitory effect on the proliferation of primary human T lymphocytes stimulated by anti-CD3/CD28 Ab. The proliferation-suppressive actions of AC were not explained by a drug-induced reduction in cell viability. We observed that AC decreased production and mRNA expression of IL-2 and IFN-γ and activation of NF-AT in human T lymphocytes induced by anti-CD3/CD28 Ab.

Apart from *A. lappa*, AC is found in various plants such as *Bardanae fructus, Saussurea medusa, Torreya nucifera* and *Lepomea cairica*. AC prevents leukocytes from recruitment into the inflamed tissue [21]. AC blocks TNF-α production by impairments of AP-1 activation [9]. The present study demonstrated that AC suppressed proliferation and IL-2 and IFN-γ production in primary human T lymphocytes activated by anti-CD3/CD28 Ab. AC is a potent inducer of apoptosis for HL-60 T leukemia cells, MH60 B lymphoma cells and SW480 colon cancer cells [22]. Thus, we could not rule out the possibility that AC inhibited the proliferation of primary human T lymphocytes via the apoptosis pathway. The possible inhibitory effect of DMSO on primary human T lymphocytes was also studied in these experiments. The cell proliferation and viability were not changed by DMSO. Therefore, the inhibitory function of AC was unlikely related to DMSO.

Interaction of T lymphocytes with antigens initiates a cascade of genes expression such as IL-2 and IFN-γ mRNA inducing the resting T cells to proliferate [23]. This study showed that AC inhibited IL-2 and IFN-γ productions in primary human T lymphocytes stimulated by anti-CD3/CD28 Ab. The impairments of IL-2 and IFN-γ production were related to the suppression of their mRNA transcriptions by AC. Since T lymphocyte proliferation is primarily mediated by IL-2, inhibition of IL-2 production is a central mechanism of action of several immunosuppressants such as CsA. This study also demonstrated that CsA inhibited IL-2 and IFN-γ gene expression and cell proliferation in primary human T lymphocytes induced by anti-CD3/CD28 Ab, suggesting that AC actions are similar to those of CsA which induces arrest activation and proliferation of T cells by inhibiting IL-2 transcription [14]. Furthermore, the preliminary data from immunofluorescence staining indicated that AC had no effect on IL-2 receptor expression in primary human T lymphocytes activated by anti-CD3/CD28 Ab (data not shown), suggesting that the reduction of proliferation in AC-treated T lymphocytes was not caused by down-regulation of IL-2 receptor expression. Failure to produce IL-2 and IFN-γ may be the reason why primary human T lymphocytes do not proliferate.

NF-AT is a major player in the control of T lymphocytes activation and proliferation [2]. After anti-CD3/CD28 Ab stimulation, calcium-dependent phosphatase calcineurin binds to NF-AT, dephosphorylates NF-AT and causes nuclear import of NF-AT. The binding domain of NF-AT is Rel similarity domain located in numerous cytokine promoters. IL-2 and IFN-γ gene expressions in T lymphocytes are controlled by NF-AT-dependent promoters/enhancers [24]. This study found that AC decreased NF-AT activation. NF-AT is a target for the immunosuppressants CsA and FK506 which are efficient inhibitors of T cell activation [14]. This study also demonstrated that CsA blocked NF-AT activation, suggesting that AC inhibited IL-2 and IFN-γ production and cell proliferation in primary human T lymphocytes by modulation of NF-AT activation. Interleukin-10 is mainly produced by regulatory T lymphocytes and regulates other immune cells [24]. We also showed that AC (25 μM) did not affect IL-10 production in primary human T lymphocytes induced by anti-CD3/CD28 Ab (453 ± 88 vs. 412 ± 75pg/ml).

7.5 CONCLUSION

AC inhibited T lymphocyte proliferation and decreased the gene expression of IL-2, IFN-γ and NF-AT.

REFERENCES

1. Kuo YC, Yang NS, Chou CJ, Lin LC, Tsai WJ: Regulation of cell proliferation, gene expression, production of cytokines and cell cycle progression in primary human T lymphocytes by piperlactam S isolated from Piper kadsura. Mol Pharmacol 2000, 58:1057-1066.
2. Rao A, Luo C, Hogan PG: Transcription factors of the NFAT family: regulation and function. Annu Rev Immunol 1997, 15:707-747.
3. Rochman Y, Spolski R, Leonard WJ: New insights into the regulation of T cells by gamma (c) family cytokines. Nat Rev Immunol 2009, 9:480-490.
4. Kuo YC, Weng SC, Chou CJ, Chang TT, Tsai WJ: Activation and proliferation signals in primary human T lymphocytes inhibited by ergosterol peroxide isolated from Cordyceps cicadae. Br J Pharmacol 2003, 140:895-906.
5. Hoyer KK, Dooms H, Barron L, Abbas AK: Interleukin- in the development and control of inflammatory disease. Immunol Rev 2008, 226:19-28.

6.　Liu CP, Kuo YC, Lin YL, Liao JF, Shen CC, Chen CF, Tsai WJ: (S)-Armepavine inhibits human peripheral blood mononuclear cells activation by regulating Itk and PLCγ activation in a PI3K-dependent manner. J Leukoc Biol 2007, 81:1276-1286.

7.　Holetz FB, Pessini GL, Sanches NR, Cortez DA, Nakamura CV, Filho BP: Screening of some plants used in the Brazilian folk medicine for the treatment of infectious diseases. Mem Inst Oswaldo Cruz 2002, 97:1027-1031.

8.　Zhao F, Wang L, Liu K: *In vitro* anti-inflammatory effects of arctigenin, a lignan from *Arctium lappa* L., through inhibition on iNOS pathway. J Ethnopharmacol 2009, 122:457-462.

9.　Cho MK, Jang YP, Kim YC, Kim SG: Arctigenin, a phenylpropanoid dibenzylbutyrolactone lignan, inhibits MAP kinases and AP-1 activation via potent KK inhibition: the role in TNF-alpha inhibition. Int Immunopharmacol 2004, 4:1419-1429.

10.　Matsumoto T, Hosono-Nishiyama K, Yamada H: Antiproliferative and apoptotic effects of butyrolactone lignans from *Arctium lappa* on leukemic cells. Planta Med 2006, 72:276-278.

11.　Kim SH, Jang YP, Sung SH, Kim CJ, Kim JW, Kim YC: Hepatoprotective dibenzylbutyrolactone lignans of Torreya nucifera against CCl4-induced toxicity in primary cultured rat hepatocytes. Biol Pharm Bull 2003, 26:1202-1205.

12.　Liu S, Chen K, Schliemann W, Strack D: Isolation and identification of arctiin and arctigenin in leaves of Burdock (Arcticum lappa L.) by polyamide column chromatography in combination with HPLC-ESI/MS. Phytochem Anal 2005, 16:86-89.

13.　Wu MH, Tsai WJ, Don MJ, Chen YC, Kuo YC: Tanshinlactone A from Salvia miltiorrhiza modulates interleukin-2 and interferon-γ gene expression. J Ethnopharmacol 2007, 113:210-217.

14.　Schreiber SL, Crabtree GR: The mechanism of action of cyclosporin A and FK 506. Immunol Today 1992, 13:136-142.

15.　Chen YC, Tsai WJ, Wu MH, Lin LC, Kuo YC: Suberosin inhibits human peripheral blood mononuclear cells proliferation through the modulation of NF-AT and NF-κB transcription factors. Br J Pharmacol 2007, 150:298-312.

16.　Seko Y, Cole S, Kasprzak W, Shapiro BA, Ragheb JA: The role of cytokine mRNA stability in the pathogenesis of autoimmune disease. Autoimmun Rev 2006, 5:299-305.

17.　Crabtree GR: Contingent genetic regulatory events in T lymphocyte activation. Science 1989, 243:355-361.

18.　Lin CC, Lu JM, Yang JJ, Chuang SC, Ujiie T: Anti-inflammatory and radical scavenge effects of Articum lappa. Am J Chin Med 1996, 24:127-137.

19.　Iwakami S, Wu JB, Ebizuka Y, Sankawa U: Platelet activating factor (PAF) antagonists contained in medicinal plants: lignans and sesquiterpenes. Chem Pharm Bull (Tokyo) 1992, 40:1196-1198.

20.　Knipping K, van Esch ECAM, Wijering SC, van der Heide S, Dubois AE, Garsen J: *In vitro* and in vivo anti-allergic effects of *Arctium lappa*. Exp Biol Med 2008, 233:1469-1477.

21.　Kang HS, Lee JY, Kim CJ: Anti-inflammatory activity of arctigenin from Forsythiae fructus. J Ethnopharmacol 2008, 116:305-312.

22. Yoo JH, Lee HJ, Kang K, Jho EH, Kim CY, Baturen D, Tunsag J, Nho CW: Lignans inhibit cell growth via regulation of Wnt/beta-catenin signaling. Food Chem Toxicol 2010, 48:2247-2252.

23. Arai K, Lee F, Miyajima A: Cytokines: Coordinators of immune and inflammatory response. Annu Rev Biochem 1990, 59:783-836.

24. Serfling E, Berberich-Siebelt F, Chuvpilo S, Jankevics E, Klein-Hessling S, Twardzik T, Avots A: The role of NF-AT transcription factors in T cell activation and differentiation. Biochim Biophys Acta 2000, 1498:1-18.

PART II

TARGETING IMPORTANT DISEASES USING NATURAL PRODUCTS (TK OR NON-TK BASED)

CHAPTER 8

A NEW DAWN FOR THE USE OF TRADITIONAL CHINESE MEDICINE IN CANCER THERAPY

HARENDRA S. PAREKH, GANG LIU, AND MING Q. WEI

8.1 INTRODUCTION

Reports of therapeutic success with traditional Chinese medicine (TCM) have until very recently been met with much scepticism and pessimism by the West, due in-part to the sheer lack of available credible and rigorous clinical data and at claims that a given TCM can remedy common ailments and be just as efficacious in eliminating life threatening diseases, such as cancer. The tide is now beginning to turn on this negative outlook, aided by the ever-increasing migration of people and along with them knowledge (based upon ancestral cultural influences) from two of the world's fasting growing populations, China and India, to the West [1]. This translation to the West of ancient complementary and alternative medicine formularies and their ever-increasing integrative role in the armoury against cancer means that their presence and place in modern medicine can no longer be overlooked, by regulatory authorities and clinicians alike, as being merely anecdotal.

This chapter was originally published under the Creative Commons Attribution License. Parekh HS, Liu G, and Wei MQ. A New Dawn for the Use of Traditional Chinese Medicine in Cancer Therapy. Molecular Cancer 8,21 (2009). doi:10.1186/1476-4598-8-21.

The age-old holistic approach employed by Chinese practitioners proposes that a multitude of events are key to returning a patient to a healthy state; where cancer therapy is concerned these primarily include an interplay between the induction of apoptosis/cell-cycle arrest, inhibition of angiogenesis, overcoming multidrug resistance (MDR), and boosting the immune system (Figure 1). Following an extensive review of the literature we describe the detailed molecular basis of a proven group of TCM, and highlight reported synergies when administered alongside so-called 'conventional therapies' in tumour cell regulation and in bringing about homeostasis.

The many physiological growth control mechanisms that regulate cell proliferation and tissue homeostasis are linked to apoptosis and it follows that resistance developed to this 'programmed cell death' can be directly linked to prolonged tumour cell survival and resistance to therapy [2,3]. The processes resulting in apoptosis are mediated by extrinsic (via death receptors) or intrinsic (via mitochondrial) pathways and although their paths are not mutually exclusive, evidence suggests the latter certainly predominates where TCM is concerned [4]. Here we look in some detail at two of the primary mechanisms—'apoptosis' and 'angiogenesis' in the context of TCM, proposed to be key avenues responsible for imparting therapeutic efficacy against a wide range of cancers.

8.1.1 MOLECULAR BASIS OF TCM: APOPTOSIS

Apoptosis is guided by a range of complex multi-step, multi-pathway programs that eventuate in the breakdown of cellular DNA leading to cell death [5]. And by far the most emphasized and reported endpoint in TCM trials to-date have been those of cell cycle arrest and apoptosis [6,7]. The cascade of intracellular events triggering cell death have been identified to involve activation or suppression of a number of key receptors, genes and enzymes [8]. The mitochondria, a cell's energy source, is recognized as playing a central role in the sustained survival of cells and many of the triggers to apoptosis are known to act here, either directly or indirectly [9,10].

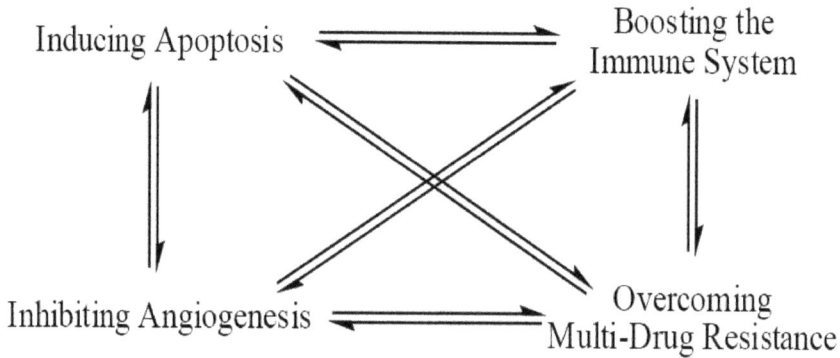

FIGURE 1: The complex interplay between the primary mechanisms of TCM.

8.1.2 APOPTOSIS BY THE 'CASPASE' EFFECT

Of the pro-apoptotic enzymes implicated in TCM activity the family of cysteine proteases, commonly termed 'caspases' are key players with their role and function extensively reviewed elsewhere [2,3,10]. Briefly, caspases are divided into two broad groups, the 'initiators' and the 'executioners' and once activated they go on to activate other pro-caspases that trigger apoptosis. The primary role of 'initiator' caspases (caspase-8, -9 & -10) is the processing and activation of both pro-enzymes (procaspase-8, -9 & -10) and 'executioner' caspases (mainly caspase-3, -6, & -7) [2]. Pro-caspases are inactive forms of their cousins, the caspases, and any processing of these pro-enzymes is regarded as a reliable marker for caspase activation, and so apoptosis. It is the result of 'executioner' caspases cleaving each other that triggers an amplifying proteolytic cascade, effecting cleavage/degradation of cellular substrates—these aptly named 'death' substrates are responsible for signalling biochemical and morphological changes that eventuate in cell death [11].

8.1.3 APOPTOSIS BY NF-KB

Cellular stress is invoked by an imbalance in a cell's redox state. Nuclear factor-κB (NF-κB) is a key regulatory molecule, activated when a cell experiences oxidative stress [12]. It is well-documented that tumour necrosis factor-α (TNF-α) and the closely related tumour necrosis factor-related apoptosis ligand (TRAIL) along with lipopolysaccharides, interleukins (IL) and UV or IR radiation all impart cellular stress that triggers the NF-κB cascade [13,14]. NF-κB ordinarily resides in the cytosol of non-stressed cells, non-covalently bound to the family of inhibitory-κB (IκB) proteins which function to mask the nuclear localization signal (NLS) present on NF-κB. When the redox balance of the cell is perturbed by extracellular stimuli, IκBs are rapidly degraded exposing the NLS. The consequence is transfer of NF-κB to the nucleus where it regulates gene expression, the products of which are directly involved in tumorigenesis [15,16].

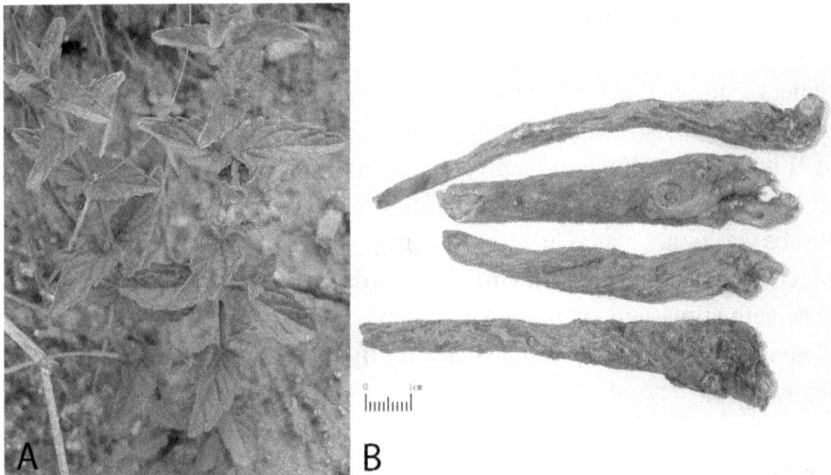

FIGURE 2: Plant (A) and root (B) of Scutellaria Baicalensis ('golden root') where root scale is shown as 1 cm.

8.1.4 APOPTOSIS BY TCM

Numerous studies have been aimed at deciphering the precise molecular basis for a variety of TCM and those most noteworthy are discussed below.

The root of *Scutellaria baicalensis* (Figure 2), commonly referred to as 'Baikal skullcap', 'Huang qin' or the 'Golden Root', is probably one of the most widely used herbs in TCM preparations with its flavonoid-rich elements considered to impart anti-inflammatory, anti-viral, anti-bacterial and anti-neoplastic activity [17-20].

It is also one of the most widely studied by researchers, being used either alone or more often in combination with other TCM for a range of cancers (*in vitro* and in vivo), namely of the prostate, breast, lung, liver and ovaries [6,21-23]. The roots chief therapeutic ingredient is baicalin, although it is converted to baicalein by intestinal gut flora with this latter bioactive firmly considered to be the primary active constituent responsible for its pro-apoptotic and anti-proliferative effects [21]. Extensive studies reveal that other flavonoids present within the herb e.g. neobaicalein, wogonin and wogonoside are also at work and that their co-synergies most likely contribute to the observed efficacy [24]. The principle mechanism of action of *Scutellaria baicalensis* is via the inhibition of eicosanoid synthesis—being important mediators of pro-inflammatory (cyclooxygenase-2 (Cox-2)) and tumour cell proliferatory (lipoxygenase) markers [25]. Simultaneous inhibition of Cox-2 and 12-lipooxygenase has been shown to result in both reduced inflammation and tumorigenesis [25,26]. The role of baicalein against cell proliferation in PC-3 and DU145 prostate cancer cell lines is that of cell cycle arrest (at G_0-G_1) while also inducing apoptosis—confirmed via detection of caspase-3, at concentrations typical for administration to humans [27].

Further evidence of TCM acting via caspase activation and NF-κB also exists with Takrisodokyeum (TRSDY)—comprising 12 herbs in various proportions [28]. Caspase-3 activity assays conducted by Kwon et al on promyelocytic leukeamic cells (HL-60) cells pre-treated with TRSDY revealed that apoptotic cell death was indeed caspase-3 induced [27]. Its activation resulting in classical apoptotic signs including DNA fragmentation, chromatin condensation and plasma membrane blebbing [29,30]. Introduction of a caspase-3 inhibitor resulted in no detectable caspase-3 production and the downfield cleavage of cellular death substrates was also absent. It was further identified that oxidative stress by way of hydrogen peroxide generation was a co-contributor to apoptosis in the same population of cells. In an attempt to elucidate which of caspase-3 or hydrogen peroxide was generated first, cells were pre-treated with an antioxidant and scavenger, quenching any oxidative agent. Levels of caspase-3 were found to be negligible in this case, strengthening the hypothesis that caspase-3 activation does not take place in these cells without prior oxidative stress [31,32]. Whether intracellular events leading to apoptosis follow this sequence of events in other cancer cell lines using this or other TCM is yet to be determined although parallel studies using other TCM do concur that activity is via selective members of the caspase family, namely caspase-3 [33-36].

TRAIL has received considerable attention by researchers since the discovery that most cancer cells are sensitive to its apoptotic effect but that normal cells confer resistance to it [37]. The potential of TRAIL as a realistic future therapy against cancer was further encouraged by the discovery that conventional therapy, namely chemotherapy or γ-irradiation can sensitize cells previously resistant to TRAIL [38-40]. The bioactive Triptolide (PG490)—extracted from the TCM *Tripterygium wilfordii* has been studied extensively for anti-inflammatory and immunosuppressive activity, being shown to sensitize various types of tumour cells to apoptosis induced by TRAIL, TNF-α and chemotherapy [41-44]. A study conducted by Frese et al evaluating PG490 suggests that it sensitizes previously resistant Calu-1 lung cancer cell lines to TRAIL-induced apoptosis while sparing normal human bronchial epithelial cells [42]. PG490-mediated sensitization of the cells to TRAIL requires activation of a family of extracellular-regulated protein kinases (ERK's), namely ERK-1. Located in the intracellular environment ERK-1 is thought to be the crucial link bridging the process that follows death receptor activation and precedes caspase activation. TRAIL, acting via death receptors (TRAIL-R1 & R2) forms a death-inducing signalling complex (DISC); this then recruits an 'initiator', caspase-8, which begins a cascade of protease activation enlisting the 'executioner'—caspase-3, promoting cleavage of death substrates with the end-point being cell death. [45-47]. Carter et al confirmed the role of PG490 in apoptosis and went further to highlight that mitochondria, and not the death receptor, predominate in PG490 activity in mouse embryonic fibroblasts, due to caspase-9 activation [48]. This contradicted the findings of Frese et al where caspase-8 was found to be the key pro-enzyme in triggering apoptosis highlighting that mechanistic variability indeed exists with TCM as would be expected, thus caution must be taken when making any broad claims relating to their precise mechanism of action [42]. Synergistic induction of apoptosis has also been observed when chemotherapeutic agents are employed together with PG490, further corroborating the case for TCM use with conventional anticancer agents [48].

All cancer cells possess an elevated apoptotic threshold and although the therapeutic interventions of chemotherapy and γ-irradiation are crucial they are commonly plagued with resistance, resulting in a cycle of remission and relapse. The ever-rising incidence of resistance to chemotherapy suggests an increase in this apoptotic threshold and so the challenge is whether it can be reduced sufficiently to break the cycle at the point of remission. Advances made in recognizing and activating the key molecules involved in apoptotic pathways are certainly very encouraging from the perspective of eradicating a tumour although resistance to these interventions are also emerging [49]. The growing acceptance of TCM as a real adjunct therapy makes it an invaluable tool in the fight against many cancers and it holds much promise especially in cases where resistance to therapy is prevalent.

8.1.5 MOLECULAR BASIS OF TCM: ANGIOGENESIS

Angiogenesis—the creation of a healthy vascularised network by a tumour is a key underlying process in the induction and establishment of cancer [50]. It, like apoptosis, involves multi-step biochemical interactions that require activation of cell-signalling pathways, supply of nutrients and a host immune response. A range of TCM such as the Chinese wormwood (*Artemisia absinthium*—Figure 3), turmeric (*Curcuma longa*—Figure 4) and *Scutellaria baicalensis* are commonly employed by traditional practitioners and studies demonstrate that their actions are at least in-part achieved by blocking the critical process of tumour vascularisation [51]. In order for cancer cells to grow and develop a healthy network of blood vessels high sources of nutrients and oxygen are vital. The rapidly dividing cells are subject to a hypoxic environment, so failure to set-up this fundamental framework results in stunted growth of the tumour ($\leq$ 1–2 mm) and development of necrosis at its core [52,53]. Starving an established tumour of its blood supply involves an intervention in the complex angiogenic cascade, of which vascular endothelial growth factor (VEGF) is the most reported biomarker [54]. VEGF production is considered essential for angiogenesis and cancer metastasis, with high titres being indicative of a poor prognosis [55]. A wide array of oncogenes (e.g. ras, HER-2, p53 and C-jun) and growth factors (EGF, TGF, IGF and PDGF) have been identified as up-regulating VEGF-mRNA and so TCM that inhibits their expression and production, respectively, are also considered invaluable tools in cancer therapy.

Artemisinin, an active constituent of Chinese wormwood (*Artemisia absinthium*—Figure 3) is a potent antimalarial, however more recently it has been shown to possess anti-angiogenic properties, acting by lowering both VEGF and its receptor (VEGF-R2(in embryo), KDR(in humans) and flk-1(in mice)) in tumour and endothelial cells in a dose-dependent manner [56-59].

Phytochemicals have long been used as 'lead compounds' to generate drugs with better pharmacokinetic profiles and reduced toxicity in vivo. Artesunate (ART) and dihydro-ART are semi-synthetic derivatives of artemisinin with demonstrable activity against a wide range of cancer cell lines including KML-562 (chronic myeloid leukaemia), HeLa (cervical cancer) and HO-8910 (ovarian cancer) [60-62]. Human umbilical vein endothelial cells (HUVECs) are commonly employed alongside cancer cell assays to assess the extent to which angiogenesis is induced by way of new micro-vessel tube formation. Studies using this model show that dihydro-ART has significant anti-angiogenic activity compared to ART and prevents new-microvessel formation by 70–90% *in vitro* [61]. Along with the low toxicity profile associated with these agents their future role to complement treatment regimes is encouraging and warrants further investigation.

Curcumin (*Curcuma longa*—Figure 4), the principle curcuminoid in turmeric and widely used culinary spice is cytotoxic to cancer cells on a number of levels with a proven synergy when used in combination with

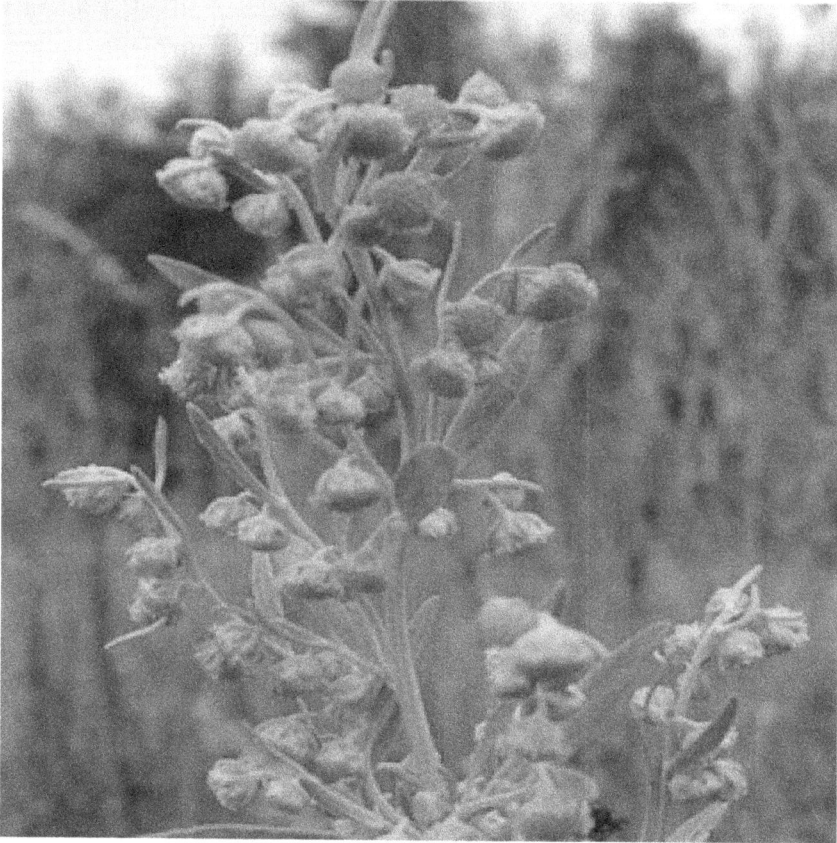

FIGURE 3: Plant of *Artemisia absinthium* ('Chinese wormwood').

chemotherapy/radiotherapy [63-65]. Its angioinhibitory action has been substantiated in a number of cancer cell lines including that of the breast where it was found to inhibit two major angiogenic factors, VEGF and b-FGF (basic-fibroblast growth factor) [66,67]. Besides this it also impedes tumour cell invasion, a property found to diminish circulating but not established metastases. It does this via downregulation of matrix metallo-proteinases (MMP), most notably MMP-2 & MMP-9 – responsible for the invasive growth property of tumours [68-70]. In Ehrlich ascites tumour (EAT) cells a time-dependent inhibition of VEGF and key growth factor angiopoietin was observed, combined with an anti-proliferative effect on

HUVECs, this being attributed directly to VEGF and NF-κB inhibition [71,72]. Other reported actions of curcumin include inhibition of epidermal growth factor receptor (EGFR) and intracellular signalling tyrosine kinases, the latter of which are known to promote angiogenesis through gene activation of cyclooxygenase-2, IL-2 and MMPs [73-75]. Derivatives of curcumin have also being investigated with preliminary findings pointing towards an increase in antitumor activity, although further corroborative studies are necessary to confirm these findings [76-78].

TCM often possess quite distinct and specialised modes of action, and consequently tumours normally resistant to conventional chemotherapy are reported to be more susceptible to TCM therapy [79]. They have demonstrable and often direct inhibitory effects on tumour cell growth and proliferation, affecting different stages of the cell growth cycle and mitotic phase [80]. Herbal compounds such as paclitaxel (Taxol®) and its derivatives suppress microtubule depolymerization, thus terminating cell mitosis [81]. As a result these, and compounds including harringtonine (*Cephalotaxus hainanensis*) and camptothecin (*Camptotheca acuminata*) with similar mechanisms of action are already commonly used in the clinic as anticancer agents for a variety of cancers [82]. The mechanism of action of camptothecin (*Camptotheca acuminata*) being to inhibit

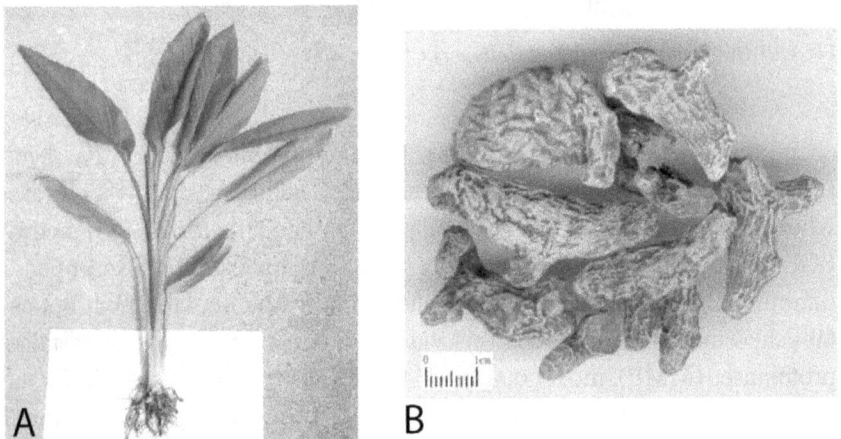

FIGURE 4: Plant (A) and root (B) of Curcuma longa ('curcumin') where root scale is shown as 1 cm.

DNA topoisomerase I, consequently affecting DNA replication; paclitaxel is a mitotic spindle inhibitor (spindle poison), which can also bind with tubulin and prevent the normal physiological process of microtubule depolymerization.

Anticancer properties of the TCM elemene (*Rhizoma zedoariae*) and oridonin (*Rabdosia rubescens*) lend themselves to being co-administered with conventional chemotherapeutic agents (e.g. doxorubicin and 5-flu-orouracil (5-FU)) to impart a synergistic anti-tumour effect. Combining elemene (*Rhizoma zedoariae*) with the pyrimidine base analogue 5-FU, resulted in significantly higher tumour growth inhibitive effects [83]. The anti-tumour activity of another TCM, 'half-flag' (*Pteris semipinnata* L.—Figure 5) was also significant, being shown to inhibit DNA production in HL-60 cells by 41% when combined with 5-FU, compared to only 10% in cells treated with the TCM alone. Half-flag also improved the anticancer efficiency of several other chemotherapeutic drugs when used concomitantly [84].

Similarly, derivatives of the herbal compound berbamine (*Berberis amurensis*), namely EBB (O-(4-ethoxy-butyl)-berbamine) when combined with cyclophosphamide and mitomycin-C respectively enhanced the antitumor capacity, while also significantly improving patients' quality of life [85]. Zhang and co-workers tested 20 natural flavonoid compounds in breast cancer cell lines discovering they assist in the intracellular accumulation of anthracycline drugs while also reversing anthracene resistance [86,87]. Kim SW et al., reported that ginsenoside-Rg3 (*Panax ginsenoside* Rg3) promotes Rhodamine-123 accumulation in vincristine-resistant KBV20C human fibroblast cancer cells, reversing vincristine resistance acquired by a variety of cells [88].

The discovery that single components within TCM have the potential to overcome multidrug resistance developed by tumour cells opens the door to new avenues of multi-drug/TCM therapy. These findings justify and moreover pave the way for them to be used alongside conventional drugs, where significant resistance to therapy has already developed.

Although only one clinical trial using TCM was reported up until 2001 it was poorly controlled and any conclusions drawn were deemed unreliable, it is noteworthy however that given the very recent attention being received by TCM a re-analysis study has since been conducted [89,90].

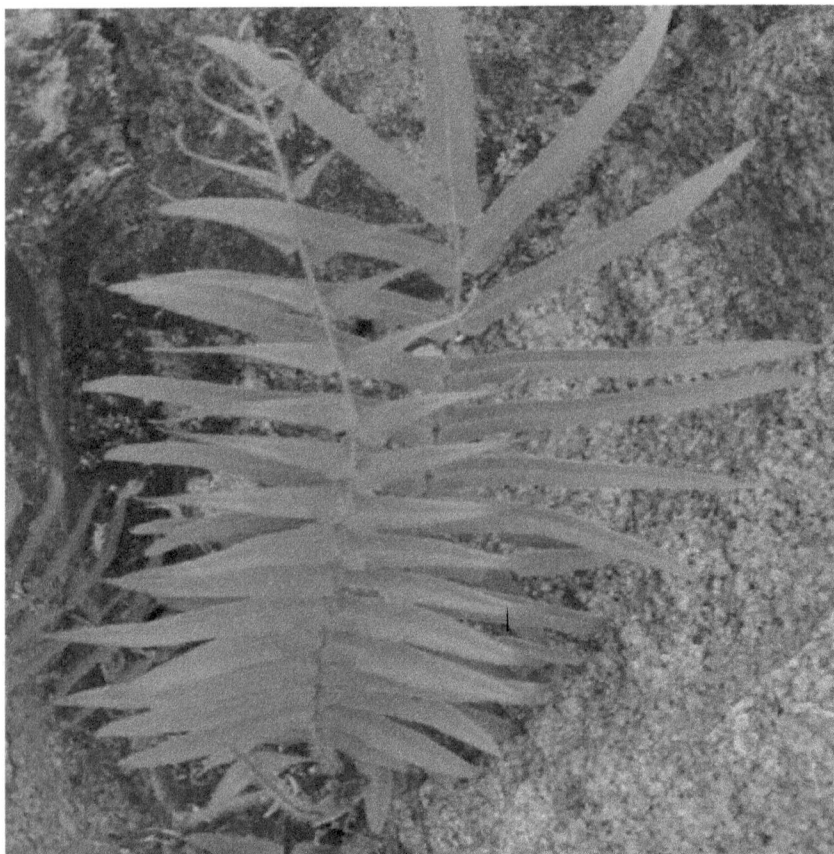

FIGURE 5: Plant of Pteris semipinnata L. ('half-flag').

This raises the call for more well-defined, robust and regulated clinical trials on TCM to ensure reliable data is generated which would enable regulatory authorities and clinicians alike to make well-informed decisions when considering their incorporation into western formularies.

8.2 CONCLUSION

In treating diseases/illnesses of a systemic nature the typical route of TCM administration is oral. This is deemed a far from optimal approach in cancer patients given patient-to-patient variability when formulating TCM, the unpredictable absorption profile of the various bioactives across the gastrointestinal tract together with compliance issues. Furthermore, the challenge of ensuring batch-to-batch reproducibility of any given formulation remains, although the adoption of cutting-edge genetic/chemical fingerprinting in conjunction with micro-array-based cell line testing offers unique solutions to this. With modern techniques of isolation, characterisation and functionalisation of compounds along with *in vitro*/in vivo testing now common place within research facilities where drug discovery and delivery is a focus, the drive to engineer well-defined, targeted drug delivery systems offers a new dawn for this very traditional practice of medicine [91-93]. By identifying potent bioactives derived from TCM as discussed above, and tailoring formulations that encapsulate/incorporate them into cutting-edge drug delivery systems for parenteral administration one can envision overcoming the shortfalls that have prevented TCM being accepted by the West as a real adjunct/alternative to conventional cancer therapies. With a library of over 250,000 individual therapeutic compounds at our disposal, many of which have yet to be successfully isolated and tested for both safety and efficacy, there are certainly challenges that lay ahead—the scope and scale of which could well revolutionise drug discovery and delivery in the fight against cancer, for many decades to come.

REFERENCES

1. Taiwan: time to end the exile Lancet 1999, 354:2093-2093.
2. Igney FH, Krammer PH: Death and anti-death: Tumour resistance to apoptosis. Nature Reviews Cancer 2002, 2:277-288.
3. Schmitz I, Kirchhoff S, Krammer PH: Regulation of death receptor-mediated apoptosis pathways. Int J Biochem Cell Biol 2000, 32:1123-1136.
4. Kwon K-B, Park B-H, Ryu D-G: Chemotherapy through mitochondrial apoptosis using nutritional supplements and herbs: A brief overview. J Bioenerg Biomembr 2007, 39:31-34.
5. Klein G: Cancer, apoptosis, and nonimmune surveillance. Cell Death Differ 2004, 11:13-17.
6. Ruan W-J, Lai M-D, Zhou J-G: Anticancer effects of Chinese herbal medicine, science or myth? Journal of Zhejiang University, Science, B 2006, 7:1006-1014.

7. Luk JM, Wang X, Liu P, Wong K-F, Chan K-L, Tong Y, Hui C-K, Lau GK, Fan S-T: Traditional Chinese herbal medicines for treatment of liver fibrosis and cancer: from laboratory discovery to clinical evaluation. Liver Int 2007, 27:879-890.
8. Green DR, Evan GI: A matter of life and death. Cancer Cell 2002, 1:19-30.
9. Petit PX, Susin SA, Zamzami N, Mignotte B, Kroemer G: Mitochondria and programmed cell death: Back to the future. FEBS Lett 1996, 396:7-13.
10. Bossy-Wetzel E, Green DR: Apoptosis: checkpoint at the mitochondrial frontier. Mutation Research, DNA Repair 1999, 434:243-251.
11. Rathmell JC, Thompson CB: The central effectors of cell death in the immune system. Annu Rev Immunol 1999, 17:781-828.
12. Janssen-Heininger YMW, Poynter ME, Baeuerle PA: Recent advances towards understanding redox mechanisms in the activation of nuclear factor kb. Free Radical Biology & Medicine 2000, 28:1317-1327.
13. Baeuerle PA, Henkel T: Function and activation of NF-kappa B in the immune system. Annu Rev Immunol 1994, 12:141-179.
14. Baeuerle PA, Rupec RA, Pahl HL: Reactive oxygen intermediates as second messengers of a general pathogen response. Pathologie Biologie 1996, 44:29-35.
15. Pahl HL: Activators and target genes of Rel/NF-kappa B transcription factors. Oncogene 1999, 18:6853-6866.
16. Shishodia S, Aggarwal BB: Nuclear factor-kappa B activation: A question of life or death. J Biochem Mol Biol 2002, 35:28-40.
17. Li BQ, Fu T, Gong WH, Dunlop N, Kung HF, Yan YD, Kang J, Wang JM: The flavonoid baicalin exhibits anti-inflammatory activity by binding to chemokines. Immunopharmacology 2000, 49:295-306.
18. Chi YS, Lim H, Park H, Kim HP: Effects of wogonin, a plant flavone from Scutellaria radix, on skin inflammation: in vivo regulation of inflammation-associated gene expression. Biochem Pharmacol 2003, 66:1271-1278.
19. Yu HQ, Rafi MM, Ho CT: Targeting inflammation using Asian herbs. In Herbs: Challenges in Chemistry and Biology. Edited by Ho CT. Oxford: Oxford University Press; 2006::266-280.
20. Tan BKH, Vanitha J: Immunomodulatory and antimicrobial effects of some traditional Chinese medicinal herbs: A review. Curr Med Chem 2004, 11:1423-1430.
21. Nelson PS, Montgomery B: Unconventional therapy for prostate cancer: Good, bad or questionable? Nature Reviews Cancer 2003, 3:845-858.
22. Po LS, Chen ZY, Tsang DSC, Leung LK: Baicalein and genistein display differential actions on estrogen receptor (ER) transactivation and apoptosis in MCF-7 cells. Cancer Lett 2002, 187:33-40.
23. Powell CB, Fung P, Jackson J, Dall'Era J, Lewkowicz D, Cohen I, Smith-McCune K: Aqueous extract of herb Scutellaria barbatae, a Chinese herb used for ovarian cancer, induces apoptosis of ovarian cancer cell lines. Gynecol Oncol 2003, 91:332-340.
24. Ye F, Xui L, Yi JZ, Zhang WD, Zhang DY: Anticancer activity of Scutellaria baicalensis and its potential mechanism. J Altern Complement Med 2002, 8:567-572.
25. Pidgeon GP, Kandouz M, Meram A, Honn KV: Mechanisms controlling cell cycle arrest and induction of apoptosis after 12-lipoxygenase inhibition in prostate cancer cells. Cancer Res 2002, 62:2721-2727.

26. Burnett BP, Jia Q, Zhao Y, Levy RM: A medicinal extract of Scutellaria baicalensis and Acacia catechu acts as a dual inhibitor of cyclooxygenase and 5-lipoxygenase to reduce inflammation. J Med Food 2007, 10:442-451.

27. Chan FL, Choi HL, Chen ZY, Chan PSF, Huang Y: Induction of apoptosis in prostate cancer cell lines by a flavonoid, baicalin. Cancer Lett 2000, 160:219-228.

28. Kwon K-B, Kim E-K, Shin B-C, Seo E-A, Park J-W, Kim J-S, Park B-H, Ryu D-G: Induction of apoptosis by takrisodokyeum through generation of hydrogen peroxide and activation of caspase-3 in HL-60 cells. Life Sci 2003, 73:1895-1906.

29. Sahara S, Aoto M, Eguchi Y, Imamoto N, Yoneda Y, Tsujimoto Y: Acinus is a caspase-3-activated protein required for apoptotic chromatin condensation. Nature 1999, 401:168-173.

30. Sebbagh M, Renvoize C, Hamelin J, Riche N, Bertoglio J, Breard J: Caspase-3-mediated cleavage of ROCK I induces MLC phosphorylation and apoptotic membrane blebbing. Nat Cell Biol 2001, 3:346-352.

31. Kwon KB, Kim EK, Han MJ, Shin BC, Park YK, Kim KS, Lee YR, Park JW, Park BH, Ryu DG: Induction of apoptosis by Radix Paeoniae alba extract through cytochrome c release and the activations of caspase-9 and caspase-3 in HL-60 cells. Biol Pharm Bull 2006, 29:1082-1086.

32. DiPietrantonio AM, Hsieh T-C, Wu JM: Activation of caspase 3 in HL-60 cells exposed to hydrogen peroxide. Biochem Biophys Res Commun 1999, 255:477-482.

33. Sung HJ, Choi SM, Yoon Y, An KS: Tanshinone IIA, an ingredient of Salvia miltiorrhiza bunge, induces apoptosis in human leukemia cell lines through the activation of caspase-3. Exp Mol Med 1999, 31:174-178.

34. Yoon Y, Kim YO, Jeon WK, Park JH, Sung HJ: Tanshinone IIA isolated from Salvia miltiorrhiza bunge induced apoptosis in HL60 human premyelocytic leukemia cell line. J Ethnopharmacol 1999, 68:121-127.

35. Lee H, Kim YJ, Kim HW, Lee DH, Sung M-K, Park T: Induction of apoptosis by Cordyceps militaris through activation of caspase-3 in leukemia HL-60 cells. Biol Pharm Bull 2006, 29(4):670-674.

36. Liu WK, Cheung FWK, Che C-T: Stellettin A Induces Oxidative Stress and Apoptosis in HL-60 Human Leukemia and LNCaP Prostate Cancer Cell Lines. J Nat Prod 2006, 69:934-937.

37. Walczak H, Miller RE, Ariail K, Gliniak B, Griffith TS, Kubin M, Chin W, Jones J, Woodward A, Le T, et al.: Tumoricidal activity of tumor necrosis factor related apoptosis-inducing ligand in vivo. Nat Med 1999, 5:157-163.

38. Nagane M, Pan GH, Weddle JJ, Dixit VM, Cavenee WK, Huang HJS: Increased death receptor 5 expression by chemotherapeutic agents in human gliomas causes synergistic cytotoxicity with tumor necrosis factor-related apoptosis-inducing ligand in vitro and in vivo. Cancer Res 2000, 60:847-853.

39. Chinnaiyan AM, Prasad U, Shankar S, Hamstra DA, Shanaiah M, Chenevert TL, Ross BD, Rehemtulla A: Combined effect of tumor necrosis factor-related apoptosis-inducing ligand and ionizing radiation in breast cancer therapy. Proc Natl Acad Sci USA 2000, 97:1754-1759.

40. Keane MM, Ettenberg SA, Nau MM, Russell EK, Lipkowitz S: Chemotherapy augments TRAIL-induced apoptosis in breast cell lines. Cancer Res 1999, 59:734-741.

41. Kupchan SM, Bryan RF, Gilmore CJ, Dailey RG, Court WA: Tumor inhibitors .74. triptolide and tripdiolide, novel antileukemic diterpenoid triepoxides from tripteryg-ium-wilfordii. J Am Chem Soc 1972, 94:7194-5.

42. Frese S, Pirnia F, Miescher D, Krajewski S, Borner MM, Reed JC, Schmid RA: PG490-mediated sensitization of lung cancer cells to Apo2L/TRAIL-induced apop-tosis requires activation of ERK2. Oncogene 2003, 22:5427-5435.

43. Lee KY, Chang WT, Qiu DM, Kao PN, Rosen GD: PG490 (triptolide) cooperates with tumor necrosis factor-alpha to induce apoptosis in tumor cells. J Biol Chem 1999, 274:13451-13455.

44. Chang WT, Kang JJ, Lee KY, Wei K, Anderson E, Gotmare S, Ross JA, Rosen GD: Triptolide and chemotherapy cooperate in tumor cell apoptosis – A role for the p53 pathway. J Biol Chem 2001, 276:2221-2227.

45. Sprick MR, Weigand MA, Rieser E, Rauch CT, Juo P, Blenis J, Krammer PH, Walczak H: FADD/MORT1 and caspase-8 are recruited to TRAIL receptors 1 and 2 and are essential for apoptosis mediated by TRAIL receptor 2. Immunity 2000, 12:599-609.

46. Kischkel FC, Lawrence DA, Chuntharapai A, Schow P, Kim KJ, Ashkenazi A: Apo2L/TRAIL-dependent recruitment of endogenous FADD and caspase-8 to death receptors 4 and 5. Immunity 2000, 12:611-620.

47. Walczak H, Krammer PH: The CD95 (APO-1/Fas) and the TRAIL (APO-2L) apop-tosis systems. Exp Cell Res 2000, 256:58-66.

48. Carter BZ, Mak DH, Schober WD, McQueen T, Harris D, Estrov Z, Evans RL, Andreeff M: Triptolide induces caspase-dependent cell death mediated via the mito-chondrial pathway in leukemic cells. Blood 2006, 108:630-637.

49. Daniel PT: A TRAIL to Chinese herbal medicine. Blood 2006, 108:3634.

50. Folkman J, Bach M, Rowe JW, Davidoff F, Lambert P, Hirsch C, Goldberg A, Hiatt HH, Glass J, Henshaw E: Tumor angiogenesis – therapeutic implications. N Engl J Med 1971, 285:1182.

51. Yance DR Jr, Sagar SM: Targeting angiogenesis with integrative cancer therapies. Integr Cancer Ther 2006, 5:9-29.

52. Shweiki D, Itin A, Soffer D, Keshet E: Vascular endothelial growth-factor induced by hypoxia may mediate hypoxia-initiated angiogenesis. Nature 1992, 359:843-845.

53. Shima DT, Deutsch U, Damore PA: Hypoxic induction of vascular endothelial growth-factor (VEGF) in human epithelial-cells is mediated by increases in messen-ger-RNA stability. FEBS Lett 1995, 370:203-208.

54. Risau W: Mechanisms of angiogenesis. Nature 1997, 386:671-674.

55. Toi M, Matsumoto T, Bando H: Vascular endothelial growth factor: its prognostic, predictive, and therapeutic implications. Lancet Oncol 2001, 2:667-673.

56. Efferth T, Dunstan H, Sauerbrey A, Miyachi H, Chitambar CR: The anti-malarial artesunate is also active against cancer. Int J Oncol 2001, 18:767-773.

57. Efferth T, Davey M, Olbrich A, Rucker G, Gebhart E, Davey R: Activity of drugs from traditional Chinese medicine toward sensitive and MDR1- or MRP1-overex-pressing multidrug-resistant human CCRF-CEM leukemia cells. Blood Cells Mol-ecules and Diseases 2002, 28:160-168.

58. Mueller MS, Runyambo N, Wagner I, Borrmann S, Dietz K, Heide L: Randomized controlled trial of a traditional preparation of Artemisia annua L. (Annual Worm-wood) in the treatment of malaria. Trans R Soc Trop Med Hyg 2004, 98:318-321.

59. Chen HH, Zhou HJ, Wu GD, Lou XE: Inhibitory effects of artesunate on angiogenesis and on expressions of vascular endothelial growth factor and VEGF receptor KDR/flk-1. Pharmacology 2004, 71:1-9.

60. Zhou H-J, Wang W-Q, Wu G-D, Lee J, Li A: Artesunate inhibits angiogenesis and downregulates vascular endothelial growth factor expression in chronic myeloid leukemia K562 cells. Vascul Pharmacol 2007, 47:131-138.

61. Chen HH, Zhou HJ, Fan X: Inhibition of human cancer cell line growth and human umbilical vein endothelial cell angiogenesis by artemisinin derivatives *in vitro*. Pharmacol Res 2003, 48:231-236.

62. Efferth T, Sauerbrey A, Olbrich A, Gebhart E, Rauch P, Weber HO, Hengstler JG, Halatsch ME, Volm M, Tew KD, et al.: Molecular modes of action of artesunate in tumor cell lines. Mol Pharmacol 2003, 64:382-394.

63. Narayan S: Curcumin, A Multi-Functional Chemopreventive Agent, Blocks Growth of Colon Cancer Cells by Targeting β-Catenin-Mediated Transactivation and Cell-Cell Adhesion Pathways. J Mol Histol 2004, 35:301-307.

64. Sen S, Sharma H, Singh N: Curcumin enhances Vinorelbine mediated apoptosis in NSCLC cells by the mitochondrial pathway. Biochem Biophys Res Commun 2005, 331:1245-1252.

65. Khafif A, Hurst R, Kyker K, Fliss Dan M, Gil Z, Medina Jesus E: Curcumin: a new radio-sensitizer of squamous cell carcinoma cells. Otolaryngol Head Neck Surg 2005, 132:317-321.

66. Arbiser JL, Klauber N, Rohan R, Van Leeuwen R, Huang M-T, Fisher C, Flynn E, Byers HR: Curcumin is an in vivo inhibitor of angiogenesis. Molecular Medicine 1998, 4:376-383.

67. Shao ZM, Shen ZZ, Liu CH, Sartippour MR, Go VL, Heber D, Nguyen M: Curcumin exerts multiple suppressive effects on human breast carcinoma cells. Int J Cancer 2002, 98:234-240.

68. Stetler-Stevenson WG, Yu AE: Proteases in invasion: matrix metalloproteinases. Semin Cancer Biol 2001, 11:143-153.

69. Stetler-Stevenson WG, Seo D-W: Matrix metalloproteinases in tumor progression. Cancer Metastasis – Biology and Treatment 2006, 8:143-158.

70. Chen H-W, Yu S-L, Chen JJW, Li H-N, Lin Y-C, Yao P-L, Chou H-Y, Chien C-T, Chen W-J, Lee Y-T, Yang P-C: Anti-invasive gene expression profile of curcumin in lung adenocarcinoma based on a high throughput microarray analysis. Mol Pharmacol 2004, 65:99-110.

71. Gururaj AE, Belakavadi M, Venkatesh DA, Marme D, Salimath BP: Molecular mechanisms of anti-angiogenic effect of curcumin. Biochem Biophys Res Commun 2002, 297:934-942.

72. Bachmeier BE, Nerlich AG, Iancu CM, Cilli M, Schleicher E, Vene R, Dell'Eva R, Jochum M, Albini A, Pfeffer U: The chemopreventive polyphenol Curcumin prevents hematogenous breast cancer metastases in immunodeficient mice. Cell Physiol Biochem 2007, 19:137-152.

73. Reddy S, Aggarwal BB: Curcumin is a noncompetitive and selective inhibitor of phosphorylase-kinase. FEBS Lett 1994, 341:19-22.

74. Dorai T, Cao YC, Dorai B, Buttyan R, Katz AE: Therapeutic potential of curcumin in human prostate cancer. III. Curcumin inhibits proliferation, induces apoptosis,

and inhibits angiogenesis of LNCaP prostate cancer cells in vivo. Prostate 2001, 47:293-303.

75. Leu TH, Su SL, Chuang YC, Maa MC: Direct inhibitory effect of curcumin on Src and focal adhesion kinase activity. Biochem Pharmacol 2003, 66:2323-2331.

76. Kim JH, Shim JS, Lee SK, Kim KW, Rha SY, Chung HC, Kwon HJ: Microarray-based analysis of anti-angiogenic activity of demethoxycurcumin on human umbilical vein endothelial cells: Crucial involvement of the down-regulation of matrix metalloproteinase. Jpn J Cancer Res 2002, 93:1378-1385.

77. Shim JS, Kim DH, Jung HJ, Kim JH, Lim D, Lee SK, Kim KW, Ahn JW, Yoo JS, Rho JR, et al.: Hydrazinocurcumin, a novel synthetic curcumin derivative, is a potent inhibitor of endothelial cell proliferation. Bioorg Med Chem 2002, 10:2987-2992.

78. John VD, Kuttan G, Krishnankutty K: Anti-tumour studies of metal chelates of synthetic curcuminoids. J Exp Clin Cancer Res 2002, 21:219-224.

79. Shi Z-M, Tian J-H: Correlative factors for cancer response evaluation treated by TCM. Shanghai Journal of Traditional Chinese Medicine 2006, 40:16-18.

80. Li Y, Ming Y-W: Molecular mechanism of Chinese anti-tumor herbal medicine. Chinese Journal of Information on TCM 2005, 12:95-96.

81. Kaye SB: Progress in the treatment of ovarian cancer. Anticancer Drugs 1999, 10:S29-S32.

82. Wang S-Z, Yang J-Y: Development of Clinical Applications for Anti-tumor Botanicals and Semi-Synthetic Medicine. Journal of Xin Jiang Medical University 2001, 24:183-184.

83. Zheng X, He M-X, Bin L, et al.: Effects of elemene combined with chemotherapy drugs on the growth of cancer cells. Cancer Prevention and Control Research 1998, 25:220-221.

84. Li J, Liang N, Mo L, He C, Zhang X: Effect of compound 6F isolated from Pteris semipinnata on cell cycle and synthesis of DNA, RNA and protein of lung adenocarcinoma cell. Chinese Pharmacology 1999, 15:49-51.

85. Zhang J, Mao Q, Xu N, Chen J: Effect of berbamine derivative (EBB) on anticancer and immune function of tumor-bearing mice. Chinese Herbal Journal 1998, 29:243-246.

86. Chen J-L, Jiang S, Yang R-F, Liu F-S, Sun X-M: Mechanism of drug resistance and reversal with ligustrazine and cyclosporin A in cisplatin-induced human epithelial ovarian cancer resistant cell line 3Ao/cDDP. Chinese Journal of Cancer Research 2000, 12:197-203.

87. Kim S-H, Yeo G-S, Lim Y-S, Kang C-D, Kim C-M, Chung B-S: Suppression of multidrug resistance via inhibition of heat shock factor by quercetin in MDR cells. Exp Mol Med 1998, 30:87-92.

88. Kim S-W, Kwon H-y, Chi D-W, Shim J-H, Park J-D, Lee Y-H, Pyo S, Rhee D-K: Reversal of P-glycoprotein-mediated multidrug resistance by ginsenoside Rg3. Biochem Pharmacol 2003, 65:75-82.

89. Grossarth-Maticek R, Kiene H, Baumgartner SM, Ziegler R: Use of Iscador, an extract of European mistletoe (Viscum album), in cancer treatment: Prospective

nonrandomized and randomized matched-pair studies nested within a cohort study. Altern Ther Health Med 2001, 7:57.

90. Grossarth-Maticek R, Ziegler R: Randomised and non-randomised prospective controlled cohort studies in matched-pair design for the long-term therapy of breast cancer patients with a mistletoe preparation (Iscador): A re-analysis. Eur J Med Res 2006, 11:485-495.

91. Parekh HS: The advance of dendrimers – a versatile targeting platform for gene/drug delivery. Curr Pharm Des 2007, 13:2837-2850.

92. Petrak K: Essential properties of drug-targeting delivery systems. Drug Discov Today 2005, 10:1667-1673.

93. Wang MD, Shin DM, Simons JW, Nie S: Nanotechnology for targeted cancer therapy. Expert Rev Anticancer Ther 2007, 7:833-837.

CHAPTER 9

ANTI CANCER EFFECTS OF CURCUMIN: CYCLE OF LIFE AND DEATH

GAURISANKAR SA AND TANYA DAS

9.1 INTRODUCTION

Cancers arise by an evolutionary process as somatic cells mutate and escape the restraints that normally rein in their untoward expansion. Consequently, multiple mechanisms have arisen to forestall uncontrolled cell division. Some of these are devices within the cell, such as those that limit cell-cycle progression, whereas others are social signals that prompt a cell to remain within its supportive microenvironment. In combination, these tumor-suppressing mechanisms are remarkably effective and can discriminate between neoplastic (abnormally growing) and normal cellular states and efficiently quell the former without suppressing the latter.

It is interesting to note that many, perhaps all, networks that drive cell proliferation harbor intrinsic growth-suppressive properties. Such innate inhibitory functions obscure any immediate selective advantage that mutations in such pathways might otherwise confer. Because no single pathway confers a net growth advantage, any proto-cancer cell acquiring any single oncogenic mutation is effectively trapped in an evolutionary cul-de-

This chapter was originally published under the Creative Commons Attribution License. Sa G and Das T. Anti Cancer Effects of Curcumin: Cycle of Life and Death. Cell Division 3,14 (2008). doi:10.1186/1747-1028-3-14.

sac. By contrast in normal cells, coordinated extra-cellular cues activate multiple pathways in concert. In this way the inherent growth-suppressive activity of each pathway is gated by another, thereby unlocking the cell's proliferative potential. However, de-regulation of one or more of these activities may ultimately lead to cancer.

It is acknowledged that cancer results from the interaction of genetic susceptibility and environmental exposures. It is, therefore, not very unexpected that there are striking variations in the risk of different cancers by geographic area. These geographical variations indicate that there is clearly a strong environmental component to the risk differences. These patterns reflect in one hand prevalence of specific risk factors and on the other raise the possibility of presence of anti-cancer agents in the diet differentially depending on the food habit. Supporting both, migrant populations from high-risk parts of the world show a marked diminution in risk when they move to a lower risk area [1]. There is growing evidence that populations with greater reliance on fruits and vegetables in the diet experience a reduced risk for the major cancers [2]. The major classes of phytochemicals with disease-preventing functions are antioxidants, detoxifying agents and immunity-potentiating agents. Such dietary phytochemicals include curcumin (diferuloylmethane), a major naturally-occurring phenolic compound obtained from the rhizome of the plant *Curcuma longa*, which is used as a spice or yellow coloring agent for foods or drugs [3,4]. This phytochemical has long been known to have broad antioxidant properties [5]. Because curcumin can suppress cancer cell proliferation, induce apoptosis, inhibit angiogenesis, suppress the expression of anti-apoptotic proteins while protecting immune system of the tumor bearer—it may have untapped therapeutic value [3,6,7].

Recent studies using gene-array approach indicate that in any given type of cancer 300–500 normal genes have been altered/modified somehow to result in the cancerous phenotype. Although cancers are characterized by the deregulation of cell signaling pathways at multiple steps, most current anticancer therapies involve the modulation of a single target. The ineffectiveness, lack of safety, and high cost of mono-targeted therapies have led to a lack of faith in these approaches. As a result, many pharmaceutical companies are increasingly interested in developing multitargeted therapies. Many plant-based products, however, accomplish multi-targeting naturally and, in addition, are inexpensive and safe compared to synthetic agents. However, because pharmaceutical companies are not usually able to secure intellectual property rights to plant-based products, the development of plant-based anticancer therapies has not been prioritized. Nonetheless, curcumin, a plant-based product, has shown significant promise against cancer and other inflammatory diseases.

In the present review we discuss how alterations in the cell cycle control contribute to the malignant transformation of normal cells and provide an overview of how curcumin targets cell cycle regulators to assert its anti-neoplastic effects. The purpose of the current article is to present an appraisal of the current level of knowledge regarding the potential of curcumin as an agent for the chemoprevention of cancer via an understanding of its mechanism of action at the level of cell cycle regulation.

9.1.1 CANCER: CYCLE OUT OF HAND

Cell proliferation and cell death are such diametrically opposed cellular fates that how the two are linked and interdependent processes was a great surprise [8,9]. There is little mechanistic overlap between the machineries driving proliferation and apoptosis. Rather, the two processes are coupled at various levels through the individual molecular players responsible for orchestrating cell expansion. Importantly, the same players are often targets for oncogenic mutations, and in many instances, mutations that drive proliferation cooperate with those that uncouple proliferation from apoptosis during transformation and tumorigenesis [10,11]. But, although the phenomenon of oncogene-induced apoptosis is now generally accepted as an innate tumor-suppressive mechanism, we have only recently begun to glimpse the diversity and complexity of mechanisms by which oncogenic lesions engage the cell suicide machinery.

In normal cells there is a finely controlled balance between growth promoting and growth restraining signals such that proliferation occurs only when required. The balance tilts when increased cell numbers are required, e.g., during wound healing and during normal tissue turn over [12]. Proliferation and differentiation of cells during these processes occur in ordered manner and cease when no longer required. In tumor cells this

process disrupts, continued cell proliferation occurs and loss of differentiation may be found. In addition, the normal process of programmed
cell death that exists in normal cells may no longer operate [12]. In other
words, a normal cell becomes malignant when the cellular proliferation
is no longer under normal growth control. There are of course other characteristics that cancer cell may possess, such as angiogenesis, metastasis
and suppression of apoptosis. But at the end the uncontrolled proliferation of the cell is at the heart of the disease. Therefore to understand
cancer we need to transpire our knowledge on cell proliferation and its
control.

The process of replicating DNA and dividing a cell can be described
as a series of coordinated events that compose a "cell division cycle".
The mammalian cell cycle has been divided into a series of sequential
phases. The G1, S, G2, and M phases are sequentially transitioned in
response to growth factor or mitogenic stimulation (Figure 1). The DNA
synthetic (S phase) and mitotic (M phase) phases are preceded by gap
phases (G1, G2). Cell proliferation is tightly regulated by multiple interactions between molecules in normal cells. One molecular system
senses growth-promoting conditions and sends a signal to a second set
of molecules that actually regulates cell division. In addition, cells are
equipped with signaling pathway that can sense unfavorable conditions
for proliferation. This pathway antagonizes the proliferative signaling
pathway and can directly block cell division [13-15]. Loss of integrity
of these signaling pathways due to mutations can result in a hyper-proliferative state of cells, manifested as cancer [9,10]. Therefore, cancer
is a disease of deregulated cell proliferation. It is becoming clear that
many external signals including both those that stimulate growth, such
as growth factors, and those that inhibit growth, such as DNA damaging
agents, control cell proliferation through regulating the cell cycle. Thus,
elucidating the machinery of cell cycle progression and its regulation by
these signals is essential for understanding and controlling cell proliferation. Recent advances in our understanding of the cell cycle machinery
in the last years have demonstrated that disruption of normal cell cycle
control is frequently observed in human cancer [10,15].

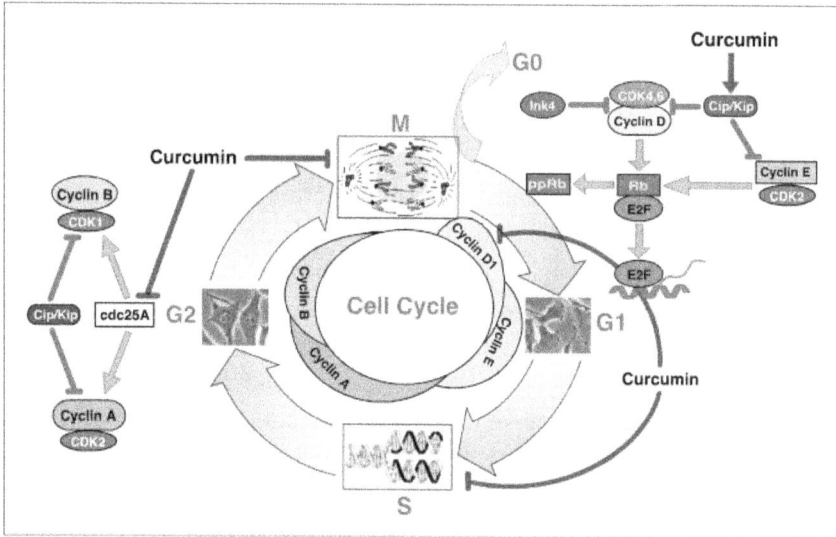

FIGURE 1: The cell division cycle and its control. The cell cycle is divided into four distinct phases (G1, S, G2, and M). The progression of a cell through the cell cycle is promoted by CDKs, which are positively and negatively regulated by cyclins and CKis, respectively. As shown, cyclin D isoforms interact with CDK4 and CDK6 to drive the progression of a cell through G1. Cyclin D/CDK4,6 complexes phosphorylate pRb, which releases E2F to transcribe genes necessary for cell cycle progression. The association of cyclin E with CDK2 is active at the G1-S transition and directs entry into S-phase. The INK4s bind and inhibit cyclin D-associated kinases (CDK4 and CDK6). The kinase inhibitor protein group of CKi, p21Cip1/Waf-1, p27Kip1, and p57Kip2, negatively regulate cyclin D/CDK4,6 and cyclin E/CDK2 complexes. S-phase progression is directed by the cyclinA/CDK2 complex, and the complex of cyclin A with Cdk1 is important in G2. CDK1/cyclin B is necessary for the entry into mitosis. Curcumin modulates CKis, CDK-cyclin and Rb-E2F complexes to render G1-arrest and alters CDK/cyclin B complex formation to block G2/M transition.

9.1.2 CYCLIN-DEPENDENT PATHWAY: THE FUEL OF CELL CYCLE

At least two types of cell cycle control mechanisms are recognized: a cascade of protein phosphorylations that relay a cell from one stage to the next and a set of checkpoints that monitor completion of critical events and delay progression to the next stage if necessary. The first type of control involves a highly regulated kinase family [13-15]. Kinase activation generally requires association with a second subunit that is transiently expressed at the appropriate period of the cell cycle; the periodic "cyclin" subunit associates with its partner "cyclin-dependent kinase" (CDK) to create an active complex with unique substrate specificity. Regulatory phosphorylation and dephosphorylation fine-tune the activity of CDK-cyclin complexes, ensuring well-delineated transitions between cell cycle stages. The orderly progression through G1 phase of the cell cycle is regulated by the sequential assembly and activation of three sets of cyclin-CDK complexes (Figure 2), the D cyclins (D1, D2 and D3) and CDK4 or CDK6, cyclin E and CDK2, cyclin A and CDK2 [14,15]. Genetic aberrations in the regulatory circuits that govern transit through the G1 phase of the cell cycle occur frequently in human cancer, and deregulated over-expression of cyclin D1 is one of the most commonly observed alterations that may serve as a drive oncogene through its cell-cycle regulating function [16]. In normal cells *cyclin D1* expression is tightly regulated by mitogenic signals involving Ras pathway [17]. Increased cyclin D1 abundance occurs relatively early during tumorigenesis [18]. In most cancer types cyclin D1 over-expression results from induction by oncogenic signals, rather than a clonal somatic mutation or rearrangement in the cyclin D1 gene [19]. Tissue culture-based experiments evidenced cyclin D1 functions as a collaborative oncogene that enhances oncogenic transformation of other oncogenes (i.e., *Ras, Src, E1A*) [20,21]. Targeted expression of cyclin D1 or cyclin E induce mammary tumors [22,23]. The cyclin D- and E-dependent kinases contribute sequentially to the phosphorylation of the retinoblastoma gene susceptibility product (pRB), canceling its ability to repress E2F transcription factors and activating genes required for S phase entry [13,14].

Although the RB-1 gene was first identified through its role in a rare pediatric cancer, subsequent tumor studies have shown that this gene is sporadically mutated in a wide range of cancers [24]. In addition to direct mutation of the RB-1 gene, its encoded protein (pRB) is functionally inactivated in many tumor cells either by viral proteins that bind to pRB, or through changes in a regulatory pathway that controls the activity of pRB. Current mutation data indicates that nearly all tumor cells contain mutations or gene silencing events that effectively lead to inactivation of pRB. This establishes that pRB is necessary for restricting entry into the cell

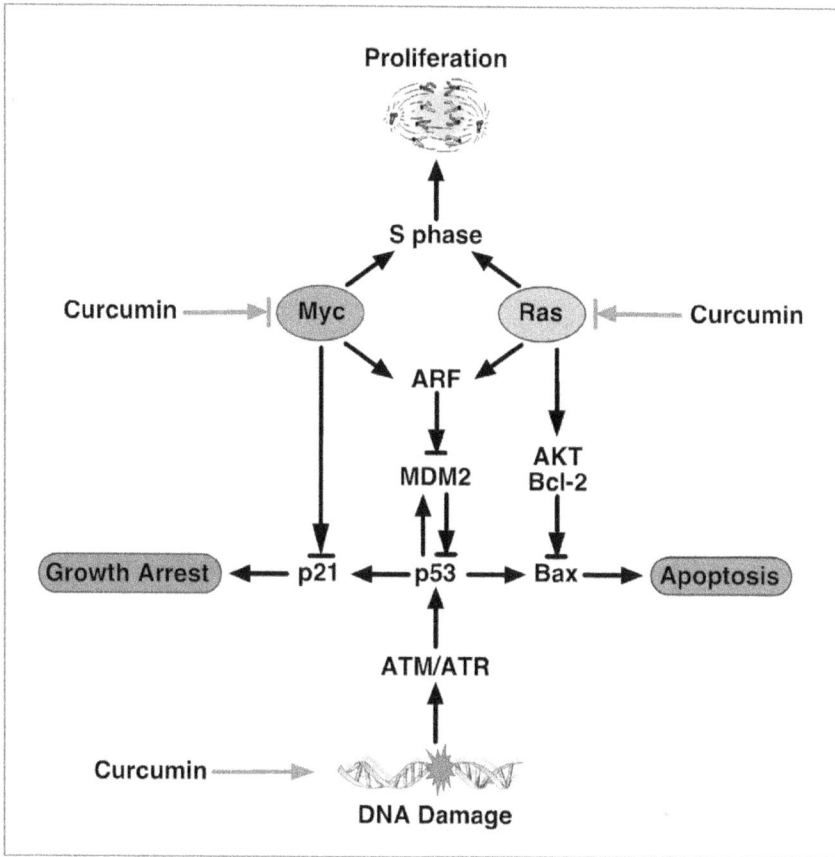

FIGURE 2: The ARF-p53 circuit in tumour development and therapy. Activation of Myc and Ras can force proliferation or trigger apoptosis. These oncogenic signals engage the tumor-suppressor network at many points, including through the ARF-p53 circuit shown here. Which components contribute most to tumor suppression depends on context. For example, Myc activates p53 to promote apoptosis while interfering with its ability to induce growth arrest by p21. Conversely, Ras activates p53 to promote growth arrest while suppressing apoptosis. This simplified view helps explain why, despite the potential of p53 to control several processes; apoptosis is primarily responsible for p53-mediated tumor suppression. DNA damage and oncogene signaling engage the tumor-suppressor network at different points and, as such, DNA-damage signaling relies more on p53 than on ARF to elicit an anti-proliferative response. Such a model explains why loss of ARF or p53 confers similar advantages during Myc-induced tumorigenesis but not following treatment with DNA-damaging drugs such as curcumin. Here, drug resistance is an unselected trait conferred by p53 mutations that provides a unique advantage as the tumor encounters a new environment (e.g., chemotherapy).

cycle and preventing cancer. This cyclin-CDK-mediated pathway leading to G1-S transition is known as "cyclin-dependent pathway". Regulation of G1-CDK activity is affected by their association with inhibitory proteins, called CDK inhibitors (CKi) [25]. So far, two families of CKi have been defined based on their structure and CDK targets: the Ink4 family and the Cip/Kip family [26]. The inhibitors of Ink4 family (p15^{Ink4b}, p16^{Ink4a}, p18^{Ink4c} and p19^{Ink4d}) bind to monomeric Cdk4 and Cdk6 but not to Cdk2, thereby precluding the association of these Cdks to cyclins D [27]. Conversely, the members of Cip/Kip family, that include p21$^{Cip1/Waf-1}$, p27^{Kip1} and p57^{Kip2}, all contain characteristic motifs at their N-terminal moieties that able them to bind both CDK and cyclins (Figure 1) [26,28]. It can thus be envisaged from the above discussion that any deregulation of this cyclin-dependent pathway can jeopardize the normal cell cycle progression and also that alteration of such deregulation can be one of the targets of cancer therapy. Therefore, the regulation of G1-S and G2-M transition could be an effective target to control the growth and proliferation of cancer cells, and facilitate their apoptotic death.

9.1.3 P53: THE MASTER REGULATOR

Besides "cyclin-dependent pathway", as a tumor suppressor, p53 has a central role in cell cycle regulation. However, this second type of cell cycle regulation, checkpoint control, is more supervisory. It is not an essential part of the cell cycle progression machinery. Cell cycle checkpoints sense flaws in critical events such as DNA replication and chromosome segregation [29]. When checkpoints are activated, for example, by under-replicated or damaged DNA, signals are relayed to the cell cycle-progression machinery. These signals cause a delay in cell cycle progression, until the danger of mutation has been averted. Because checkpoint function is not required in every cell cycle, the extent of checkpoint function is not as obvious as that of components integral to the process, such as CDKs. Researches conducted in the last two decades have firmly established the importance of p53 in mediating the cell cycle arrest that occurs following DNA damage, thus acting as a molecular "guardian of genome" (Figure 2) [8,30,31]. However, during the same time, the role of p53 in mediating apoptosis has become increasingly less clear, even as the number of putative pro-apoptotic proteins trans-activated by p53 has increased [8]. Numerous studies have analyzed the pattern of genes induced after p53 activation using global technologies such as SAGE, DNA array, Suppression Subtractive Hybridization or by cloning functional p53-binding sites. These studies emphasize the heterogeneity of the p53 response that is highly variable depending on the cell type, the nature and amount of DNA damage, the genetic background of the cells and the amount of p53 protein. Similarly unclear is how p53 makes a choice between cell-cycle arrest and apoptosis raising the possibility that p53 alone is not responsible for this crucial decision. An important function of p53 is to act as a transcription factor by binding to a p53-specific DNA consensus sequence in responsive genes, which would be expected to increase the synthesis of p21^{Cip1} or Bax [8,30,31].

Up-regulation of p21^{Cip1}/p21^{Waf-1} results in the inhibition of cell cycle progression from G1 to S phase of cell cycle [32]. Interestingly, at Cip1, p53 pathway meets cyclin-dependent pathway. p21^{Cip1} binds to cyclin-CDK complex, inhibits kinase activity and blocks cell cycle progression [32]. However, the underlying mechanism is still not yet fully revealed. Since the stabilization of another member of CKi family, p27^{Kip1}, by phosphorylation prevents inhibition of Cdk/cyclin complexes in the ternary complex and blocks cell cycle progression [26,33,34], similar mechanism might be operative in case of p21^{Cip1}. The available evidence suggests that Cip1-PCNA complexes block the role of PCNA as a DNA polymerase processivity factor in DNA replication, but not its role in DNA repair. Thus, Cip1 can act on cyclin-CDK complexes and PCNA to stop DNA replication. The removal of both Cip1 alleles from a cancerous cell line in culture that contained a wild-type p53 allele completely eliminated the DNA damage-induced G1 arrest in these cells, indicating that Cip1 is sufficient to enforce a G1 arrest in this experimental situation [35].

Another group of important regulators of apoptosis is the Bcl-2 family. These oncoproteins are classified into two groups: anti-apoptotic that inhibits apoptosis and pro-apoptotic that induces or accelerates it. The members form heterodimers to inactivate each other. The up-regulation of Bax expression and down-regulation of Bcl-2 have been demonstrated during apoptosis [32-36]. Interestingly, Bcl-2 over-expression renders cells resistant to apoptosis when it homodimerizes, whereas, up-regulation of Bax alters Bcl-2/Bax ratio in cellular microenvironment and cause release of cytochrome c from mitochondria into cytosol [37]. Cytochrome c then binds to Apaf-1 and activates caspase cascade, which is responsible for the later process of apoptosis [38]. Therefore, in one hand, deregulation of these cell cycle regulators leads to cancer and on the other any agent that can regulate these processes in cancer cells may have a role in tumor regression.

9.1.4 CELL CYCLE AND APOPTOSIS: TWO SIDES OF THE SAME COIN

The fundamental processes of progression through the cell cycle and of programmed cell death involve the complex interaction of several families of proteins in a systematic and coordinated manner. They are separate, distinct processes that are intimately related and together play an important role in the sensitivity of malignant cells to chemotherapy. The cell cycle is the mechanism by which cells divide. Apoptosis is an active, energy-dependent process in which the cell participates in its own destruction. The cell cycle and apoptosis are intimately related, as evidenced by the central role of p53, both in cell cycle arrest and in the induction of apoptosis. Another example of this intimate relation was demonstrated in human colon cancer cell lines that differ only in their p21 checkpoint status. Cells with wild-type p21, when irradiated with γ-radiation, underwent a cell cycle growth arrest followed by clonogenic survival, where as cells lacking p21, when irradiated with γ-radiation, did not undergo a cell cycle growth arrest and furthermore proceeded to apoptosis [39]. Cells that undergo a growth arrest may be protected from apoptosis and may therefore be ultimately resistant to the cytotoxic agent.

9.1.5 CURCUMIN—THE CURRY FOR CURE: OUR HYPOTHESIS

Cell cycle progression is an important biological event having controlled regulation in normal cells, which almost universally becomes aberrant or deregulated in transformed and neoplastic cells. In this regard, targeting deregulated cell cycle progression and its modulation by various natural and synthetic agents are gaining widespread attention in recent years to control the unchecked growth and proliferation in cancer cells. In fact, a vast number of experimental studies convincingly show that many phytochemicals halt uncontrolled cell cycle progression in cancer cells. Among these phytochemicals, curcumin has been identified as one of the major natural anticancer agents exerting anti-neoplastic activity in various types of cancer cells. Here we hypothesize that curcumin asserts its anti-tumor activity in cancer cells by altering the de-regulated cell cycle via (a) cyclin-dependent, (b) p53-dependent and (c) p53-independent pathways.

9.1.6 AT THE CROSSROADS OF ALTERNATIVE AND MAIN STREAM MEDICINE

Turmeric has been used for thousands of years in Ayurvedic and traditional Chinese medicine. In modern times, curcumin, the yellow pigment of the spice turmeric, continues to be used as an alternative medicinal agent in many parts of South East Asia for the treatment of common ailments such as stomachic upset, flatulence, jaundice, arthritis, sprains, wounds and skin infections among many others. Curcumin and turmeric products have been characterized as safe by health authorities such as the Food and Drug Administration (FDA) in United States of America, Food and Agriculture Organization/World Health Organization (FAO/WHO). Curcumin has entered scientific clinical trials at the phase I and II clinical trial level only in the last 10–15 years. A phase III study of gemcitabine, curcumin and celecoxib is due to open to recruitment at the Tel-Aviv Sourasky Medical Center for patients with metastatic colorectal cancer [40].

9.1.7 WHY CURCUMIN?

Curcumin is a component of turmeric; the yellow spice derived from the roots (rhizomes) of the plant *Curcuma longa*. *Curcuma longa* is a short-stemmed perennial, which grows to about 100 cm in height. It has curved leaves and oblong, ovate or cylindrical rhizomes (Figure 3). *Curcuma*

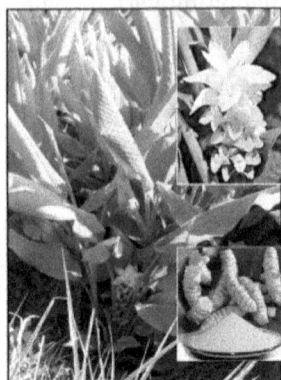

Turmeric Plant with Rhizome

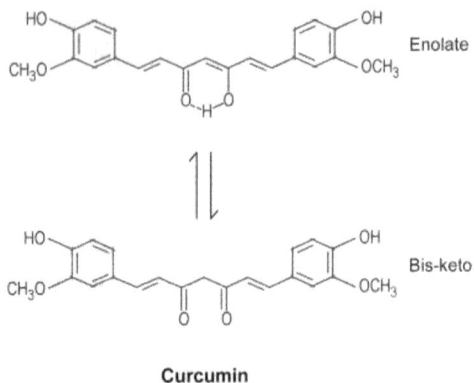

Curcumin

FIGURE 3: *Curcuma longa* plant and chemical structure of curcumin, the active ingradient of rhizome termeric. The tautomerism of curcumin is demonstrated under different physiological conditions. Under acidic and neutral conditions, the bis-keto form (bottom) is more predominant than the enolate form.

longa grows naturally throughout the Indian subcontinent and in tropical countries, particularly South East Asia. A traditional remedy in "Ayurvedic medicine" and ancient Indian healing system that dates back over 5,000 years, turmeric has been used through the ages as an "herbal aspirin" and "herbal cortisone" to relieve discomfort and inflammation associated with an extraordinary spectrum of infectious and autoimmune diseases [4].

Curcumin, chemically it is known as diferuloylmethane ($C_{21}H_{20}O_6$), has been the subject of hundreds of published papers over the past three decades, studying its antioxidant, anti-toxic, anti-inflammatory, cancer chemopreventive and potentially chemotherapeutic properties [3,4,41-44]. The pharmacology and putative anti-cancer properties of curcumin have been the subject of several review articles published since 1991, which predate a number of clinical studies of curcumin which have been completed and published within the last few years [45]. But these properties do not prove the superiority of this phytochemical over other chemotherapeutic agents that also induced apoptosis successfully in cancer cells.

Majority of chemotherapeutic agents, including those isolated from plants (such as taxol or vincristin etc.) not only induce cancer cell apoptosis but also severely damage the normal cells of the host, the effects being particularly severe in case of the immune system [46]. On the contrary, curcumin is a part of our daily food habit and its use in large quantities from ancient time has already proved that it is a safe product [4]. In fact, since curcumin preferably induces apoptosis in highly proliferating cells, death is much more pronounced in tumor cells than normal ones [47]. Report from our laboratory has shown that anticancer dose of curcumin arrests non-malignant cells in G0 phase reversibly but does not induce apoptosis in them [6]. Further studies revealed that this phytochemical protects T cells of the cancer bearer from cancer as well as chemotherapeutic agent-induced apoptosis [7,47]. The basis of this differential regulation may be attributed to its differential effects on normal and neoplastic cell cycles since deregulation of some components of cell cycle regulatory machinery can drive uncontrolled proliferation and hence neoplastic transformations.

The broad biological activity of this phytochemical, including antioxidant and metabolic effect, influences upon key signal transduction pathways of cell cycle and effectiveness in animal model systems have fostered development of translational, and clinical research programs. In pilot clinical studies in India, Taiwan, USA and UK, curcumin has been associated with regression of pre-malignant lesions of the bladder, soft palate, GI tract, cervix, and skin, and with treatment responses in established malignancy [48-52]. Doses up to 8–10 g could be administered daily to patients with pre-malignant lesions for 3 months without overt toxicity [48-50]. It cannot be assumed that diet-derived agents will be innocuous when administered as pharmaceutical formulations at doses likely to exceed those consumed in the dietary matrix. Anecdotal reports suggest that dietary consumption of curcumin up to 150 mg/day is not associated with any adverse effects in humans [44]. The epidemiological data interestingly suggest that it may be reason for the lower rate of colorectal cancer in these countries than in "developed" countries [1,2]. The preclinical data in human subjects suggest that a daily dose of 3.6 g curcumin achieves measurable levels in colorectal tissue. Efficient first-pass and some degree of intestinal metabolism of curcumin, particularly glucuronidation and sulphation, may explain its lesser systemic availability when administered via oral route [53]. So, gastrointestinal tract could represent a preferential chemoprevention target because of its greater exposure to unmetabolized bioactive curcumin from diet than other tissues. All these information not only suggest that curcumin has enormous potential in the prevention and therapy of cancer but also well justify the utility of using curcumin as an anti-tumor agent.

9.1.8 TO ARREST OR TO KILL—TWO WEAPONS OF CURCUMIN

It is now apparent that many of the phytochemicals preferentially inhibit the growth of tumor cells by inducing cell cycle arrest or apoptosis (Figure 2). The anti-tumor effect of curcumin has also been attributed in part to the suppression of cell proliferation, reduction of tumor load and induction of apoptosis in various cancer models both *in vitro* and in vivo [6,44,48,49,54-57]. Curcumin inhibits multiple levels within transcriptional network to restrict cell proliferation. It induces p53-dependent apoptosis in various cancers of colon, breast, bladder, neuron, lung, ovary etc., although both p53-dependent and -independent G2/M phase arrest by curcumin has been observed in colorectal cancer cells [6,48,49,57-61]. Curcumin promotes caspase-3-mediated cleavage of β-catenin, decreases β-catenin/Tcf-Lef transactivation capacity for c-Myc and cyclin D1 [62]. It also activates caspase-7 and caspase-9 and induces polyadenosine-5'-diphosphate-ribose polymerase cleavage through the down-regulation of NFκB in multiple myeloma cells [63]. Furthermore, curcumin inhibits EGFR activation [64], Src activity [65] and inhibits activity of some nuclear receptors [66]. Curcumin inhibitory effects upon Cox-2 and cyclin D1, mediated through NF-κB, also restrict tumor cell growth [62,67]. Induction of G2/M arrest and inhibition of Cox-2 activity by curcumin in human bladder cancer cells has also been reported [58]. It induces colon cancer cell apoptosis by JNK-dependent sustained phosphorylation of c-Jun [68] and enhances TNF-α-induced prostate cancer cell apoptosis [70]. In fact, curcumin induces apoptosis in both androgen-dependent and androgen-independent prostate cancer cells [70]. On the other hand, in breast carcinoma cells, it inhibits telomerase activity through human telomerase reverse-transcritpase [71]. In Bcr-Abl-expressing cells, G2/M cell cycle arrest, together with increased mitotic index and cellular as well as nuclear morphology resembling those described for mitotic catastrophe, was observed and preceded caspase-3 activation and DNA fragmentation leading to apoptosis [72]. Curcumin arrested cell growth at the G2/M phase and induced apoptosis in human melanoma cells by inhibiting NFκB activation and thus depletion of endogenous nitric oxide [73]. However, in mantle cell lymphoma curcumin has been found to induce G1/S arrest and apoptosis [74]. In T cell leukemia curcumin induced growth-arrest and apoptosis in association with the inhibition of constitutively active Jak-Stat pathway and NFκB [75,76]. Holy [77] reported disruption of mitotic spindle structure and induction of micronucleation in human breast cancer cells by this yellow pigment. Besides arresting growth or inducing apoptosis, curcumin also enhances differentiation by targeting PI3K-Akt pathway, Src-mediated signaling and PPAR [64,65,78]. This action of curcumin promotes cells exit from cycle. All these reports indicate that curcumin might be asserting its anti-cancer effect by modulating cancer cell cycle regulatory machineries.

9.1.9 CURCUMIN: THE MANIPULATOR OF CYCLIN PATHWAY

It is clear that curcumin spares normal cell from apoptotic induction making it a relatively safe anti-cancer agent. The question thus arises that what confers this selectivity. In an attempt to understand the basic mechanisms of carcinogenesis, it was found that, in slowly-proliferating non-malignant cells, Ras activity is stimulated to high level at G1 phase upon mitogenic challenge and leads to cyclin D1 elevation during mid to late G1 phase [13-16]. Interestingly, we found that this pattern, upon which most models of cell cycle regulation are based, does not apply to actively proliferating cancer cells. In fact, in these rapidly cycling cells, oncogenic Ras is active throughout the cell cycle during exponential growth and induces high levels of cyclin D1 expression in G2 phase that continues through mitosis to G1 phase bypassing G0 phase, a phase that regulates uncontrolled proliferation [79-81]. These results not only demonstrated that the critical signaling events upon which cell cycle progression depends take place during G1 phase in normal cells, but during G2 phase in actively growing cancer cells but also that G2 phase of cell cycle plays a critical role in controlling hyper-proliferative status of cancer cell and is thus susceptible to successful anti-cancer drug therapy.

With elegant time-lapse video-micrography and quantitative imaging approach our works with breast malignant cells and adjacent non-malignant cells indicate that curcumin did not alter the cell cycle progression of carcinoma cells, although it induced apoptosis in the same at G2 phase of cell cycle (Figure 4) while reversibly blocking non-malignant cell cycle progression without apoptosis [6]. An interesting finding in this study was that curcumin appeared to be sparing the normal epithelial cells by arresting them at the G0 phase of the cell cycle via down-regulation of cyclin D1 and its related protein kinases or up-regulation of the inhibitory protein. The experiments with cyclin D1-deregulated cells showed that curcumin did not alter cyclin D1 expression level in cancer cells, but in normal cells, where cyclin D1 expression is tightly regulated by mitogenic signaling, its expression is inhibited by curcumin. This inability of curcumin to inhibit cyclin D1 expression in cyclin D1-deregulated cells may serve as the basis for differential regulation of cancerous and normal cells. In addition, curcumin was found to inhibit the association of cyclin D1 with CDK4/CDK6 or phosphorylation of pRb in some cancer cells where the expression of cyclin D1 is not deregulated and thus arrest them at G0/G1 phase (Figure 1) [82,83]. This yellow pigment has been shown to inhibit neoplastic cell proliferation by decreasing Cdk1 kinase activity and arresting cells at G2/M check point [81]. Ectopically over-expression of cyclin D1 renders susceptibility of these cells towards curcumin toxicity [6]. These results may well explain why in cancer cells, despite up-regulation of p53 and increase in Cip1 level, there was no cell cycle arrest. In fact, the level of cyclin D1 is very high in these cells and remained unchanged upon curcumin treatment. Thus, the amount of Cip1, as up regulated by curcumin, was still not sufficient to overpower cyclin D1 and to stop cell cycle progression. On the other hand, in non-malignant cells, the level of Cip1 increased dramatically with parallel down-regulation of cyclin D1, thereby making the ratio of Cip1 to cyclin D1 > 1 and this might be one of the causes of cell cycle arrest without apoptosis [6]. The above discussion not only relates curcumin activity with cell cycle regulation but also explains the mechanism underlying the differential effect of this phytochemical in normal and malignant cells.

9.1.10 CURCUMIN REGULATING "GUARDIAN OF GENOME"

The tumor suppressor gene *p53*, acknowledged as the "guardian of genome", is situated at the crossroads of a network of signaling pathways that are essential for cell growth regulation and apoptosis [30-35]. In normal unstressed cells, these upstream pathways predominantly include the

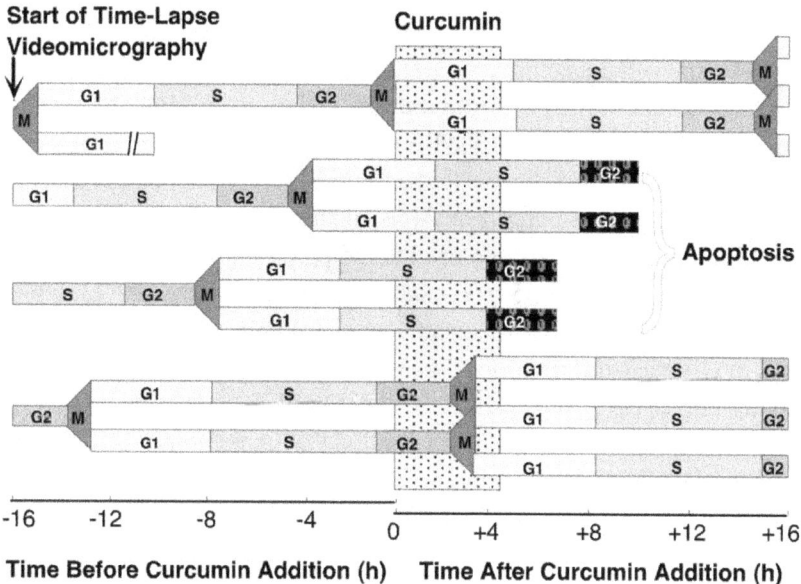

FIGURE 4: Time-lapse determination of approximate cell cycle position of curcumin-induced apoptosis. Time-lapse video-micrography was employed to monitor curcumin-induced apoptosis of breast cancer cells. Age of each cell was analyzed from a time-lapse analysis before curcumin addition. The occurrence and the time of apoptosis after curcumin addition were determined from a time-lapse analysis after addition.

binding by proteins such as Mdm2 that promote p53 degradation via the ubiquitin-26S proteasome pathway [32]. COP9 signalosome (CNS)-specific phosphorylation targets p53 to ubiquitin-26S proteasome-dependent degradation. Curcumin has been found to inhibit CSN and block Mdm2- and E6-dependent p53 degradation [84]. Furthermore, in basal cell carcinoma, curcumin promotes de novo synthesis of p53 protein or some other proteins for stabilization of p53, and hence enhances its nuclear translocation to transactivate Cip1 and Gadd45 indicating that p53-associated signaling pathway is critically involved in curcumin-mediated apoptotic cell death [56]. With time-lapse video-micrography and quantitative imaging approach we have demonstrated that in deregulated cells, curcumin induces p53 dramatically at G2 phase of cell cycle and enhances p53 DNA-binding activity resulting in apoptosis at G2 phase (Figure 4) [6,47]. On the other hand, curcumin increases p53 expression to a lower extent throughout the cell cycle in non-malignant cells [6]. In these cells, curcumin reversibly up-regulates Cip1 expressions and inactivates pRB and thus arrests them in G0 phase of cell cycle. Therefore, these cells escape from curcumin-induced apoptosis at G2 phase. Works from other laboratories also suggest that curcumin induces p53 expression in colon, breast, and other cancer cells [57-61]. Reports from our laboratory as well as from other laboratories suggest that curcumin predominantly acts in a p53-dependent manner as careful analysis of the effect of curcumin in various cells expressing wild-type or mutated p53 as well as cells transfected with dominant-negative p53, revealed that the cells expressing high levels of wild-type p53 were more sensitive to curcumin toxicity. On the other hand, p53-knock-out as well as p53-mutated cells also showed toxicity, although the apoptotic-index is lower [6,42,47].

Search for downstream of p53 revealed that in mammary epithelial carcinoma and colon adenocarcinoma cells curcumin could increase the expression of the pro-apoptotic protein Bax and decrease the anti-apoptotic protein Bcl-2/Bcl-xL through the phosphorylation at Ser15 and activation of p53 [6,85]. Our results also revealed curcumin-induced G2/M arrest and apoptosis of mammary epithelial carcinoma cells via p53-mediated Bax activation [6,47]. On the other hand, c-Abl, a non-receptor tyrosine kinase, has been reported to play an important role in curcumin-induced cell death through activation of JNK and induction of p53 [86].

All these reports indicate that curcumin can induce cancer cell killing predominantly via p53-mediated pathway, p53 not only controls apoptotic pathways but also acts as a key cell cycle regulatory protein as it can trans-activate cell cycle inhibitors like Cip1 on the event of DNA damage during proliferation and when the damage is irreparable it induces apoptosis by inducing the expression of pro-apoptotic proteins like Bax (Figure 2). So far our discussion thus clearly indicates the involvement of the guardian of genome, p53, in curcumin-induced cancer cell apoptosis via cell cycle regulation.

9.1.11 P53-INDEPENDENT PATHWAYS AND CURCUMIN

It is evident that curcumin can induce selective cancer cell killing in a p53-dependent manner, but impaired p53 expression or activity is associated with a variety of neoplastic transformations. Increasing reports are indicating that curcumin can block cell cycle progression or even apoptosis in a p53-independent manner as well, especially in the cells that lack functional p53 [83]. Curcumin induces apoptosis in p53-null lung cancer cells [61]. It induces melanoma cell apoptosis by activating caspase-8 and caspase-3 via Fas receptor aggregation in a FasL-independent manner, blocks NFκB cell survival pathway and suppresses the apoptotic inhibitor XIAP [87]. Curcumin inhibits cellular isopeptidases, and cause cell death independently of p53 in isogenic pairs of RKO and HCT 116 cells with differential p53 status [88]. It enhances the chemotherapy-induced cytotoxicity in p53-null prostate cancer cell line PC-3, via up-regulation of Cip1 and C/EBPβ expressions and suppression of NFκB activation [89]. It also induces apoptosis in multiple myloma cells by inhibiting IKK and NFκB activity [64]. Study indicates that curcumin down regulates NFκB and AP-1 activity in androgen-dependent and -independent prostate cancer cell lines [70]. Curcumin is a potent inhibitor of protein kinase C (PKC), EGF (epidermal growth factor)-receptor tyrosine kinase and IκB kinase. Subsequently, curcumin inhibits the oncogenes including *c-jun, c-fos, c-myc, NIK, MAPKs, ELK, PI3K, Akt, CDKs* and *iNOS* [63,90]. In contrast to the mentioned reports, studies by Collet et al. shows that curcumin induces JNK-dependent apoptosis of colon cancer cells and it can induce JNK-dependent sustained phosphorylation of c-jun and stimulation of AP-1 transcriptional activity [68]. The oxidized form of cancer chemopreventive agent curcumin can inactivate PKC by oxidizing the vicinal thiols present within the catalytic domain of the enzyme [90]. Recent studies indicated that proteasome-mediated degradation of cell proteins play a pivotal role in the regulation of several basic cellular processes including differentiation, proliferation, cell cycling, and apoptosis. It has also been demonstrated that curcumin-induced apoptosis is mediated through the impairment of ubiquitin-proteasome pathway [90]. All these reports suggests that curcumin can induce apoptosis or block cell cycle progression in a variety of cancer cell lines, predominantly via p53-dependent pathways, but it can also act in a p53-independent manner (Figure 5).

9.1.12 OTHER FUNCTIONS OF CURCUMIN

Curcumin inhibits angiogenesis directly and via regulation of angiogenic growth factors like vascular endothelial growth factor, basic fibroblast growth factor and epidermal growth factor, as well as the genes like angiopoietin 1 and 2, hypoxia-inducible factor-1, heme oxygenase-1, and the transcriptional factors like NF-κB [40]. Inhibition of angiogenic growth factor production and metalloproteinase generation, both integral to the formation of new vasculature, has also been influenced by curcumin in non-malignant and malignant cells growth [91,92]. Similar to the inhibition of angiogenic factors, curcumin has been shown to regulate proteins related to cell-cell adhesion, such as β-catenin, E-cadherin and APC and to inhibit the production of cytokines relevant to tumor growth, e.g. tumour necrosis factor-α (TNF-α) and interleukin-1 [93,94]. Additionally, curcumin has been shown to reduce the expression of membrane surface molecules such as intracellular adhesion molecule-1, vascular cell adhesion molecule-1 and E-selectin and matrix metaloproteases those play important roles in cellular adhesion and metastasis [3,95].

Curcumin has also been shown to quench reactive oxygen species and scavenge superoxide anion radicals and hydroxyl radicals and strongly inhibits nitric oxide (NO) production by down-regulating inducible nitric oxide synthase gene expression [96,97]. Curcumin inhibits of phase I

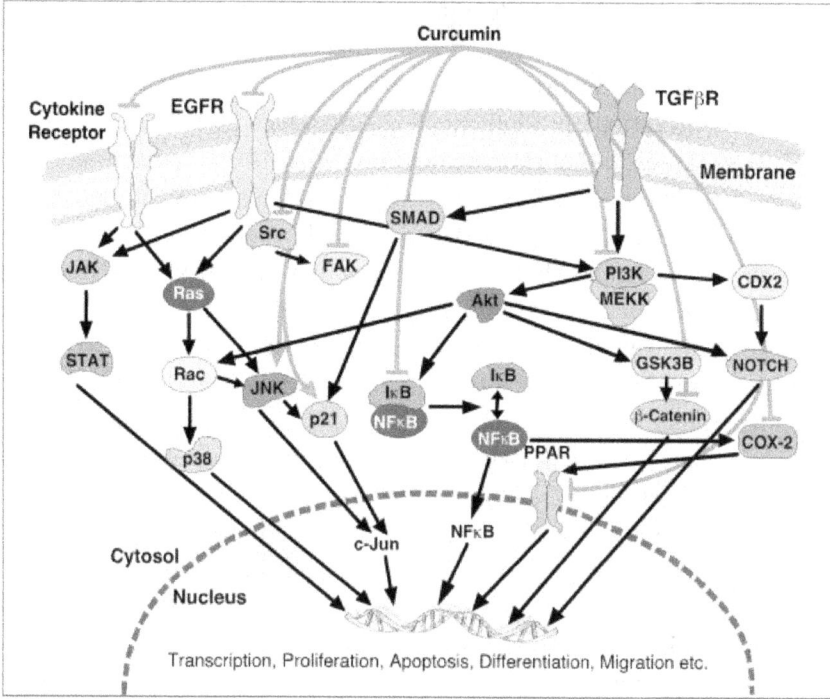

FIGURE 5: Oncogenic signaling targets many levels curcumin. Curcumin enhances apoptotic death, inhibits deregulated cellular proliferation, dedifferentiation and progression towards the neoplastic phenotype by altering key signaling molecules required for cell cycle progression. Such a network organization allows the cell to sense many aspects of the intracellular and extra-cellular milieu, yet ensures that cell death proceeds efficiently once activated. Excessive oncogenic signaling is coupled to apoptosis by a complex mechanism that targets key control points in the pathways. Blunt-head lines indicate that these molecules can be down-regulated by curcumin, where as arrow-head lines indicate that these molecules are often up-regulated by curcumin.

enzymes systems consist of cytochrome P450 isoforms, the P450 reductase, the cytochrome b5 and the epoxide hydrolase and protect from the toxic effects of chemicals and carcinogens [60]. On the other hand curcumin induces phase II enzymes (glutathione S-transferases and epoxide hydrolase), which play a protective role by eliminating toxic substances and oxidants and conferring benefit in the prevention of the early stages of carcinogenesis [98].

Curcumin can act as a potent immunomodulatory agent that can modulate the activation of T cells, B cells, macrophages, neutrophils, natural killer cells, and dendritic cells. Curcumin can also down-regulate the expression of various pro-inflammatory cytokines including TNF, IL-1, IL-2, IL-6, IL-8, IL-12, and chemokines, most likely through inactivation of the transcription factor NF-κB [99]. Interestingly, however, curcumin at low doses can also enhance antibody responses. Curcumin has been shown to activate host macrophages and natural killer (NK) cells and modulate of lymphocyte-mediated functions [100]. Studies from our laboratory showed that curcumin neutralized tumor-induced oxidative stress, restored NF-kB activity, and inhibited TNF-α production, thereby minimizing tumor-induced T-cell apoptosis [7]. Further work suggests that curcumin helps in T cell survival both in primary and effecter immune compartments of tumor-bearing hosts by normalizing perturbed of Jak-3/Stat-5 activity via restoration of IL2-receptor γc chain expression [101]. Curcumin was found to prevent tumor-induced loss of T-effector cells, reverse type-2 cytokine bias and blocks T-regulatory cell augmentation in tumor-bearing hosts via down-regulation of TGF-β in cancer cells (unpublished data). From all these observations it is suggested that curcumin may be used alone or can be combined with classical anti-tumor drugs so as to sustain the immune capacity of the host, which can be affected by the disease or the treatment or may be the both.

9.1.13 CURCUMIN—A MULTIPLE EDGED SWORD

Above discussions on the broad biological activity of this phytochemical prove our hypothesis that curcumin asserts its anti-tumor activity in cancer cells by altering the deregulated cell cycle via (a) cyclin-dependent, (b) p53-dependent and (c) p53-independent pathways. Such influences of curcumin upon key signal transduction pathways of cell cycle and effectiveness in animal model systems have qualified it as a multiple edged sword in combating the deadly disease—cancer. Given that disruption of cell cycle plays a crucial role in cancer progression, its modulation by curcumin seems to be a logical approach in controlling carcinogenesis. Most of the plant products with anticancer activity act as strong antioxidants and some of them are effective modulators of protein kinases/phosphatases that are associated with cell cycle regulation. Many of these phytochemicals are either part of the human diet or consumed as dietary supplement, and do not show adverse health effects even at large doses. Due to failure of conventional chemotherapy in advance stages of cancer and its enormous adverse effects, cancer chemoprevention by this phytochemical in a defined molecular target approach will play an important role in future in reducing cancer incidence as well as the number of deaths caused by this disease.

9.1.14 PROSPECTS FOR THE FUTURE

Previous seminal work, summarized above has demonstrated curcumin inhibition of key molecular mechanisms of tumorigenesis. Effects have been shown of common signaling intermediates that influence the tumor phenotype. Major advances in the understanding of cell cycle regulation mechanisms provided a better knowledge of the molecular interactions involved in human cancer. Moreover, the components of the cell cycle are probably involved in other non-cancerous diseases and their role must be defined. Further mechanistic work however, is required to investigate curcumin effects on switches that connect common effector pathways that regulate cell behavior, phenotype alteration and cell death or lineage commitment. Human intervention studies of curcumin, whether alone or in combination, are indicated against intermediate biomarkers and morphological stages of gastrointestinal tumorigenesis. Curcumin could thus provide a useful component of dietary or pharmacological treatment aimed at reduction of the incidence of and mortality from cancer.

REFERENCES

1. McMichael AJ, McCall MG, Hartchorne JM, Woodings TL: Patterns of gastrointestinal cancer in European migrants to Australia: the role of dietary change. Int J Cancer 1980, 5:431-437.
2. Wargovich MJ: Nutrition and cancer: the herbal revolution. Curr Opin Clin Nutr Metab Care 1999, 2:421-424.

3. Campbell FC, Collett PG: Chemopreventive properties of curcumin. Future Oncol 2005, 1:405-414.
4. Sharma RA, Gescher AJ, Steward WP: Curcumin: the story so far. Eur J Cancer 2005, 41:1955-1968.
5. Sharma OP: Antioxidant activity of curcumin and related compounds. Biochem Pharmacol 1976, 25:1811-1812.
6. Choudhuri T, Pal S, Das T, Sa G: Curcumin selectively induces apoptosis in deregulated cyclin D1-expressed cells at G2 phase of cell cycle in a p53-dependent manner. J Biol Chem 2005, 280:20059-20068.
7. Bhattacharyya S, Mandal D, Sen GS, Pal S, Banerjee S, Lahiry L, Finke JH, Tannenbaum CS, Das T, Sa G: Tumor-induced oxidative stress perturbs NFκB activity augmenting TNFα-mediated T cell death: Protection by curcumin. Cancer Res 2007, 60:362-370.
8. Lowe SW, Cepero E, Evan G: Intrinsic tumor suppression. Nature 2004, 432:307-315.
9. Evan GI, Vousden KH: Proliferation, cell cycle and apoptosis in cancer. Nature 2001, 411:342-348.
10. Sherr CJ: Cancer cell cycles. Science 1996, 274:1672-1677.
11. Danial NN, Korsmeyer SJ: Cell death: critical control points. Cell 2004, 116:205-219.
12. Hahn WC, Weinberg RA: Rules for making human tumor cells. N Engl J Med 2002, 347:1593-1603.
13. Norbury C, Nurse P: Animal cell cycles and their control. Annu Rev Biochem 1992, 61:441-470.
14. Nurse P, Masui Y, Hartwell L: Understanding the cell cycle. Nat Med 1998, 4:1103-1106.
15. Hartwell LH, Kastan MB: Cell cycle control and cancer. Science 1994, 266:1821-1828.
16. Diehl JA: Cycling to cancer with cyclin D1. Cancer Biol Thera 2002, 1:226-231.
17. Yu Q, Geng Y, Sicinski P: Specific protection against breast cancers by cyclin D1 ablation. Nature 2001, 411:1017-1021.
18. Weinstein IB: Relevance of cyclin D1 and other molecular markers to cancer chemoprevention. J Cell Biochem Suppl 1996, 25:23-28.
19. Hosokawa Y, Arnold A: Mechanism of cyclin D1 (CCND1, PRAD1) over-expression in human cancer cells: analysis of allele-specific expression. Genes Chromosomes Cancer 1998, 22:66-71.
20. Hinds PW, Dowdy SF, Eaton EN, Arnold A, Weinberg RA: Function of a human cyclin gene as an oncogene. Proc Natl Acad Sci, USA 1994, 91:709-713.
21. Al Robles, ML Rodriguez-Puebla, AB Glick, C Trempus, L Hansen, P Sicinski, RW Tennant, RA Weinberg, SH Yuspa, CJ Conti: Reduced skin tumor development in cyclin D1-deficient mice highlights the oncogenic ras pathway in vivo. Genes Dev 1998, 12:2469-2474.
22. Wang TC, Cardiff RD, Zukerberg L, Lees E, Arnold A, Schmidt EV: Mammary hyperplasia and carcinoma in MMTV-cyclin D1 transgenic mice. Nature 1994, 369:669-671.

23. Bortner DM, Rosenberg MP: Induction of mammary gland hyperplasia and carcinomas in transgenic mice expressing human cyclin E. Mol Cell Biol 1997, 17:453-459.

24. Harbour JW, Dean DC: Rb function in cell cycle regulation and apoptosis. Nat Cell Biol 2000, 2:65-67.

25. Sherr CJ, Roberts JM: CDK inhibitors: positive and negative regulators of G1-phase progression. Genes Dev 1999, 13:1501-1512.

26. Sa G, Stacey DW: P27 expression is regulated by separate signaling pathways, downstream of Ras, in each cell cycle phase. Exp Cell Res 2004, 300:427-439.

27. Ortega S, Malumbres M, Barbacid M: Cyclin D-dependent kinases, INK4 inhibitors and cancer. Biochim Biophys Acta 2002, 1602:73-87.

28. Vidal A, Koff A: Cell-cycle inhibitors: three families united by a common cause. Gene 2000, 247:1-15.

29. Elledge SJ: Cell cycle checkpoints: preventing an identity crisis. Science 1996, 274:1664-1672.

30. Hollstein M, Sidransky D, Vogelstein B, Harris CC: p53 mutations in human cancers. Science 1991, 253:49-53.

31. Polyak K, Waldman T, He T-C, Kinzler KW, Vogelstein B: Genetic determinants of p53-induced apoptosis and growth arrest. Genes Dev 1996, 10:1945-1952.

32. Levin AJ: p53, the cellular gatekeeper for growth and division. Cell 1997, 88:323-331.

33. Grimmler M, Wang Y, Mund T, Cilensek Z, Keidel EM, Waddell MB, Jäkel H, Kullmann M, Kriwacki RW, Hengst L: Cdk-inhibitory activity and stability of p27Kip1 are directly regulated by oncogenic tyrosine kinases. Cell 2007, 128:269-80.

34. Chu I, Sun J, Arnaout A, Kahn H, Hanna W, Narod S, Sun P, Tan CK, Hengst L, Slingerland J: p27 phosphorylation by Src regulates inhibition of cyclin E-Cdk2. Cell 2007, 128:281-94.

35. Miyashita T, Reed JC: Tumor suppressor p53 is a direct transcriptional activator of the human bax gene. Cell 1995, 80:293-299.

36. Das T, Sa G, Sinha P, Ray PK: Induction of cell proliferation and apoptosis: dependence on the dose of the inducer. Biochem Biophys Res Commun 1999, 260:105-110.

37. Harrington EA, Fanidi A, Evan GI: Oncogenes and cell death. Curr Opinion Genet Dev 1994, 4:120-129.

38. Liu X, Kim CN, Yang J, Jemmerson R, Wang X: Induction of apoptotic program in cell-free extracts: requirement for dATP and cytochrome c. Cell 1996, 86:147-157.

39. Waldman T, Yongyang Y, Diollehay L, Yu J, Kinzler KW, Vogelstein B, Williams J: Cell cycle arrest versus cell death in cancer therapy. Nat Med 1997, 3:1034-1036.

40. Strimpakos AS, Sharma RA: Curcumin: Preventive and therapeutic properties in laboratory studies and clinical trials. Antioxid Redox Signal 2008, 10:511-45.

41. Oyama Y, Masuda T, Nakata M, Chikahisa L, Yamazaki Y, Miura K, Okagawa M: Protective actions of 5'-n-alkylated curcumins on living cells suffering from oxidative stress. Eur J Pharmacol 1998, 360:65-71.

42. Pal S, Bhattacharya S, Choudhuri T, Datta GK, Das T, Sa G: Amelioration of immune cell number depletion and potentiation of depressed detoxification system of tumor-bearing mice by curcumin. Cancer Detection Prevention 2005, 29:470-478.

43. Sugimoto K, Hanai H, Tozawa K, Aoshi T, Uchijima M, Nagata T, Koide Y: Curcumin prevents and ameliorates trinitrobenzene sulfonic acid-induced colitis in mice. Gastroenterology 2002, 123:1912-1922.

44. Pal S, Choudhuri T, Chattopadhyay S, Bhattacharya A, Datta G, Das T, Sa G: Mechanisms of curcumin-induced apoptosis of Ehrlich's ascites carcinoma cells. Biochem Biophys Res Commun 2001, 288:658-665.

45. Ammon HP, Wahl MA: Pharmacology of *Curcuma longa*. Planta Med 1991, 57:1-7.

46. Vial T, Descotes J: Immunosuppressive drugs and cancer. Toxicology 2003, 185:229-240.

47. Choudhuri T, Pal S, Agwarwal ML, Das T, Sa G: Curcumin induces apoptosis in human breast cancer cells through p53-dependent Bax induction. FEBS Lett 2002, 512:334-340.

48. Dhillon N, Aggarwal BB, Newman RA, Wolff RA, Kunnumakkara AB, Abbruzzese JL, Ng CS, Badmaev V, Kurzrock R: Phase II trial of curcumin in patients with advanced pancreatic cancer. Clin Cancer Res 2008, 14:4491-4499.

49. Aggarwal BB, Kumar A, Bharti AC: Anticancer potential of curcumin: preclinical and clinical studies. Anticancer Res 2003, 23:363-398.

50. Cheng AL, Hsu CH, Lin JK, Hsu MM, Ho YF, Shen TS, Ko JY, Lin JT, Lin BR, Ming-Shiang W, Yu HS, Jee SH, Chen GS, Chen TM, Chen CA, Lai MK, Pu YS, Pan MH, Wang YJ, Tsai CC, Hsieh CY: Phase I clinical trial of curcumin, a chemopreventive agent, in patients with high-risk or pre-malignant lesions. Anticancer Res 2001, 21:2895-2900.

51. Kuttan R, Sudheeran PC, Josph CD: Turmeric and curcumin as topical agents in cancer therapy. Tumori 1987, 73:29-31.

52. Garcea G, Berry DP, Jones DJ, Singh R, Dennison AR, Farmer PB, Sharma RA, Steward WP, Gescher AJ: Consumption of the putative chemopreventive agent curcumin by cancer patients: assessment of curcumin levels in the colorectum and their pharmacodynamic consequences. Cancer Epidemiol Biomarkers Prev 2005, 14:120-125.

53. Ireson C, Orr S, Jones DJ, Verschoyle R, Lim CK, Luo JL, Howells L, Plummer S, Jukes R, Williams M, Steward WP, Gescher A: Characterization of metabolites of the chemopreventive agent curcumin in human and rat hepatocytes and in the rat in vivo, and evaluation of their ability to inhibit phorbol ester-induced prostaglandin E2 production. Cancer Res 2001, 61:1058-1064.

54. Huang MT, Wang ZY, Georgiadis CA, Laskin JD, Conney AH: Inhibitory effects of curcumin on tumor initiation by benzo[α]pyrene and 7,12-dimethylbenz[α]anthracene. Carcinogenesis 1992, 13:2183-2186.

55. Huang MT, Newmark HL, Frenkel KJ: Inhibitory effects of curcumin on tumorigenesis in mice. Biochem Suppl 1997, 27:326-34.

56. Jee SH, Shen SC, Tseng CR, Chiu HC, Kuo ML: Curcumin induces a p53-dependent apoptosis in human basal cell carcinoma cells. J Invest Dermatol 1998, 111:656-661.

57. Moos PJ, Edes K, Mullally JE, Fitzpatrick FA: Curcumin impairs tumor suppressor p53 function in colon cancer cells. Carcinogenesis 2004, 25:1611-1617.

58. Park C, Kim GY, Kim GD, Choi BT, Park YM, Choi YH: Induction of G2/M arrest and inhibition of cyclooxygenase-2 activity by curcumin in human bladder cancer T24 cells. Oncol Rep 2006, 15:1225-1231.

59. Liontas A, Yeger H: Curcumin and resveratrol induce apoptosis and nuclear translocation and activation of p53 in human neuroblastoma. Anticancer Res 2004, 24:987-998.

60. Pillai GR, Srivastava AS, Hassanein TI, Chauhan DP, Carrier E: Induction of apoptosis in human lung cancer cells by curcumin. Cancer Lett 2004, 208:163-170.

61. Shi M, Cai Q, Yao L, Mao Y, Ming Y, Ouyang G: Antiproliferation and apoptosis induced by curcumin in human ovarian cancer cells. Cell Biol Int 2006, 30:221-226.

62. Jaiswal AS, Marlow BP, Gupta N, Narayan S: Beta-catenin-mediated transactivation and cell-cell adhesion pathways are important in curcumin (diferuylmethane)-induced growth arrest and apoptosis in colon cancer cells. Oncogene 2002, 21:8414-8427.

63. Bharti AC, Donato N, Singh S, Aggarwal BB: Curcumin (diferuloylmethane) downregulates the constitutive activation of nuclear factor-kappa B and IkappaBalpha kinase in human multiple myeloma cells, leading to suppression of proliferation and induction of apoptosis. Blood 2003, 101:1053-1062.

64. Chen A, Xu J: Activation of PPAR{gamma} by curcumin inhibits Moser cell growth and mediates suppression of gene expression of cyclin D1 and EGFR. Am J Physiol Gastrointest Liver Physiol 2005, 288:G447-456.

65. Leu TH, Su SL, Chuang YC, Maa MC: Direct inhibitory effect of curcumin on Src and focal adhesion kinase activity. Biochem Pharmacol 2003, 66:2323-2331.

66. Nakamura K, Yasunaga Y, Segawa T, Ko D, Moul JW, Srivastava S, Rhim JS: Curcumin down-regulates AR gene expression and activation in prostate cancer cell lines. Int J Oncol 2002, 21:825-830.

67. Balasubramanyam K, Varier RA, Altaf M, Swaminathan V, Siddappa NB, Ranga U, Kundu TK: Curcumin, a novel p300/CREB-binding protein-specific inhibitor of acetyltransferase, represses the acetylation of histone/nonhistone proteins and histone acetyltransferase-dependent chromatin transcription. J Biol Chem 2004, 279:51163-51171.

68. Collett GP, Campbell FC: Curcumin induces c-jun N-terminal kinase-dependent apoptosis in HCT116 human colon cancer cells. Carcinogenesis 2004, 25:2183-2189.

69. Deeb D, Xu YX, Jiang H, Gao X, Janakiraman N, Chapman RA, Gautam SC: Curcumin (Diferuloyl-Methane) enhances tumor necrosis factor-related apoptosis-inducing ligand-induced apoptosis in LNCaP prostate cancer cells. Mol Cancer Ther 2003, 2:95-103.

70. Dorai T, Gehani N, Katz A: Therapeutic potential of curcumin in human prostate cancer-I. Curcumin induces apoptosis in both androgen-dependent and androgen-independent prostate cancer cells. Prostate Cancer Prostatic Dis 2000, 3:84-93.

71. Ramachandran C, Fonseca HB, Jhabvala P, Escalon EA, Melnick SJ: Curcumin inhibits telomerase activity through human telomerase reverse transcritpase in MCF-7 breast cancer cell line. Cancer Lett 2002, 184:1-6.

72. Wolanin K, Magalska A, Mosieniak G, Klinger R, McKenna S, Vejda S, Sikora E, Piwocka K: Curcumin affects components of the chromosomal passenger complex and induces mitotic catastrophe in apoptosis-resistant Bcr-Abl-expressing cells. Mol Cancer Res 2006, 4:457-469.

73. Zheng M, Ekmekcioglu S, Walch ET, Tang CH, Grimm EA: Inhibition of nuclear factor-kappaB and nitric oxide by curcumin induces G2/M cell cycle arrest and apoptosis in human melanoma cells. Melanoma Res 2004, 14:165-171.

74. Shishodia S, Amin HM, Lai R, Aggarwal BB: Curcumin (diferuloylmethane) inhibits constitutive NF-kappaB activation, induces G1/S arrest, suppresses proliferation, and induces apoptosis in mantle cell lymphoma. Biochem Pharmacol 2005, 70:700-701.

75. Rajasingh J, Raikwar HP, Muthia G, Johnson C, Bright JJ: Curcumin induces growth-arrest and apoptosis in association with the inhibition of constitutively active JAK-STAT pathway in T cell leukemia. Biochem Biophys Res Commun 2006, 340:359-368.

76. Tomita M, Kawakami H, Uchihara JN: Curcumin (diferuloylmethane) inhibits constitutive active NF-kappaB, leading to suppression of cell growth of human T-cell leukemia virus type I-infected T-cell lines and primary adult T-cell leukemia cells. Int J Cancer 2006, 118:765-772.

77. Holy JM: Curcumin disrupts mitotic spindle structure and induces micronucleation in MCF-7breast cancer cells. Mutat Res 2002, 518:71-84.

78. Woo JH, Kim YH, Choi YJ, Kim DG, Lee KS, Bae JH, Min DS, Chang JS, Jeong YJ, Lee YH, Park JW, Kwon TK: Molecular mechanisms of curcumin-induced cytotoxicity: induction of apoptosis through generation of reactive oxygen species, down-regulation of Bcl-XL and IAP, the release of cytochrome c and inhibition of Akt. Carcinogenesis 2003, 24:1199-1208.

79. Sa G, Hitomi M, Harwalkar J, Stacey A, Chen G, Stacey DW: Ras is active throughout the cell cycle, but is able to induce cyclin D1 only during G2 phase. Cell Cycle 2002, 1:50-58.

80. Sa G, Guo Y, Stacey DW: Regulation of S phase initiation by p27Kip1 in NIH3T3 cells. Cell Cycle 2005, 4:618-627.

81. Hitomi M, Stacey DW: Cellular ras and cyclin D1 are required during different cell cycle periods in cycling NIH 3T3 cells. Mol Cell Biol 1999, 19:4623-4632. P

82. Mukhopadhyay A, Banerjee S, Stafford LJ, Xia CX, Liu M, Aggarwal BB: Curcumin induced suppression of cell proliferation correlates with downregulation of cyclin D1 expression and CDK4-mediated retinoblastoma protein phosphorylation. Oncogene 2002, 21:8852-8862.

83. Park MJ, Kim EH, Park IC, Lee HC, Woo SH, Lee JY, Hong YJ, Rhee CH, Choi SH, Shim BS, Lee SH, Hong SI: Curcumin inhibits cell cycle progression of immortalized human umbilical vein endothelial (ECV304) cells by up-regulating cyclin-dependent kinase inhibitor, p21WAF1/CIP1, p27KIP1 and p53. Int J Oncol 2002, 21:379-383.

84. Bech-Otschir D, Kraft R, Huang X: COP9 signalosome-specific phosphorylation targets p53 to degradation by the ubiquitin system. EMBO J 2001, 20:1630-1639. P

85. Song G, Mao YB, Cai QF, Yao LM, Ouyang GL, Bao SD: Curcumin induces human HT-29 colon adenocarcinoma cell apoptosis by activating p53 and regulating apoptosis-related protein expression. Braz J Med Biol Res 2005, 38:1791-1798.

86. Kamath R, Jiang Z, Sun G, Yalowich JC, Rajasekaran B: c-Abl kinase regulates curcumin-induced cell death through activation of c-Jun N-terminal kinase. Mol Pharmacol 2007, 71:61-72.

87. Bush JA, Cheung KJ Jr, Li G: Curcumin induces apoptosis in human melanoma cells through a Fas receptor/caspase-8 pathway independent of p53. Exp Cell Res 2001, 271:305-314.

88. Mullally JE, Fitzpatrick FA: Pharmacophore model for novel inhibitors of ubiquitin isopeptidases that induce p53-independent cell death. Mol Pharmacol 2002, 69:351-358.

89. Chen J, Huang CY, Guan JY, Lu SH, Pu YS: Curcumin enhances cytotoxicity of chemotherapeutic agents in prostate cancer cells by inducing p21WAF1/CIP1 and C/EBPβ expressions and suppressing NF-κB activation hour. The prostate 2002, 51:211-218.

90. Lin JK: Suppression of protein kinase C and nuclear oncogene expression as possible action mechanisms of cancer chemoprevention by curcumin. Arch Pharm Res 2004, 27:683-692.

91. Choi H, Chun YS, Kim SW, Kim MS, Park JW: Curcumin inhibits hypoxia-inducible factor-1 by degrading aryl hydrocarbon receptor nuclear translocator: a mechanism of tumor growth inhibition. Mol Pharmaco 2006, 70:1664-1671.

92. Mohan R, Sivak J, Ashton P, Russo LA, Pham BQ, Kasahara N, Raizman MB, Fini ME: Curcuminoids inhibit the angiogenic response stimulated by fibroblast growth factor-2, including expression of matrix metalloproteinase gelatinase B. J Biol Chem 2000, 275:10405-10412.

93. Lala PK, Chakraborty C: Role of nitric oxide in carcinogenesis and tumour progression. Lancet Oncol 2001, 2:149-56.

94. Bae MK, Kim SH, Jeong JW, Lee YM, Kim HS, Kim SR, Yun I, Bae SK, Kim KW: Curcumin inhibits hypoxia-induced angiogenesis via down-regulation of HIF-1. Oncol Rep 2006, 15:1557-1562.

95. Park CH, Hahm ER, Park S, Kim HK, Yang CH: The inhibitory mechanism of curcumin and its derivative against beta-catenin/Tcf signaling. FEBS Lett 2005, 579:2965-2971.

96. Khopde M, Priyadarsini KI, Venkatesan P, Rao MN: Free radical scavenging ability and antioxidant efficiency of curcumin and its substituted analogue. Biophys Chem 1999, 80:85-91.

97. Graziewicz M, Wink DA, Laval F: Nitric oxide inhibits DNA ligase activity: potential mechanisms for NO-mediated DNA damage. Carcinogenesis 1996, 17:2501-2505.

98. Mori Y, Tatematsu K, Koide A, Sugie S, Tanaka T, Mori H: Modification by curcumin of mutagenic activation of carcinogenic N-nitrosamines by extrahepatic cytochromes P-450 2B1 and 2E1 in rats. Cancer Sci 2006, 97:896-904.

99. Jagetia GC, Aggarwal BB: "Spicing up" of the immune system by curcumin. J Clin Immunol 2007, 27:19-35.

100. Bhaumik S, Jyothi MD, Khar A: Differential modulation of nitric oxide production by curcumin in host macrophages and NK cells. FEBS Lett 2000, 483:78-82.

101. Bhattacharyya S, Mandal D, Saha B, Sen GS, Das T, Sa G: Curcumin prevents tumor-induced T cell apoptosis through Stat-5a-mediated Bcl-2 induction. J Biol Chem 2007, 282:15954-15964.

CHAPTER 10

COMPARATIVE STUDY OF THE ANTIOXIDANT AND REACTIVE OXYGEN SPECIES SCAVENGING PROPERTIES IN THE EXTRACTS OF THE FRUITS OF *TERMINALIA CHEBULA, TERMINALIA BELERICA,* AND *EMBLICA OFFICINALIS*

BIBHABASU HAZRA, RHITAJIT SARKAR, SANTANU BISWAS, AND NRIPENDRANATH MANDAL

10.1 BACKGROUND

Oxidative stress plays an important role in the pathogenesis of various diseases such as atherosclerosis, alcoholic liver cirrhosis and cancer etc. Oxidative stress is initiated by reactive oxygen species (ROS), such as superoxide anion (O^{-2}), perhydroxy radical (HOO^-) and hydroxyl radical ($HO\cdot$). These radicals are formed by a one electron reduction process of molecular oxygen (O_2). ROS can easily initiate the lipid peroxidation of the membrane lipids, causing damage of the cell membrane of phospholipids, lipoprotein by propagating a chain reaction cycle [1,2]. Thus, antioxidants defense systems have coevolved with aerobic metabolism to

This chapter was originally published under the Creative Commons Attribution License. Hazra B, Sarkar R, Biswas S, and Mandal N. Comparative Study of the Antioxidant and Reactive Oxygen Species Scavenging Properties in the Extracts of the Fruits of Terminalia chebula, Terminalia belerica, *and* Emblica officinalis. BMC Complementary and Alternative Medicine **10,**20 (2010). doi:10.1186/1472-6882-10-20.

counteract oxidative damage from ROS. Most living species have efficient defense systems to prevent themselves against oxidative stress induced by ROS [3]. Recent investigations have shown that the antioxidant properties of plants could be correlated with oxidative stress defense and different human diseases and aging process etc [4]. In this respect flavonoids and other polyphenolic compounds have received the greatest attention.

The fruits of *Terminalia chebula* Retz, *Terminalia belerica* Roxb, and *Emblica officinalis* Gaertn are widely used in the Indian traditional system of medicine [5]. The half ripe fruit of *T. belerica* and the pericarp of *T. chebula* fruit were reported to be purgative [5]. The fruit of *T. chebula* was traditionally used to cure asthma, urinary disorders, heart disease and it has cardiotonic activity [6,7]. In Ayurveda, the fruit of *E. officinalis* is used as a cardiotonic, cerebral and intestinal tonic [8], and it is also reported to have anticancer properties [9,8]. The fruit of *E. officinalis* is a rich source of vitamin C, a well-known antioxidant [10]. The crude extract of *E. officinalis* was reported to counteract the hepatotoxic and renotoxic effects of metals [11] due to antioxidant properties.

This present study is aimed to assess the antioxidant capacity of the 70% methanol extracts of *T. chebula*, *T. belerica* and *E. officinalis* fruits, through their measurement of activities in scavenging of different free radicals including hydroxyl, superoxide, nitric oxide, hydrogen peroxide, peroxynitrite, singlet oxygen, hypochlorous acid, phenol, flavonoid and ascorbic acid content and total antioxidant activity with ABTS and DPPH.

10.1 METHODS

10.1.1 CHEMICALS

2,2'-azinobis-(3-ethylbenzothiazoline-6-sulfonic acid) (ABTS) was obtained from Roche diagnostics, Mannheim, Germany. 6-hydroxy-2,5,7,8-tetramethylchroman-2-carboxylic acid (Trolox) was obtained from Fluka, Buchs, Switzerland. Potassium persulfate ($K_2S_2O_8$), 2-deoxy-2-ribose, mannitol, sodium nitroprusside (SNP), lipoic acid 5,5'-dithiobis-2-nitrobenzoic acid (DTNB), 1-chloro-2,4-dinitrobenzene (CDNB), glutathione reduced and quercetin were obtained from Sisco Research Laboratories Pvt. Ltd, Mumbai, India. Folin-ciocalteu reagent, xylenol orange and N, N-dimethyl-4-nitrosoaniline were obtained from Merck, Mumbai, India. Gallic acid, 1,1-Diphenyl-2-Picrylhydrazyl (DPPH) and curcumin were obtained from MP Biomedicals, France. Catalase was obtained from Hi-Media Laboratories Pvt. Ltd, Mumbai, India. Evans blue was purchased from BDH, England. Diethylene-triamine-pentaacetic acid (DTPA) was obtained from Spectrochem Pvt. Ltd, Mumbai, India. Thiobarbituric acid (TBA) was obtained from Loba Chemie, Mumbai, India.

10.1.2 PLANT MATERIAL

The fruits of *T. chebula*, *T. belerica* and *E. officinalis* were collected from Bankura district of West Bengal, India. The plant was identified by the Central Research Institute (Ayurveda), Kolkata, India, where specimens of each plant were deposited (Table 1).

TABLE 1: Voucher specimen number of three plants

Sl. No.	Plant	Specimen No.
1.	*Terminalia chebula*	CRHS 113/08
2.	*Terminalia belerica*	CRHS 114/08
3.	*Emblica officinalis*	CRHS 115/08

10.1.3 ANIMALS

Male Swiss albino mice (20 ± 2 g) were purchased from Chittaranjan National Cancer Institute (CNCI), Kolkata, India and were maintained under a constant 12-h dark/light cycle at an environmental temperature of $22 \pm 2°C$. The animals were fed with normal laboratory pellet diet and water ad libitum. The institutional animal ethics committee approved all experimental procedure.

10.1.4 EXTRACTION

The powder (100 g) of the individual normal air-dried fruits of *T. chebula*, *T. belerica* and *E. officinalis* were stirred using a magnetic stirrer with a 7:3 mixture of methanol: water (500 ml) for 15 hours; the mixture was then centrifuged at 2850 × g and the supernatant decanted. The process was repeated by adding the solvent with the precipitated pellet. The supernatants were collected, concentrated in a rotary evaporator [250-200 mbar at 37°C] and lyophilized. The yields for the plants materials were 5.6 g, 3.7 g and 4.2 g for *T. chebula*, *T. belerica* and *E. officinalis*, respectively. The dried extracts were stored at -20°C until use.

10.1.5 IN VITRO ANTIOXIDANT ASSAY

10.1.5.1 TOTAL ANTIOXIDANT ACTIVITY

Antioxidant capacity was measured based on the scavenging of ABTS.+ radical cation by the sample in comparison to trolox standard [12]. ABTS solution was mixed with potassium persulfate and incubated for 12-16 h in dark to generate ABTS.+ radical cation. Then 10 μl sample solution was mixed with 1 ml ABTS.+ solution and the absorbance was measured at $\lambda =$ 734 nm. All experiments were repeated six times. The percentage inhibition of absorbance was calculated and plotted as a function of concentration of standard and sample to determine the trolox equivalent antioxidant concentration (TEAC). To calculate the TEAC, the gradient of the plot for the sample was divided by the gradient of the plot for trolox.

10.1.5.2 DPPH RADICAL SCAVENGING ASSAY

The complementary study for the antioxidant capacity of the fruit extract was confirmed by the DPPH scavenging assay according to Mahakunakorn et al. [13], with slight modification. Different concentrations (0-100 µg/ml) of the extracts and the standard trolox were mixed with equal volume of ethanol. Then 50 µl of DPPH solution (1 mM) was pipetted into the previous mixture and stirred thoroughly. The resulting solution was kept standing for 2 minutes before the optical density (OD) was measured at λ = 517 nm. The measurement was repeated with six sets. The percentage radical scavenging activity was calculated from the following formula:

% scavenging [DPPH] = $[(A_0 - A_1)/A_0]$ * 100

Where A_0 was the absorbance of the control and A_1 was the absorbance in the presence of the samples and standard.

10.1.5.3 HYDROXYL RADICAL SCAVENGING ASSAY

The scavenging assay for hydroxyl radical was performed by a standard method [12]. Hydroxyl radical was generated by the Fenton reaction using a Fe^{3+}-ascorbate-EDTA-H_2O_2 system. The assay quantifies the 2-deoxyribose degradation product, by its condensation with TBA. All tests were carried out six times. Mannitol, a classical. OH scavenger, was used as a standard compound. Percent inhibition was evaluated by the following equation:

% inhibition = $[(A_0 - A_1)/A_0]$ * 100

Where A_0 was the absorbance of the control and A_1 was the absorbance in the presence of the samples and standard.

10.1.5.4 SUPEROXIDE RADICAL SCAVENGING ASSAY

Measurements of superoxide anion scavenging activities of the samples and standard quercetin were done based on the reduction of NBT according to a previously described method [12]. Superoxide radical is generated by a non-enzymatic system of phenazine methosulfate-nicotinamide adenine di-nucleotide (PMS/NADH). These radicals reduce nitro blue tetrazolium (NBT) into a purple colored formazan which was measured spectrophotometrically at $\lambda = 562$ nm. All tests were performed six times. The percentage inhibition of superoxide anion generation was calculated using the following formula:

% inhibition $= [(A_0 - A_1)/A_0] * 100$

Where A_0 was the absorbance of the control and A_1 was the absorbance in the presence of the samples and standard.

10.1.5.5 NITRIC OXIDE RADICAL SCAVENGING ASSAY

Sodium nitroprusside (SNP) gives rise to nitric oxide that under interaction with oxygen produce nitrite ions measured by Griess Illosvoy reaction [12]. The chromophore generated was spectrophotometrically measured at $\lambda = 540$ nm against blank sample. All tests were performed six times. Curcumin was used as a standard. The percentage inhibition of nitric oxide radical generation was calculated using the following formula:

% inhibition $= [(A_0 - A_1)/A_0] * 100$

Where A_0 was the absorbance of the control and A_1 was the absorbance in the presence of the samples and standard.

10.1.5.6 HYDROGEN PEROXIDE SCAVENGING ASSAY

FOX-reagent method was used to determine this activity of the sample and the reference compound sodium pyruvate, as previously described [12]. The absorbance of the ferric-xylenol orange complex was measured at $\lambda =$

560 nm. All tests were carried out six times. The percentage of scavenging of hydrogen peroxide of fruit extracts and standard compound:

% scavenged $[H_2O_2] = [(A_0 - A_1)/A_0] * 100$

where A_0 was the absorbance of the control, and A_1 was the absorbance in the presence of the sample of fruit extracts and standard.

10.1.5.7 PEROXYNITRITE SCAVENGING ASSAY

Peroxynitrite (ONOO⁻) synthesis was done 12 hrs before the assay, according to Beckman et al [14]. Acidic solution (0.6 M HCl) of 5 ml H_2O_2 (0.7 M) was mixed with 5 ml of 0.6 M KNO_2 on an ice bath for 1 s and 5 ml of ice-cold 1.2 M NaOH was added to the reaction mixture. Excess H_2O_2 was adsorbed by granular MnO_2 and the reaction mixture was left at -20°C. The concentration of the peroxynitrite solution was measured spectrophotometrically at $\lambda = 302$ nm ($\varepsilon = 1670$ M^{-1} cm^{-1}).

Evans blue bleaching assay was used to measure the peroxynitrite scavenging activity [12]. The percentage of scavenging of ONOO⁻ was calculated by comparing the results of the test and blank samples. All tests were performed six times. Gallic acid was used as reference compound. The percentage of scavenging of peroxynitrite anion was calculated using the following equation:

% scavenged $[ONOO^-] = [(A_0 - A_1)/A_0] * 100$

where A_0 was the absorbance of the control, and A_1 was the absorbance in the presence of the sample of fruit extracts and standard.

10.1.5.8 SINGLET OXYGEN SCAVENGING ASSAY

Singlet oxygen ($^1O_2$) production, and at the same time, its scavenging by the samples and the reference compound lipoic acid can be monitored by

N, N-dimethyl-4-nitrosoaniline (RNO) bleaching, using a earlier reported method [12]. Singlet oxygen was generated by a reaction between NaOCl and H_2O_2 and the bleaching of RNO was read at $\lambda = 440$ nm. All tests were performed six times. Singlet oxygen scavenging was calculated by the following formula:

$$\% \text{ of scavenging} = [(A_0 - A_1)/A_0] * 100$$

where A_0 was the absorbance of the control, and A_1 was the absorbance in the presence of the sample of fruit extracts and standard.

10.1.5.9 HYPOCHLOROUS ACID SCAVENGING ASSAY

According to a previously described method [12], hypochlorous acid (HOCl) was prepared just before the experiment by adjusting the pH of a 10% (v/v) solution of NaOCl to pH 6.2 with 0.6 M H_2SO_4 and the concentration of HOCl was determined by taking the absorbance at $\lambda = 235$ nm using the molar extinction coefficient of 100 M^{-1} cm^{-1}. The scavenging activities of the fruit extracts and the standard, ascorbic acid, a potent HOCl scavenger was evaluated by measuring the decrease in the absorbance of catalase at $\lambda = 404$ nm. All tests were performed six times. The percentage of scavenging of HOCl was calculated using the following equation:

$$\% \text{ scavenged [HOCl]} = [(A_0 - A_1)/A_0] * 100$$

where A_0 was the absorbance of the control, and A_1 was the absorbance in the presence of the sample of fruit extracts and standard.

10.1.6 REDUCING POWER ASSAY

The Fe^{3+}-reducing power of the extract was determined by a standard method [12]. In a phosphate buffer solution (0.2 M, pH 6.6), different concentrations (0.0-0.4 mg/ml) of the extract were mixed with potassium hexacyanoferrate (0.1%), followed by incubation. After incubation, the upper portion of the solution was diluted, and $FeCl_3$ solution (0.01%) was added. The reaction mixture was left for 10 min at room temperature for colour development and the absorbance was measured at $\lambda = 700$ nm. All tests were performed six times. A higher absorbance of the reaction mixture indicated greater reducing power. Ascorbic acid was used as a positive control.

10.1.7 DETERMINATION OF TOTAL PHENOLIC CONTENT

The amount of total phenolics present in the fruit extract was determined using Folin-Ciocalteu (FC) reagent by a formerly reported method [12]. A gallic acid standard curve ($R^2 = 0.9468$) was used to measure the phenolic content.

10.1.8 DETERMINATION OF TOTAL FLAVONOID CONTENT

The amount of total flavonoids was determined with aluminium chloride ($AlCl_3$) according to a known method [12]. The flavonoid content was calculated from quercetin standard curve ($R^2 = 0.9947$).

10.1.9 DETERMINATION OF ASCORBIC ACID CONTENT

The amount of total ascorbic acid was determined with ferroin complexation method with minor modification [15]. To 1 ml solution of the sample, 100 μl of $3.3*10^{-3}$ M Iron (III)-phen colour reagent was added and the pH was adjusted to 4.5 with 20% sodium acetate. The absorbance was measured at $\lambda = 512$ nm and subsequently the ascorbate content was calculated from ascorbic acid standard curve ($R^2 = 0.9554$).

10.1.10 IN VIVO ANTIOXIDANT ASSAY

10.1.10.1 EXPERIMENTAL DESIGN

Mice were randomly divided into ten groups containing six animals in each group. Group I animals served as control and administered a single daily dose of normal saline. Groups II, III and IV received the *T. chebula* extract at a dose of 10, 50 and 100 mg/kg body weight, respectively. Groups V, VI and VII were given *T. belerica* extract at a dose of 10, 50 and 100 mg/kg body weight, respectively. The other three groups (Group VIII, IX and X) were administered *E. officinalis* extract at the same dose. The treatments were carried out orally for 7 days and on the 8th day all the animals were sacrificed by cervical dislocation. The liver was immediately removed and after washing with ice-cold saline it was homogenized in 10 volume of 0.1 M phosphate buffer (pH 7.4) containing 5 mM EDTA and 0.15 M NaCl, and centrifuged at 8000 g for 30 min at 4°C. The supernatant was collected and used for the assay of enzyme activities. Protein concentration was estimated according to Lowry method [16] using BSA as standard.

10.1.10.2 ASSAY OF ANTIOXIDANT ENZYMES

Superoxide dismutase (SOD) was assayed by measuring the inhibition of the formation of blue colored formazan at 560 nm according to the technique of Kakkar et al. [17]. Catalase (CAT) activity was measured by following the decrease in H_2O_2 concentration spectrophotometrically over time at 240 nm according to a previously described method [18]. Glutathione-S-transferase (GST) was determined by the method of Habig and Jacoby [19] based on the formation of GSH-CDNB conjugate and increase in the absorbance at 340 nm. Reduced glutathione (GSH) level was measured spectrophotometrically at 412 nm by the method of Ellman [20].

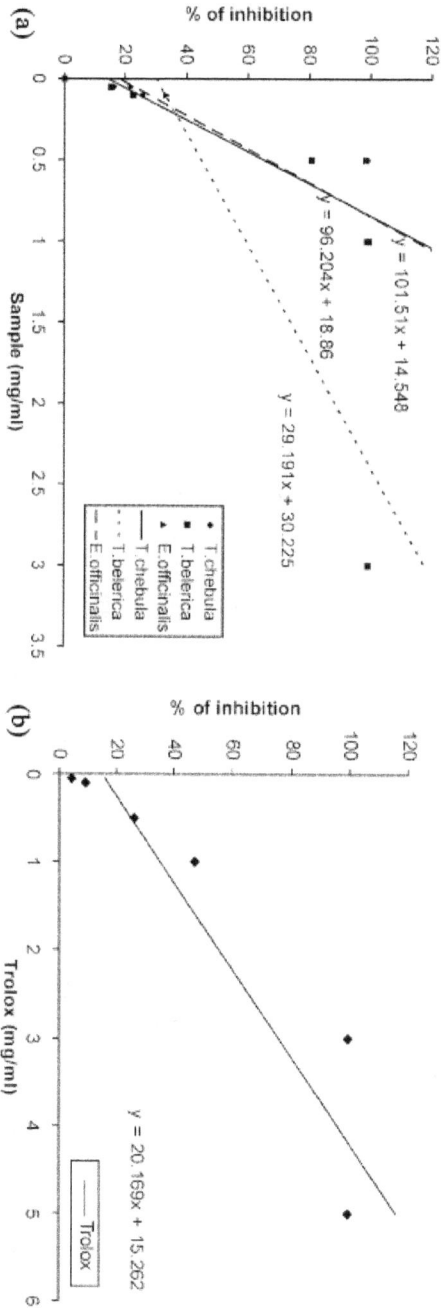

FIGURE 1: Total antioxidant activity. Total antioxidant activity of plant extract and trolox. Effect of (a) *T. chebula*, *T. belerica* and *E. officinalis* extracts and (b) reference compound trolox on ABTS radical cation decolorization assay. The percentage of inhibition was plotted against concentration of sample. All data are expressed as mean ± S.D. (n = 6).

TABLE 2: Comparison of the antioxidant and free radical scavenging capacities of 70% methanolic crudes of *Terminalia chebula, Terminalia belerica* and *Emblica officinalis*.

Name of Assay	70% methanolic crudes of			Standard	Values of Standard compounds
	Terminalia chebula	*Terminalia belerica*	*Emblica officinalis*		
TEAC Values	4.52 ± 0.12	1.01 ± 0.03	4.10 ± 0.17	—	—
† Phenolic content	127.60 ± 0.001	133.00 ± 0.003	215.60 ± 0.004	—	—
‡ Flavonoid content	219.30 ± 0.01	138.30 ± 0.01	176.00 ± 0.01	—	—
§ Ascorbic acid content	46.74 ± 1.10	45.25 ± 0.75	71.08 ± 1.63	—	—
♣ IC_{50} values of the extracts for free radical scavenging capacity for:					
DPPH	1.73 ± 0.07***	1.45 ± 0.02***	1.43 ± 0.03***	Ascorbic acid	5.29 ± 0.28
Hydroxyl (OH.)	72.02 ± 8.99***	203.25 ± 1.87**	382.02 ± 7.88***	Mannitol	571.45 ± 20.12
Superoxide (O2⁻)	13.42 ± 0.22***	18.18 ± 1.39***	13.82 ± 0.19***	Quercetin	42.06 ± 1.35
Nitric oxide (NO.)	33.28 ± 4.56***	40.83 ± 4.40***	33.89 ± 2.94***	Curcumin	90.82 ± 4.75
Peroxynitrite (ONOO.⁻)	1.27 ± 0.07***	0.99 ± 0.10**	0.83 ± 0.03NS	Gallic acid	0.88 ± 0.06
Singlet oxygen ($^1O_2$)	424.50 ± 24.70***	233.12 ± 48.68***	490.42 ± 159.59**	Lipoic acid	46.15 ± 1.16
Hypochlorous acid (HOCl)	433.60 ± 15.45**	271.51 ± 13.70***	420.58 ± 31.97***	Ascorbic acid	235.96 ± 5.75

† *Phenolic content (mg/ml Gallic acid equivalent per 100 mg plant extract)*
‡ *Flavonoid content (mg/ml Quercetin equivalent per 100 mg plant extract)*
§ *Ascorbic acid content (mg/ml Ascorbic acid per 100 mg plant extract)*
♣ IC_{50} *Values are in μg/ml (except for Peroxynitrite scavenging assay where values are expressed in mg/ml). Each value represents mean ± S.D. (n = 6)*
* $p < 0.05$; ** $p < 0.01$; *** $p < 0.001$; NS = Non significant

10.1.11 STATISTICAL ANALYSIS

All data were reported as the mean ± SD of six measurements. The statistical analysis was performed by KyPlot version 2.0 beta 15 (32 bit). The IC_{50} values were calculated by the formula, $Y = 100*A1/(X + A1)$ where $A1 = IC_{50}$, Y = response ($Y = 100\%$ when $X = 0$), X = inhibitory concentration. The IC_{50} values were compared by paired t test (two-sided). $p < 0.05$ was considered significant.

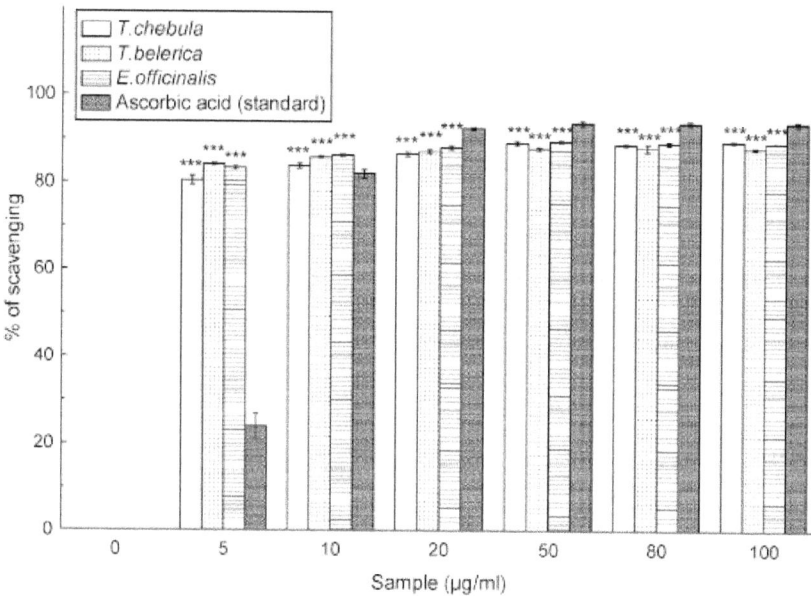

FIGURE 2: DPPH scavenging activity. Effect of the *T. chebula*, *T. belerica* and *E. officinalis* extracts and standard ascorbic acid on DPPH radical scavenging study. The data is expressed as % scavenging of DPPH radicals. The results are mean ± S.D. of six parallel measurements. ***$p < 0.001$ vs 0 µg/ml.

10.2 RESULTS

10.2.1 TOTAL ANTIOXIDANT ACTIVITY

The total antioxidant capacity of the extract was calculated from the decolorization of ABTS.+, upon interaction with the extract or standard trolox that suppressed the absorbance of the ABTS .+ radical cation and the results, expressed as percentage inhibition of absorbance, are shown in Figure 1(a) and 1(b), respectively. The TEAC value of the extracts of *T. chebula*, *T. belerica* and *E. officinalis* were 4.52 ± 0.12, 1.01 ± 0.03 and 4.10 ± 0.17, respectively.

10.2.2 DPPH SCAVENGING ACTIVITY

As is evident in the Figure 2 and the IC_{50} value of the samples, following the order *T. chebula*, *T. belerica* & *E. officinalis* (1.73 ± 0.07 µg/ml, 1.45 ± 0.02 µg/ml & 1.43 ± 0.03 µg/ml) in comparison to the ascorbic acid (5.29 ± 0.28 µg/ml) standard (Table 2) to scavenge the radical, it can be put forward as a fact that the extracts truly work as antioxidant.

10.2.3 HYDROXYL RADICAL SCAVENGING ASSAY

This assay shows the abilities of the extracts and standard mannitol to scavenge hydroxyl radical, as shown in Figure 3. The IC_{50} values (Table 2) of the extracts (in the order *T. chebula*, *T. belerica* and *E. officinalis*) and standard in this assay were 72.02 ± 8.99 µg/ml, 203.25 ± 1.87 µg/ml, 382.02 ± 7.88 µg/ml and 571.45 ± 20.12 µg/ml, respectively.

10.2.4 SUPEROXIDE RADICAL SCAVENGING ASSAY

Figure 4 shows the abilities of the fruit extracts and the reference compound quercetin to quench superoxide radicals in the PMS-NADH reaction

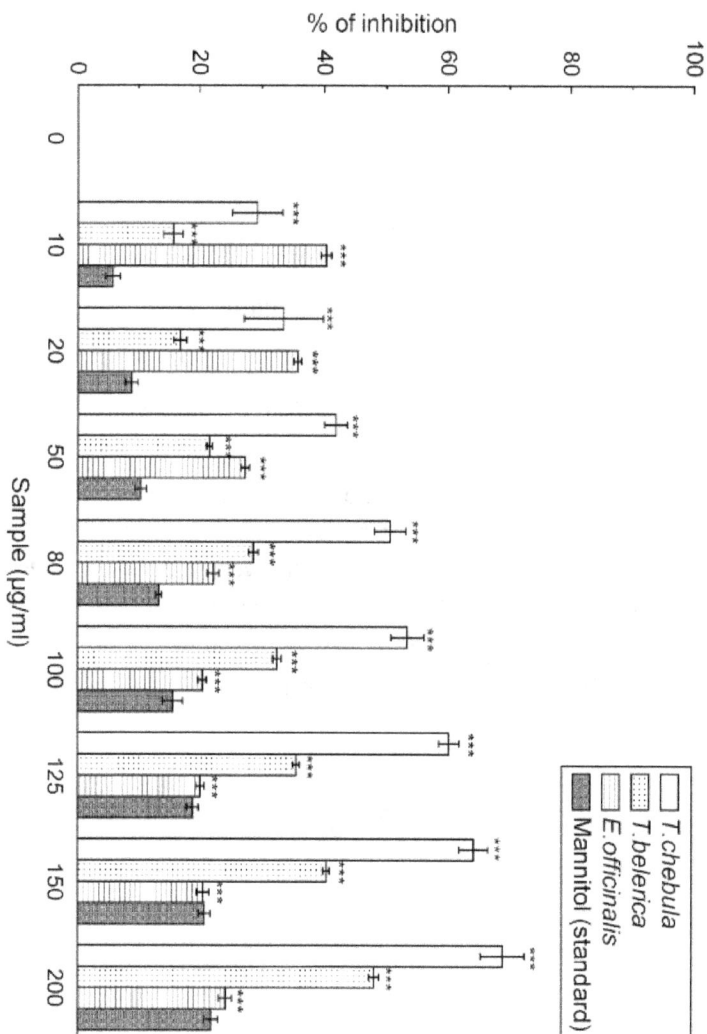

FIGURE 3: Hydroxyl radical scavenging assay. Hydroxyl radical scavenging activity of the *T. chebula*, *T. belerica* and *E. officinalis* extracts and the reference compound mannitol. The data represent the percentage of inhibition of deoxyribose degradation. The results are mean ± S.D. of six parallel measurements. ***p < 0.001 vs 0 μg/ml.

mixture. The IC_{50} values (Table 2) of the fruit extracts, in the order as mentioned above and quercetin were 13.42 ± 0.22 µg/ml, 18.18 ± 1.39 µg/ml, 13.82 ± 0.19 µg/ml and 42.06 ± 1.35 µg/ml, respectively.

10.2.5 NITRIC OXIDE RADICAL SCAVENGING ASSAY

As evident from Figure 5, the extracts of *T. chebula*, *T. belerica* and *E. officinalis* also caused considerable dose-dependent scavenging of nitric oxide in comparison to the reference compound curcumin, which is also reflected in their respective IC_{50} values (Table 2) of 33.28 ± 4.56 µg/ml, 40.83 ± 4.40 µg/ml, 33.89 ± 2.94 µg/ml and 90.82 ± 4.75 µg/ml for the extracts in the aforesaid order and curcumin.

10.2.6 PEROXYNITRITE SCAVENGING ASSAY

Figure 6 shows the peroxynitrite scavenging activity of the fruit extracts in a concentration dependent manner. The calculated IC_{50} values for *T. chebula*, *T. belerica* and *E. officinalis* were 1.27 ± 0.07 mg/ml, 0.99 ± 0.10 mg/ml and 0.83 ± 0.03 mg/ml, repetively in comparison to that of the reference compound gallic acid ($IC_{50} = 0.88 \pm 0.06$ mg/ml) (Table 2) indicating that the samples are not as potent scavenger of peroxynitrite as gallic acid, except *E. officinalis*.

10.2.7 HYDROGEN PEROXIDE SCAVENGING ASSAY

Hydrogen peroxide scavenging activity of the extracts of *T. chebula*, *T. belerica* and *E. officinalis* showed no substantial result compared to the standard sodium pyruvate ($IC_{50} = 3.24 \pm 0.30$ mg/ml) and the IC_{50} values of the same were found to be much higher than can be represented. So, no figure or IC_{50} values were provided.

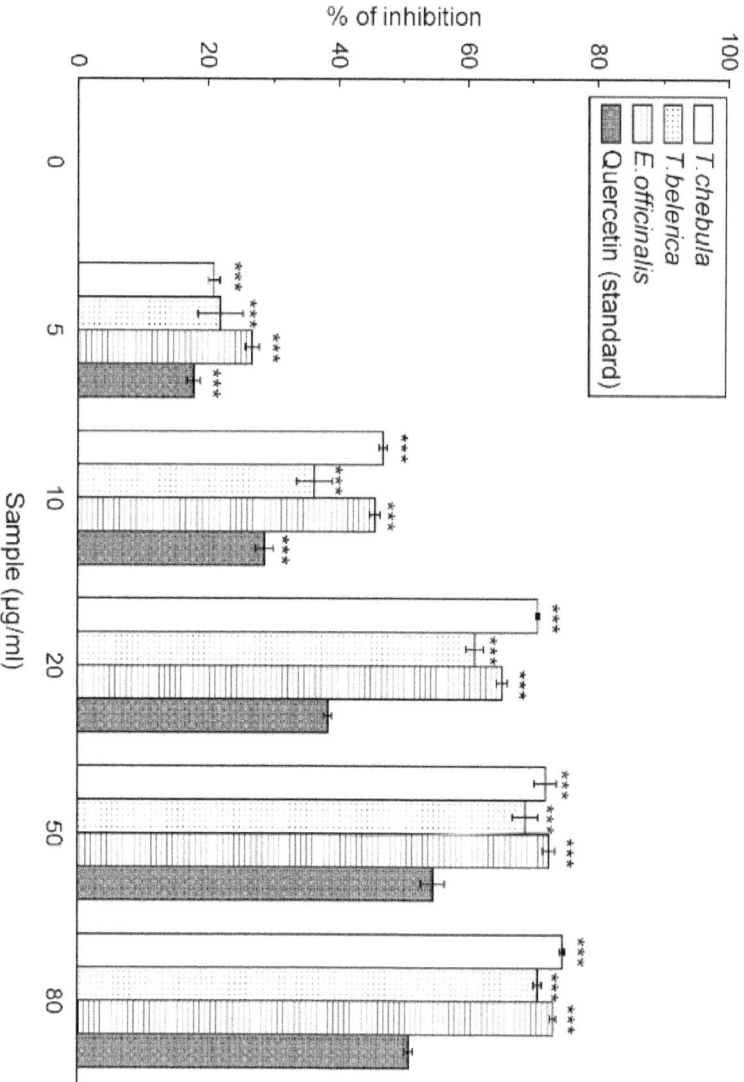

FIGURE 4: Superoxide radical scavenging assay. Scavenging effect of *T. chebula*, *T. belerica* and *E. officinalis* plant extracts and standard quercetin on superoxide radical. The data represents the percentage of superoxide radical inhibition. All data are expressed as mean ± S.D. (n = 6). ***p < 0.001 vs 0 µg/ml.

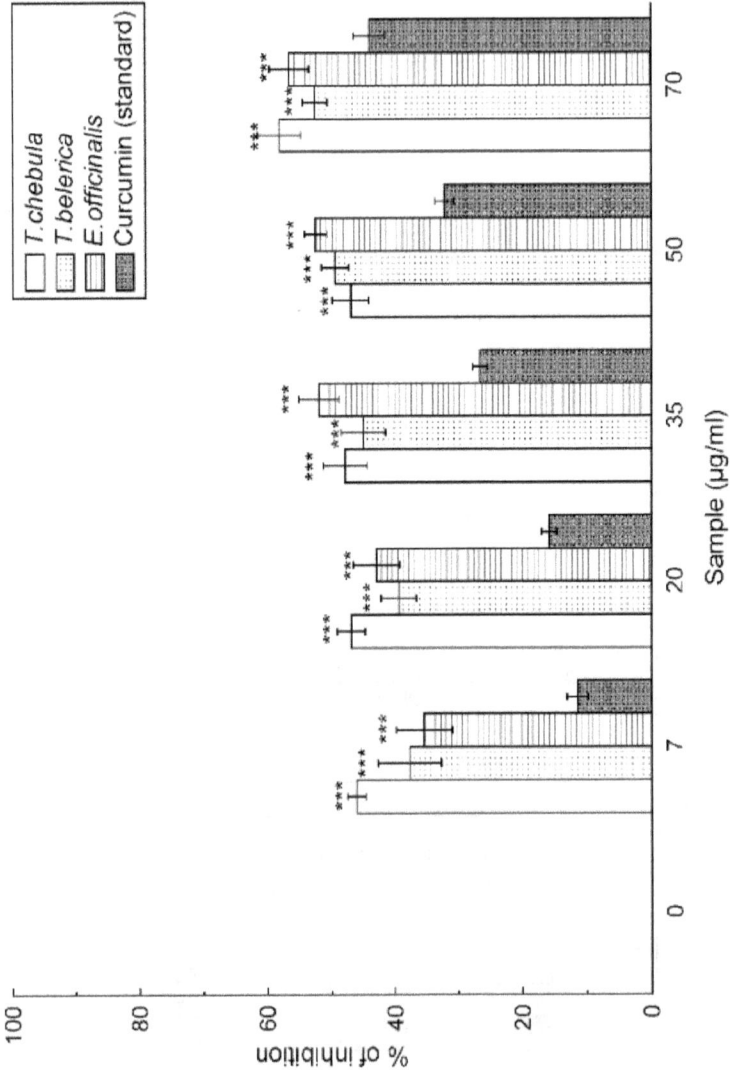

FIGURE 5: Nitric oxide radical scavenging assay. The nitric oxide radical scavenging activity of *T. chebula, T. belerica* and *E. officinalis* extracts and standard curcumin. The data represents the % of nitric oxide inhibition. Each value represents mean ± S.D. (n = 6). ***p < 0.001 vs 0 μg/ml.

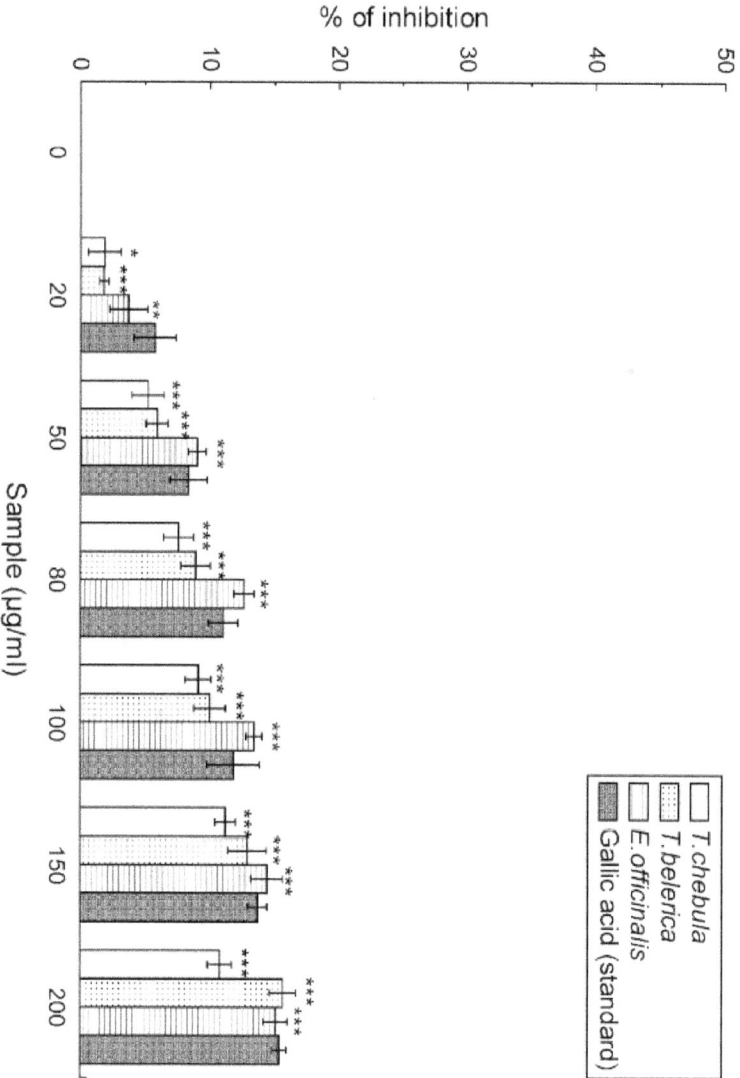

FIGURE 6: Peroxynitrite anion scavenging assay. The peroxynitrite anion scavenging activity of *T. chebula*, *T. belerica* and *E. officinalis* plant extracts and standard gallic acid. Each value represents mean ± S.D. (n = 6). *p < 0.05, **p < 0.01 and ***p < 0.001 vs 0 μg/ml.

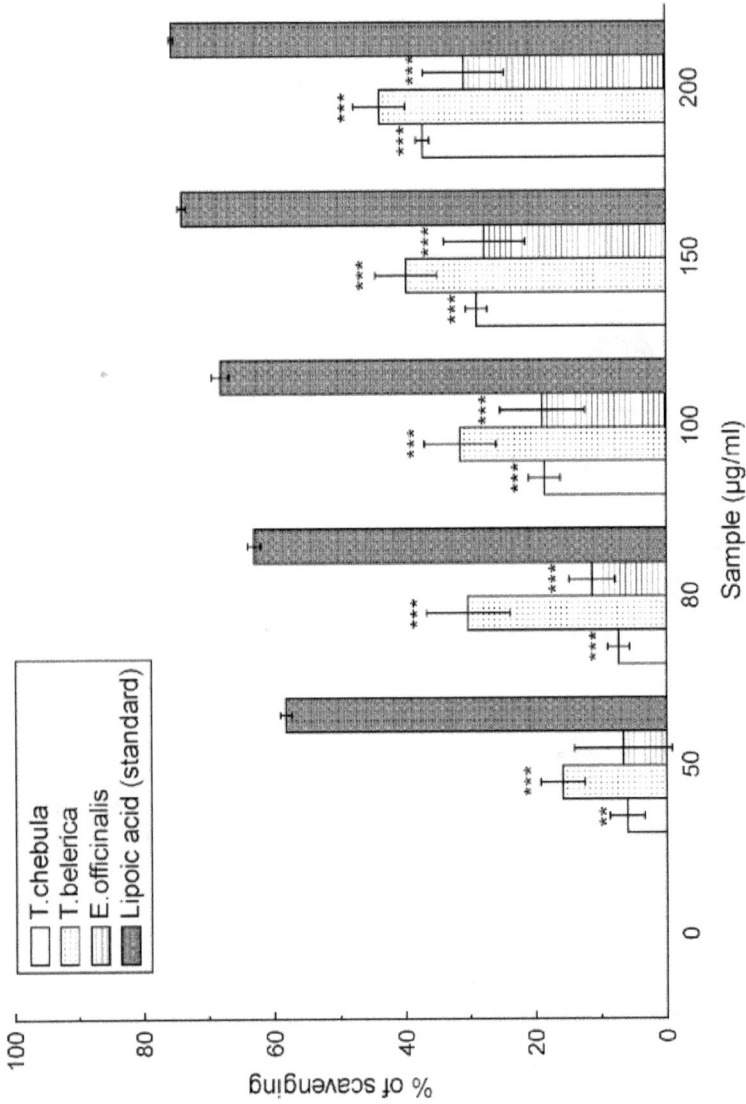

FIGURE 7: Singlet oxygen scavenging assay. Effect of *T. chebula, T. belerica* and *E. officinalis* plant extracts and standard lipoic acid on the scavenging of singlet oxygen. The results are mean ± S.D. of six parallel measurements. **p < 0.01 and ***p < 0.001 vs 0 μg/ml.

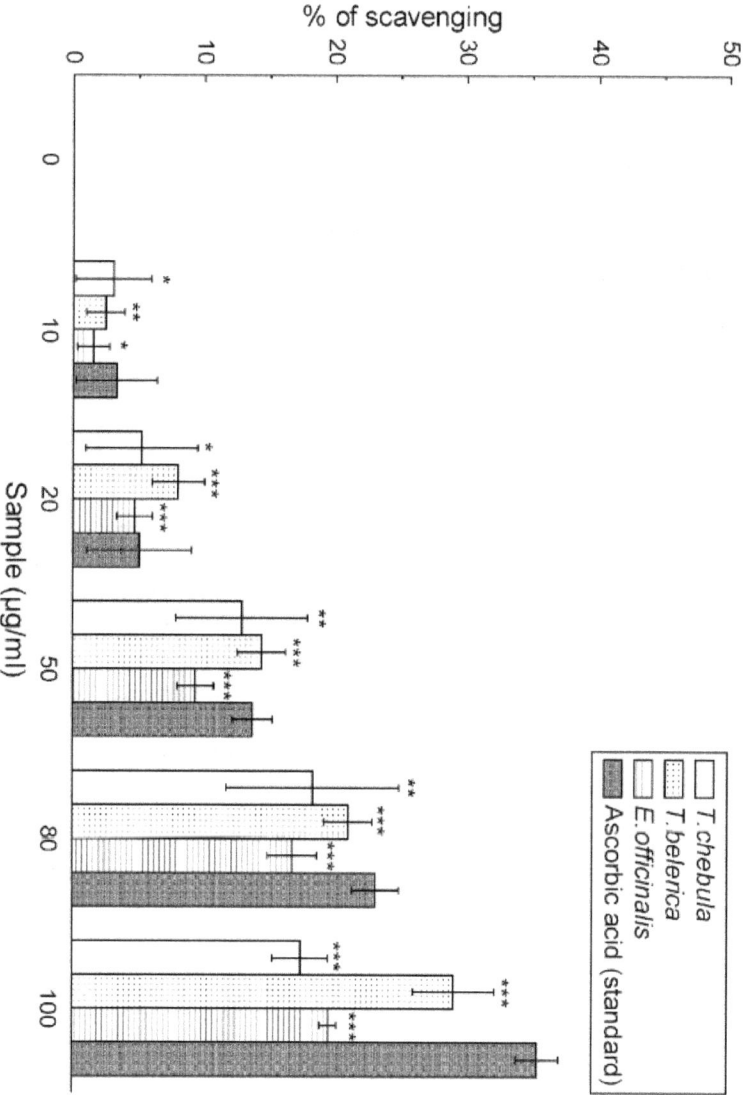

FIGURE 8: HOCl scavenging assay. Hypochlorous acid scavenging activity of *T. chebula*, *T. belerica* and *E. officinalis* plant extracts and standard ascorbic acid. All data are expressed as mean ± S.D. (n = 6). **p < 0.01 and ***p < 0.001 vs 0 μg/ml.

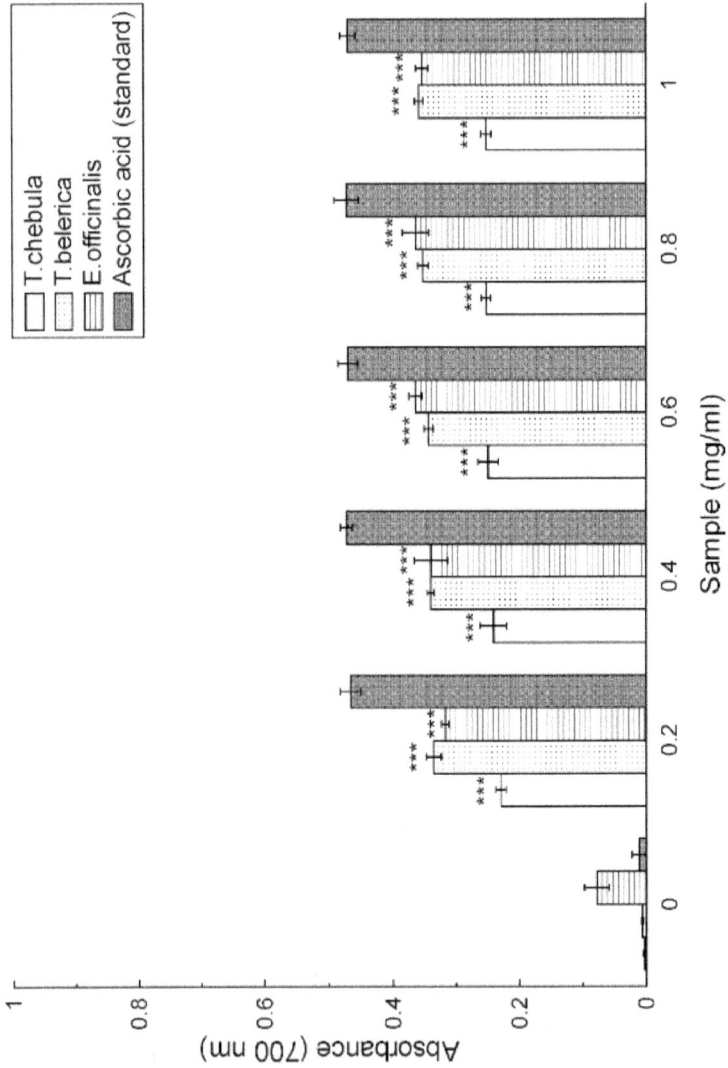

FIGURE 9: Reducing power assay. The reductive ability of *T. chebula*, *T. belerica* and *E. officinalis* extracts and standard Ascorbic acid. The absorbance (A700) was plotted against concentration of sample. Each value represents mean ± S.D. (n = 6). *** $p < 0.001$ vs 0 mg/ml.

10.2.8 SINGLET OXYGEN SCAVENGING ASSAY

The *T. chebula*, *T. belerica* and *E. officinalis* extracts also showed a moderate dose-dependent scavenging effect of singlet oxygen species with IC_{50} values (Table 2) of 424.50 ± 24.70 µg/ml, 233.12 ± 48.68 µg/ml and 490.42 ± 159.59 µg/ml, respectively (Figure 7). Lipoic acid was used as a reference compound and 46.15 ± 1.16 µg/ml lipoic acid was needed for 50% inhibition.

10.2.9 HYPOCHLOROUS ACID SCAVENGING ASSAY

Figure 8 shows how effectively the *T. chebula*, *T. belerica* and *E. officinalis* extracts dose-dependently scavenge hypochlorous acid compared to that of ascorbic acid. The 50% inhibition concentration values of the extracts in the above order ($IC_{50} = 433.60 \pm 15.45$ µg/ml, 271.51 ± 13.70 µg/ml, 420.58 ± 31.97 µg/ml) and ascorbic acid ($IC_{50} = 235.96 \pm 5.75$ µg/ml) as seen in Table 2 also corroborates the data.

10.2.10 REDUCING POWER ASSAY

As illustrated in Figure 9, Fe^{3+} to Fe^{2+} transformation in the presence of *T. chebula*, *T. belerica* and *E. officinalis* extracts and reference compound ascorbic acid was performed to measure the reductive capability. Throughout the concentration range (0.0–1.0 mg/ml), the fruits extracts and the standard showed nearly the same trend in their reductive capability, although all the extracts exhibiting lower activity than the standard.

10.2.11 DETERMINATION OF TOTAL PHENOLIC, FLAVONOID AND ASCORBIC ACID CONTENT

The phenolic and flavonoid compounds along with the subsequent ascorbic acid contents of the extracts may contribute directly to antioxidative action. The total phenolic content of 70% methanolic extracts of *T.*

chebula, T. belerica and *E. officinalis* were 127.60 ± 0.001 mg/ml, 133.00 ± 0.003 mg/ml and 215.60 ± 0.004 mg/ml gallic acid equivalent per 100 mg fruit extract, respectively, whereas the flavonoid contents were 219.30 ± 0.01 mg/ml, 138.30 ± 0.01 mg/ml, 176.00 ± 0.01 mg/ml quercetin per 100 mg fruit extract, following the above order. In case of the ascorbic acid content determination, 46.74 ± 1.10 mg/ml, 45.25 ± 0.75 mg/ml and 71.08 ± 1.63 mg/ml ascorbic acid were found to be present in 100 mg fruit extracts of *T. chebula, T. belerica* and *E. officinalis*, respectively.

10.2.12 CORRELATION BETWEEN THE TOTAL PHENOLIC OR FLAVONOID CONTENTS WITH THE ANTIOXIDANT ACTIVITY

As showed in Figure 10(a), the total phenolic content of *E. officinalis* significantly correlated with antioxidant activity (R = 0.9972, p < 0.05), whereas the correlation coefficients for *T. chebula* and *T. belerica* were found to be greater than 0.9 (R = 0.9960 and R = 0.9921 respectively with p > 0.05) which proved that the phenolic contents of these plants highly attributed their antioxidant activity. The correlation coefficient of *T. chebula* for flavonoid contents with its antioxidant capacity was highly significant (R = 0.9990, p < 0.05), whereas the flavonoid contents of *T. belerica* and *E. officinalis* were highly (R = 0.9219, p > 0.05) and reasonably (R = 0.8914, p > 0.05) correlated with their antioxidant activity (Figure 10(b)). In general, the results showed that the total phenolic and flavonoid content in individual fruits was highly correlated with antioxidant activity.

10.2.13 EFFECT ON ENZYME ACTIVITY

In order to investigate whether these antioxidant activities of fruit extracts are mediated by an increase in antioxidant enzymes, the activities of SOD, CAT, GST and GSH (Table 3) were measured individually for the three plants through oral administration in mice. The activity of SOD is significantly enhanced by all three fruit extracts in a dose dependent manner. With the increasing doses of the fruit extracts, the CAT activity was also increased for each plant, in comparison to the control, as is evident from

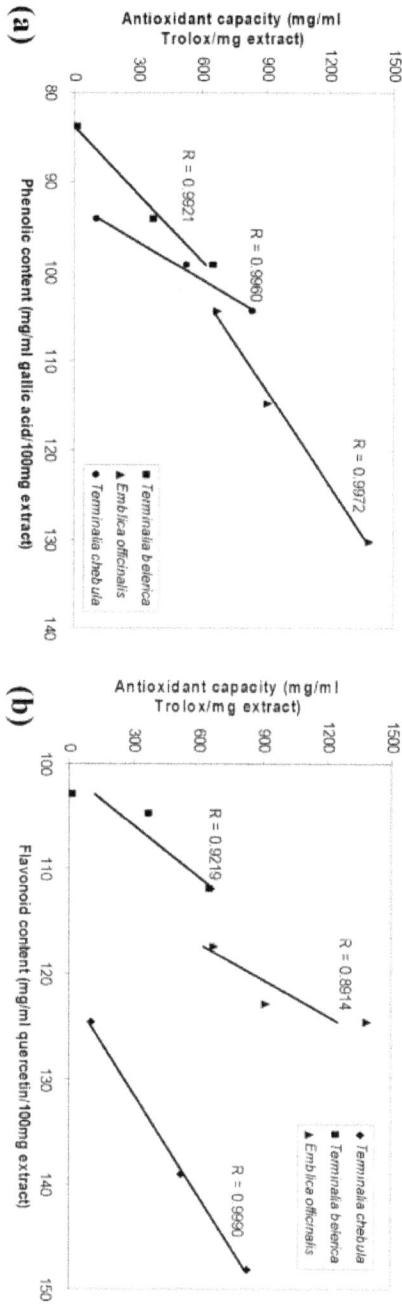

FIGURE 10: Correlation of antioxidant activity with phenolic and flavonoid contents. The relationship between (a) total phenolic content or (b) total flavonoid content in individual fruit and their antioxidant capacity. The correlation analyses were described as linear correlation coefficient (R). The differences were considered statistically significant if p < 0.05.

the results. The results also showed that there was a considerable dose-dependent effect of the fruit extracts in the gradual enhancement of the GST activity in the treated mice than the control ones. Similarly, we find a gradual increase in the GSH activity procured by the fruit extracts with their increasing concentrations for the dose treated mice compared to the control.

TABLE 3: Effect of the methanolic extract of the fruits of *Terminalia chebula*, *Terminalia belerica* and *Emblica officinalis* on the activities of antioxidant enzymes and reduced glutathione content in liver of normal mice

Tested Samples		SOD (U/mg protein)	CAT (U/mg protein)	GST (U/mg protein)	GSH (μg/mg protein)
Control	Group I	1.28 ± 0.35	0.29 ± 0.16	0.09 ± 0.04	2.8 ± 0.7
Terminalia chebula	Group II	$2.33 \pm 0.24***$	0.51 ± 0.22	0.11 ± 0.07	3.35 ± 0.5
	Group III	$3.14 \pm 0.37***$	0.74 ± 0.4	$0.26 \pm 0.05**$	$3.52 \pm 0.5*$
	Group IV	$3.75 \pm 0.27***$	$1.08 \pm 0.23*$	$0.37 \pm 0.04***$	3.51 ± 0.2
Terminalia belerica	Group V	$2.61 \pm 0.22***$	0.43 ± 0.06	0.15 ± 0.1	3.42 ± 0.3
	Group VI	$3.62 \pm 0.24***$	0.65 ± 0.2	$0.67 \pm 0.15*$	4 ± 0.1
	Group VII	$3.89 \pm 0.15***$	$0.66 \pm 0.1**$	0.71 ± 0.3	4.04 ± 0.12
Emblica officinalis	Group VIII	$2.31 \pm 0.18**$	0.33 ± 0.2	0.14 ± 0.2	3.04 ± 0.07
	Group IX	$4.01 \pm 0.17***$	$1.02 \pm 0.15**$	$0.41 \pm 0.15*$	3.85 ± 0.2
	Group X	$4.56 \pm 0.18***$	$1.06 \pm 0.1**$	$0.64 \pm 0.1**$	4.13 ± 0.1

Group I: Control group; Groups II, III and IV represent mice treated orally with the T. chebula extract in the doses of 10, 50 and 100 mg/kg body weight, respectively; Groups V, VI and VII contain mice treated orally with the T. belerica extract in a dose of 10, 50 and 100 mg/kg body weight, respectively; Groups VIII, IX and X represent mice treated orally with the E. officinalis extract in a dose of 10, 50 and 100 mg/kg body weight, respectively. Results are expressed as mean ± SD for six mice in each group.
$*p < 0.05$, $**p < 0.01$, $***p < 0.001$ compared to control.

10.3 DISCUSSION

Antioxidants are compounds that prevent the oxidation of essential biological macromolecules by inhibiting the propagation of the oxidizing chain reaction. Keeping in mind the adverse effects of synthetic antioxidants, researchers have channelled their interest in isolating natural antioxidants [21] which are very effective to control the oxidative stress and hence prevent the initiation of disease propagation. Interestingly, quite a few studies on the antioxidant properties of the three plant materials, viz., *T. chebula* [22,23], *T. belerica* [24,25] and *E. officinalis* [26,27] have been done earlier. However, this study provides a definitive report about the free radical scavenging capacity of *T. chebula*, *T. belerica* and *E. officinalis*, since the antioxidant activity of a drug may depend on the free radical scavenging activity [28].

ABTS.+ is a blue colored chromophore which is reduced to ABTS on a concentration dependant manner upon addition of the fruit extract. The results are compared with trolox and the TEAC value demonstrates the extracts as a potent antioxidant, with their TEAC values following the order *T. chebula* > *E. officinalis* > *T. belerica*. The effect of the fruit extract in the scavenging assay of DPPH radical furthermore assured the fact that the extracts smoothly act as antioxidants, since the study on TEAC and DPPH scavenging can be observed as complementary to each other [29], although it followed the order *T. belerica* > *E. officinalis* > *T. chebula*.

The most detrimental of the free radicals formed in biological systems is the hydroxyl radical that causes enormous damage on biomolecules of the living cells [30]. As the extracts or standard mannitol is added to the Fenton reaction mixture the hydroxyl radicals are scavenged and thereby sugar damage can be blocked. The results, as can be found from Figure 3 and Table 2, indicate that the fruit extracts are better hydroxyl radical scavengers than standard mannitol, with *T. chebula* being the best in comparison to *T. belerica* and *E. officinalis*.

Superoxide anion is also another harmful reactive oxygen species as it damages cellular components in biological systems [31]. The ability of the fruit extracts and the reference compound quercetin to quench superoxide radicals from reaction mixture is reflected in the decrease of the absorbance at $\lambda = 560$ nm. From the results (Figure 4 & Table 2), it can be put forward that the fruit extracts are more potent scavenger of superoxide radical than the standard quercetin with a decreasing order of *T. chebula* > *E. officinalis* >*T. belerica.*

Nitric oxide radicals play important roles in various types of inflammatory conditions including juvenile diabetes, multiple sclerosis, arthritis and ulcerative colitis [32,33]. The nitric oxide generated from sodium nitroprusside reacts with oxygen to form nitrite anion that is well restrained by the extracts. The scavenging activities of the extracts and curcumin proved that the nitric oxide scavenging activity of the former is better than the latter, with *T. chebula* and *E. officinalis* showing nearly the same activity, which is better that that of *T. belerica.*

Furthermore, the lethal consequence of NO increases significantly upon reaction with superoxide radical resulting in the formation of highly reactive peroxynitrite anion (ONOO⁻), especially its protonated form, peroxynitrous acid (ONOOH). ONOO⁻ has added to the pathogenesis of diseases such as heart disease, Alzheimer's disease, and atherosclerosis [34,35]. However, as revealed in Figure 6, highly considerable results were obtained for the scavenging effects of the studied extracts, which illustrated similar result to the standard gallic acid in the order *E. officinalis* > *T. belerica* > *T. chebula.*

Hydrogen peroxide is a weak oxidizing agent and can inactivate a few enzymes directly, usually by oxidation of essential thiol (-SH) groups. It can cross cell membrane rapidly, once inside the cell, H_2O_2 can probably react with Fe^{2+} and possibly Cu^{2+} ions to form hydroxyl radical and this may be the origin of many of its toxic effects [36]. From the results, it appeared that H_2O_2 scavenging activity of the fruit extracts is very negligible compared to standard sodium pyruvate.

A high energy form of oxygen, singlet oxygen is generated in the skin upon UV-radiation and it induces hyperoxidation, oxygen cytotxicity and decreases the antioxidant activity [37]. The higher IC_{50} values (Table 2) of the studied extracts than the reference compound lipoic acid indicated that the extracts of the fruits of *T. chebula, T. belerica* and *E. officinalis*, with *T. belerica* being the most effective among them, have singlet oxygen scavenging activity but poor compared to standard lipoic acid, as also found in Figure 7.

Hypochlorous acid is another harmful ROS. At the sites of inflammation, the oxidation of Cl⁻ ions by the neutrophil enzyme myeloperoxidase results in the production of this ROS [38], which breaks down the heme prosthetic group and inactivates the antioxidant enzyme catalase. The obtained results (Figure 8) indicate that the standard ascorbic acid is a comparable scavenger to the fruit extracts (Table 2). So, it is anticipated that *T. chebula*, *T. belerica* and *E. officinalis* are efficient scavengers of HOCl, with *T. belerica* being the most effective, just like in case of singlet oxygen.

The reducing capacity of a compound may serve as a significant indicator of its potential antioxidant activity. However, the activity of antioxidants has been attributed to various mechanisms such as prevention of chain initiation, decomposition of peroxides, reducing capacity and radical scavenging [39]. As shown in figure 9, the reducing power of the fruit extracts were compared with standard ascorbic acid and it was found that reducing capacity of the fruit extracts were although not better than standard, yet showed considerable activity with *E. officinalis* as the best among the three studied extracts.

The results indicate that the fruit extracts contain significant amount of flavonoids and phenolic content, in the order *T. belerica* > *E. officinalis* > *T. chebula* and *E. officinalis* > *T. belerica* > *T. chebula* for the flavonoid and phenolic contents, respectively. Both of these compounds have good antioxidant potential and their effects on human nutrition and health are considerable. The mechanism of action of flavonoids is through scavenging or chelating process [40]. Phenolic contents are also very important plant constituents because of their scavenging ability due to their hydroxyl groups [41]. Moreover, ascorbic acid acting as a chain breaking antioxidant impairs with the formation of free radicals in the process of formation of intracellular substances throughout the body, including collagen, bone matrix and tooth dentine [42]. From the results, the trend for the ascorbic acid content was found to be *E. officinalis* > *T. chebula* > *T. belerica*.

We also observed that treating mice with total extracts of medicinal plants increased the activity of all antioxidant enzymes examined, including SOD, CAT, GST and GSH. These enzymes are modulated in various diseases by free radical attack, thus maintaining the balance between the rates of radical generation and scavenging. It is of particular interest to note that SOD catalyzes the breakdown of O_2. to O_2 and H_2O_2, and thus prevents the formation of OH., and thereby, has been implicated as an essential defense against the potential oxygen toxicity. SOD catalyzes the breakdown of endogenous cytotoxic superoxide radicals to H_2O_2 which is further degraded by CAT. Thus, they play a crucial role in maintaining the physiological levels of O_2 and H_2O_2. GSH, in conjunction with GST, has a basic role in cellular defense against deleterious free radicals and other oxidant species [43]. GST catalyzes the conjugation of thiol group of glutathione to electrophilic substrates, and thereby detoxifies endogenous compounds such as peroxidized lipids [44]. The present study supports the antioxidant potency of the fruit extract as evidenced by the increased level of these antioxidant systems in extract treated mice.

10.4 CONCLUSIONS

The results from various free radical scavenging systems revealed that all the fruit extracts were individually strong antioxidants, with some varying scavenging activities for different ROS at different magnitudes of potency. Furthermore, evaluation of in vivo antioxidant activity of these fruit extracts has also provided interesting results that might be beneficial for the pharmacological use of these plants in clinical trials. The wide use of these fruits in the Indian indigenous system of medicine as anti-inflammatory and antihepatotoxic may be in part due to their antioxidant potency. Further, the isolation of the compounds responsible for the antioxidant activity has to be taken up which may result in modern drugs from these plants. Also the studies on antioxidant activity of the well known Ayurvedic formulation, Triphala, a mixture of these fruits, should be carried out and that is in progress.

REFERENCES

1. Braca A, Sortino C, Politi M, Morelli I, Mendez J: Antioxidant activity of flavonoids from Licania licaniaeflora. J Ethnopharmacol 2002, 79:379-381.
2. Maxwell SR: Prospects for the use of antioxidant therapies. Drugs 1995, 49:345-361.

3. Niki E, Shimaski H, Mino M: Antioxidantism-free radical and biological defense Gakkai Syuppn Center, Tokyo 1994, :3-16.
4. Finkel T, Holbrook NJ: Oxidants, oxidative stress and the biology of ageing. Nature 2000, 408:239-247.
5. Chopra RN, Nayar SL, Chopra IC: Glossary of Indian Medicinal Plants. CSIR, New Delhi, India 1956, :106.
6. Reddy VRC, Kumari SVR, Reddy BM, Azeem MA, Prabhakar MC, Appa Rao AVN: Cardiotonic activity of the fruit of *Terminalia chebula*. Fitoterapia 1990, LXI:517-525.
7. Lee HS, Won NH, Kim KH, Lee H, Jun W, Lee KW: Antioxidant effects of aqueous extract of *Terminalia chebula* in vivo and *in vitro*. Biol Pharm Bull 2005, 28:1639-1644.
8. Aslokar L, Kakkar KK, Chakre OJ: Supplement to Glossary of Indian Medicinal Plants with Active Principles. Directorate CSIR, New Delhi, India 1992, :291-293.
9. Rajarama Rao MR, Siddiqui HH: Pharmacological studies on *Emblica officinalis* Gaetn. Indian Exp Biol 1964, 2:29-31.
10. Halliwell B, Gutteridge JMC: Free radicals, ageing and disease. In Free Radicals in Biology and Medicine. Clarendon: Oxford; 1985::279-315.
11. Roy AK, Dhir H, Talukdar G: Phyllanthus emblica fruit extract and ascorbic acid modify hepatotoxic and renotoxic effects of metals in mice. Int J Pharmacog 1991, 29:117-126.
12. Hazra B, Biswas S, Mandal N: Antioxidant and free radical scavenging activity of Spondias pinnata. BMC Complement Altern Med 2008, 8:63.
13. Mahakunakorn P, Tohda M, Murakami Y, Matsumoto K, Watanabe H: Antioxidant and free radical-scavenging activity of Choto-san and its related constituents. Biol Pharm Bull 2004, 27:38-46.
14. Beckman JS, Chen H, Ischiropulos H, Crow JP: Oxidative chemistry of peroxynitrite. Methods Enzymol 1994, 233:229-240.
15. Gu X, Chen C, Zhou T: Spectrophotometric method for the determination of ascorbic acid with iron (III)-1,10-phenanthroline after preconcentration on an organic solvent-soluble membrane filter. Fresenius J Anal Chem 1996, 355:94-95.
16. Lowry OH, Roesborough MJ, Farr AL, Randall RJ: Protein measurement with Folin-Phenol reagent. J Biol Chem 1951, 193:265-275.
17. Kakkar P, Das B, Viswanathan P: A modified spectrophotometric assay of superoxide dismutase. Indian J Biochem Biophys 1984, 21:130-132.
18. Bonaventura J, Schroeder WA, Fang S: Human erythrocyte catalase: an improved method of isolation and a revalution of reported properties. Arch Biochem Biophys 1972, 150:606-617.
19. Habig WH, Jakoby WB: Glutathione S-transferases. The first enzymatic step in mercapturic acid formation. J Biol Chem 1974, 249:7130-7139.
20. Ellman GL: Tissue sulfhydryl group. Arch Biochem Biophys 1959, 82:70-77.
21. Kuo PC, Damu AG, Cherng CY, Jeng JF, Teng CM, Lee EJ, Wu TS: Isolation of a natural antioxidant, dehydrozingerone from Zingiber officinale and synthesis of its analogues for recognition of effective antioxidant and antityrosinase agents. Arch Pharm Res 2005, 28:518-528.

22. Cheng HY, Lin TC, Yu KH, Yang CM, Lin CC: Antioxidant and Free Radical Scavenging Activities of *Terminalia chebula*. Biol Pharm Bull 2003, 26:1331-1335.
23. Chattopadhyay RR, Bhattacharyya SK: *Terminalia chebula*: An update. Phcog Rev 2007, 1:151-156.
24. Sabu MC, Kuttan R: Anti-diabetic activity of some medicinal plants-relation with their antioxidant property. Amala Res Bull 2000, 20:81-86.
25. Sabu MC, Kuttan R: Antidiabetic and antioxidant activity of *Terminalia Belerica*. Roxb. Indian J Exp Biol 2009, 47:270-275.
26. Bhattacharya A, Chatterjee A, Ghoshal S, Bhattacharya SK: Antioxidant activity of tannoid principles of *Emblica officinalis* (amla). Indian J Exp Biol 1999, 37:676-680.
27. Liu Xiaoli, Zhao Mouming, Wang Jinshui, Yang Bao, Jiang Yueming: Antioxidant activity of methanolic extract of emblica fruit (Phyllanthus emblica L.) from six regions in China. J Food Compos Anal 2008, 21:219-228.
28. Ng TB, Yeung HW: Scientific basis of the therapeutic effects of Ginseng. In Folk Medicine. The Art and the Science. Edited by Steiner RP. USA: American Chem Soc Publ; 1987::139-152.
29. Lissi EA, Modak B, Torres R, Escobar J, Urzua A: Total antioxidant potential of resinous exudates from Heliotropium species, and a comparison of the ABTS and DPPH methods. Free Rad Res 1999, 30:471-477.
30. Halliwell B: Reactive oxygen species in living systems: Source, biochemistry, and role in human disease. Am J Med 1991, 91:S14-S22.
31. Robak J, Gryglewski IR: Flavonoids are scavengers of superoxide anions. Biochem Pharmacol 1988, 37:837-841.
32. Miller MJ, Sadowska-Krowicka H, Chotinaruemol S, Kakkis JL, Clark DA: Amelioration of chronic ileitis by nitric oxide synthase inhibition. The J Pharmac and Experi Thera 1993, 264:11-16.
33. Huie RE, Padmaja S: The reaction of NO with superoxide. Free Radic Res Commun 1993, 18:195-199.
34. Balavoine GG, Geletti YV: Peroxynitrite scavenging by different antioxidants. Part 1: convenient study. Nitric oxide 1999, 3:40-54.
35. Ischiropoulos H, al-Mehdi AB, Fisher AB: Reactive species in ischemic rat lung injury: contribution of peroxynitrite. Am J Physiol 1995, 269:158-164.
36. Elizabeth K, Rao MNA: Oxygen radical scavenging activity of curcumin. Int J Pharmaceut 1990, 58: 237-240
37. Halliwell B: Reactive oxygen species in living systems: source, biochemistry, and role in human disease. Am J Med 1991, 91:14-22.
38. Kochevar EI, Redmond WR: Photosensitized production of singlet oxygen. Methods Enzymol 2000, 319:20-28.
39. Aruoma OI, Halliwell B, Hoey BM, Butler J: The antioxidant action of N-acetylcysteine: Its reaction with hydrogen peroxide, hydroxyl radical, superoxide, and hypochlorous acid. Free Rad Biol Med 1989, 6:593-597.
40. Duh PD, Tu YY, Yen GC: Antioxidant activity of water extract of Harng Jyur (Chrysenthemum morifolium Ramat). Lebnes wiss Technol 1999, 32:269-277.
41. Yildirim A, Mavi A, Oktay M, Kara AA, Algur OF, Bilaloglu V: Comparison of antioxidant and antimicrobial activities of Tilia (Tilia argentea Desf Ex DC), Sage

(Savia triloba L.), and Black Tea (Camellia sinensis) extracts. J Agri Food Chem 2000, 48:5030-5034.

42. Cook NC, Samman S: Flavonoids-chemistry, metabolism, cardioprotective effects, and dietary sources. Nutr Biochem 1996, 7:66-76.

43. Beyer RE: The role of ascorbate in antioxidant protection of biomembranes: interaction with vit-E and coenzyme. Q J Bioen Biomemb 1994, 24:349-358.

44. Arivazhagan S, Balasenthil S, Nagini S: Garlic and neem leaf extracts enhance hepatic glutathione and glutathione dependent enzymes during N-methyl-Nitrosoguanidine (MNNG)-induced gastric carcinogenesis. Phytother Res 2000, 14:291-293.

45. Leaver MJ, George SG: A piscine glutathione-S-transferase which efficiently conjugates the end products of lipid peroxidation. Mar Environ Res 1998, 46:33-35.

CHAPTER 11

INHIBITION OF HIGHLY PRODUCTIVE HIV-1 INFECTION IN T CELLS, PRIMARY HUMAN MACROPHAGES, MICROGLIA, AND ASTROCYTES BY *SARGASSUM FUSIFORME*

ELENA E. PASKALEVA, XUDONG LIN, WEN LI, ROBIN COTTER, MICHAEL T. KLEIN, EMILY ROBERGE, ER K. YU, BRUCE CLARK, JEAN-CLAUDE VEILLE, YANZE LIU, DAVID Y-W LEE, AND MARIO CANKI

11.1 BACKGROUND

Macrophages and T cells are major targets for HIV-1 infection [1]. While macrophages are key cellular reservoir and a source of newly replicating HIV-1 throughout the infection, a global decline in T cell population leads to the eventual collapse of the immune system, development of clinical manifestations of AIDS, and the ultimate death of the host. Highly active antiretroviral therapy (HAART) has greatly extended the lifespan of HIV-infected individuals, however the AIDS epidemic continues to expand

This chapter was originally published under the Creative Commons Attribution License. Paskaleva EE, Lin X, Li W, Cotter R, Klein MT, Roberge E, Yu EK, Clark B, Veille J-C, Liu Y, Lee DY-W, and Canki M. Inhibition of Highly Productive HIV-1 Infection in T Cells, Primary Human Macrophages, Microglia, and Astrocytes by Sargassum fusiforme. AIDS Research and Therapy **3**,15 (2006). doi:10.1186/1742-6405-3-15.

globally and the long-term control of HIV-1 infection remains an elusive goal. Current HAART regiments, with the exception of recent fusion inhibitor (T-20), include inhibitors of two key viral enzymes, reverse transcriptase and protease [2-4]. By using combinations of reverse transcriptase and protease inhibitors in HAART, dramatic reductions in the level of chronic HIV-1 viremia have been achieved in a majority of patients [2,4]. However, both reverse transcriptase and protease inhibitors have significant clinical side effects [5-7]. Initial optimism that the natural decay of virus-producing cells in the presence of HAART would lead to eradication of virus was short-lived [8,9]. Long-term follow-up of HAART-treated individuals revealed very slow rates of decline of HIV-1 in some individuals, with continued low-level replication of virus in macrophages and T cells, and viral persistence in several tissue compartments, such as the CNS, not readily accessible to current therapies [5,9-11]. Studies in a macaque model of simian immunodeficiency virus (SIV) viral persistence in the brain, have suggested that in individuals on HAART with suppressed viral load, the CNS may act as a long-term viral reservoir [12].

HIV-1 infected human macrophages are the primary route of virus entry into the CNS [13]. Within the CNS, active virus replication is mediated by macrophages and microglia, while astrocytes are nonproductively infected [14]. The number of astrocytes in the brain ranges up to 2×10^{12}, and while only 1% of these cells may be latently infected, the total number of infected astrocytes contributing to neuropathology, may be substantial [15,16]. Brain macrophages, microglia, and astrocytes have been shown to be responsible for some of the neuropathologic manifestations of the HIV-associated dementia (HAD), which develops in about 20–30% of AIDS patients [14,17]. Although HAART has decreased frequency of HAD, it does not provide full protection or reversal of HAD [18]. Protease inhibitors and some of the nucleoside analogues used in HAART have poor CNS penetration, and drug resistance in this compartment has recently been reported, further underscoring need for discovery of new drugs [12,19,20].

Continued virus replication in the presence of HAART increases the likelihood and frequency of generating new multi-drug-resistant (MDR) HIV-1 strains, as demonstrated by the observation that approximately 20% of all new HIV-1 infections are with viruses resistant to the currently available drugs [21,22]. Consequently, concerted efforts towards the discovery and development of novel inhibitors of HIV-1 infection and replication must persist if continued viral repression and possibility of virus eradication are to be achieved.

We investigated a number of natural products, and identified *S. fusiforme* extract as a potent inhibitor of HIV-1 replication in T cells, in primary human macrophages, microglia, and astrocytes. While many natural products have been screened for anti-HIV activity [23,24], including sulfated polysaccharides derived from sea algae [25,26], *S. fusiforme* extract has not been investigated up until now [27].

11.2 RESULTS

11.2.1 S. FUSIFORME *DOES NOT INHIBIT CELL GROWTH OR VIABILITY*

To establish a non-toxic working concentration, we tested for cell growth and viability kinetics in response to treatment with *S. fusiforme* whole aqueous extract. T cells were treated with either 2 or 4 mg/ml *S. fusiforme*, 10^{-6} M ddC, or were mock treated (Fig 1). In 1G5 cells, growth kinetics remained similar, except for the highest 4 mg/ml treatment on day 7 that decreased cell growth by 19% compared to ddC treatment, indicating possible toxicity at this dose (Fig 1A). In parallel we also measured cell viability by trypan blue exclusion assay. Regardless of treatment, cell viability remained above 90%, which was comparable to mock treated cultures (Fig. 1B). We repeated this experiment with HIV-1 infected 1G5 cells, with similar results (not shown). Because of toxicity relevance in primary human cells, we also measured cell growth and viability in human peripheral blood mononuclear cells (PBMC), with similar results (Fig 1C and 1D). Cells treated with either 3 or 4.5 mg/ml *S. fusiforme* exhibited somewhat slower growth kinetics on day 6 after treatment, as compared to 1.5 mg/ml *S. fusiforme*, ddC or mock treated cells (Fig 1C). However, viability of *S. fusiforme* and ddC treated cells remained similar through day

6 of follow-up, with the overall PBMC's viability declining over time, as compared to 1G5 T cell line (compare Fig. 1D to 1B).

Based on these results we conclude that treatment with less than 4 mg/ml *S. fusiforme* extract, does not inhibit cell growth, is not toxic to cells, and is suitable for *in vitro* testing of HIV-1 inhibition in 1G5 cells.

11.2.2 S. FUSIFORME *INHIBITS HIV-1 INFECTION IN T CELLS IN A DOSE DEPENDANT MANNER*

Next, we investigated *S. fusiforme* ability to inhibit HIV-1 infection in T cells. We chose 1G5 T cells, which are stably transfected with HIV-LTR-luciferase gene construct, have low basal level of luciferase expression and are sensitive to HIV-1 tat activation, which makes them a useful tool for testing HIV-1 inhibitors [28]. Cells were treated with increasing concentrations of *S. fusiforme* extract and infected with NL4-3. On day 3 after infection, equal numbers of viable cells were analyzed for intracellular luciferase expression, and cell viability was measured by MTT uptake assay (Fig. 2). Percent HIV-1 inhibition was calculated by comparison to control infected untreated cell cultures, which expressed 18,797 relative light units (RLU) of luciferase (not shown). Treatment with 1.5, 3, and 6 mg/ml of *S. fusiforme* extract inhibited HIV-1 replication in a dose dependant manner, by 60.4, 86.7, and 92.3%, respectively (Fig. 2A). As expected, treatment with positive control HIV-1 reverse transcriptase (RT) inhibitor ddC, blocked virus replication by over 98% (not shown). In parallel, we tested for the MTT uptake by viable cells, which remained high regardless of *S. fusiforme* treatment, and was similar to ddC, as well as to viability of mock treated cells (Fig. 2B).

Based on these results we conclude that *S. fusiforme* treatment inhibits HIV-1 replication in T cells in a dose dependant manner, inhibition is similar to that achieved with ddC treatment, and treatment is not toxic to cells.

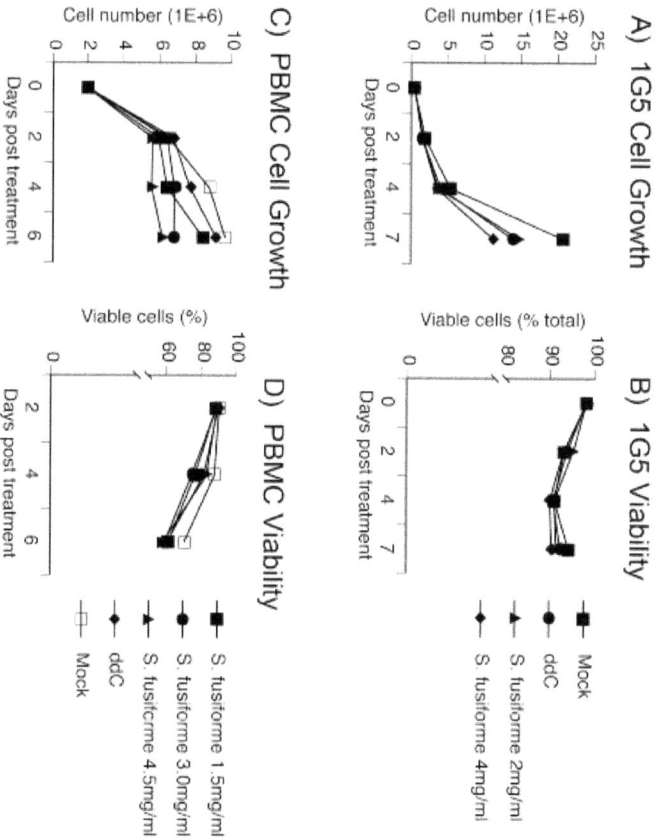

FIGURE 1: Analysis of growth kinetics and viability in T cells treated with *S. fusiforme*. 1G5 T cells were treated with 2 mg/ml or 4 mg/ml *S. fusiforme*, or with 10⁻⁶ M ddC, or were mock treated. (A) Total cell number, and (B) % viable cells from total, was monitored at the indicated time points after infection, by trypan blue exclusion assay by counting at least 200 cells each in three different fields under ×20 magnification using an Olympus BH-2 fluorescence microscope. Experiment was repeated with primary human PBMC's treated with 1.5, 3, or 4.5 mg/ml *S. fusiforme*, or with 10⁻⁶ M ddC, or mock treated, and measured (C) Total cell number, and (D) % viable cells from total. PBMC's experiments are representative of 3 separate experiments, with SEM less than 5% (not shown).

A

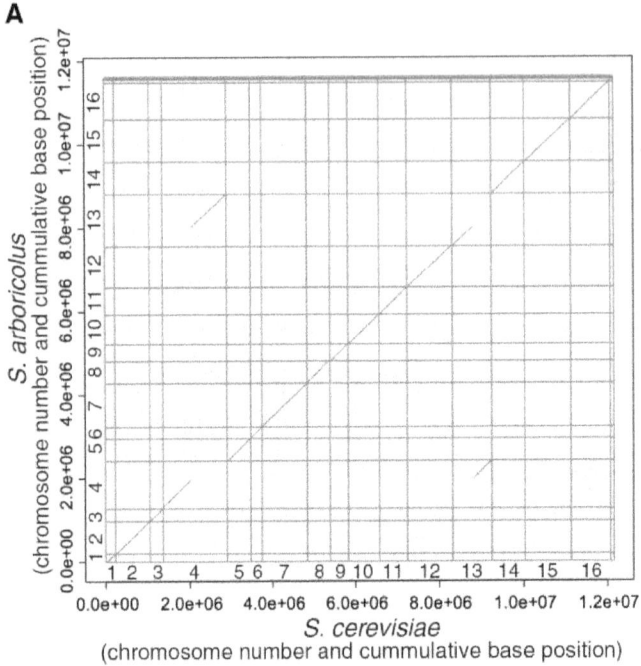

B

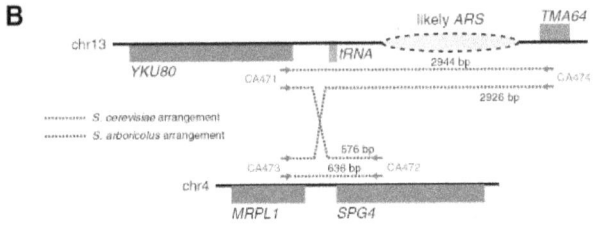

C

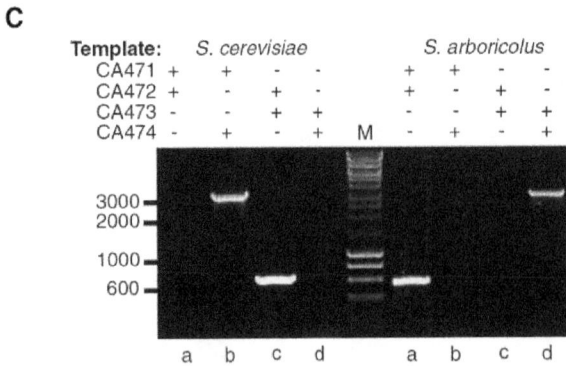

FIGURE 2: Dose response of HIV-1 inhibition and cell viability in T cells treated with *S. fusiforme*. 1G5 T cells were treated for 24 h with increasing concentrations of *S. fusiforme*, or with 10^{-6} M ddC, as indicated; then infected with CXCR4 tropic HIV-1 (NL4-3) at multiplicity of infection (moi) of 0.01 for 1.5 h, washed 3 times, and returned to culture with same concentrations of each treatment for the duration of the experiment. (A) On day 3 after infection, intracellular luciferase gene marker expression was measured from cell lysates adjusted to same number of viable cells by MTT. Percent inhibition of HIV-1 was calculated utilizing formula in the Methods section, and plotted on the Y-axis as % Inhibition. In parallel, (B) cell viability for each treatment was quantified by MTT uptake, measured at 570 nm absorbance. Data are mean +/- SD of triplicates. Representative of three separate experiments.

11.2.3 S. FUSIFORME *INHIBITION IS NON-TOXIC AND CAN BE SUSTAINED OVER EXTENDED PERIODS*

Next, we tested for the duration of HIV-1 inhibition in 1G5 T cells, treated with either 2 mg/ml *S. fusiforme* or with 10^{-6} M ddC. Infection was monitored by luciferase expression from cells equalized to same number of viable cells by MTT assay, at the indicated time points after infection (Fig. 3A). HIV-1 infection in untreated cells gradually increased from 16,110 RLU expressed on day 3, to 86,720 RLU on day 7 after infection, which demonstrated highly productive and *de novo* HIV-1 synthesis (not shown). Treatment with 2 mg/ml *S. fusiforme* inhibited this infection by 77, 99, and 99% on day 3, 5, and 7, respectively (Fig. 3A). As expected, inhibition by ddC was 99% at each time point tested. Based on these results we calculated IC_{50} to be 0.86 mg. Similar time course inhibition results were obtained in CEM T cells (not shown).

In parallel to infection kinetics, we also tested cell viability by trypan blue exclusion assay (Fig. 3B). Cell viability in *S. fusiforme* treated cultures remained high at 98, 94, and 97% viable cells on day 3, 5, and 7, respectively. Cell viability in ddC treated cultures was similar, and measured 94, 93, and 97% viable cells on day 3, 5, and 7, which was similar to mock treated cultures. This data confirm MTT viability results, which were used to equalize cells to same numbers of viable cells (not shown).

Collectively, these findings demonstrate that *S. fusiforme* inhibits infection and *de novo* HIV-1 synthesis, through day 7 of follow-up, and this treatment does not affect cell viability.

11.2.4 S. FUSIFORME *BLOCKS HIV-1 TRANSMISSION BY DIRECT CELL-TO-CELL MECHANISMS OF INFECTION*

HIV-1 infection is spread either by free viral particles, or 100 times more efficiently by direct cell-to-cell fusion [1]. Considering that *S. fusiforme* inhibits HIV-1 infection in T cells (Fig. 3), we wanted to determine its ability to block cell-to-cell mediated viral transfer. To test this, we performed two separate experiments with different cell types (Fig 4). First, we examined the ability of HIV infected CEM cells to fuse and spread infection to uninfected 1G5 cells that were either mock treated, treated with 10^{-6} M ddC only, or treated with increasing concentrations of *S. fusiforme* and ddC, or with *S. fusiforme* only. Pretreatment of 1G5 cells with 10^{-6} M ddC inhibits virus replication, and therefore serves as a control for false positive luciferase readings from free virus particle infection and replication, however it does not prevent spread of infection by cell-to-cell fusion. CEM and 1G5 cells were cocultivated for 24 h at a ratio of 1:1, and examined for cell-to-cell fusion and syncytia formation by phase contrast microcopy (A-F) or by luciferase expression (H). As expected, many large syncytia were observed in co-cultures with mock treated or only ddC treated 1G5 cells (A and B). However, 1G5 treatment with 2 mg *S. fusiforme*, with or without ddC, greatly reduced cell-to cell fusion and syncytia formation (C and E). No giant cells were detected in 1G5 cells treated with either 4 mg/ml (D and F) or with 6 mg/ml (not shown) *S. fusiforme*, with or without addition of ddC. Inhibition of viral infection by cell-to-cell fusion was also confirmed by decreased luciferase expression in *S. fusiforme* treated 1G5 cells that were cocultivated with HIV infected CEM cells (H). CEM cells do not have the HIV-LTR-luciferase gene, as 1G5 cells do, and therefore luciferase readings from cocultivated cell cultures can only arise from 1G5 cells that fused and formed giant cells with infected CEM cells. 24 h after cocultivation with untreated 1G5 cells, luciferase expression measured 1.9×10^5 RLU, which represented maximal luciferase expression in the absence of any treatment (not shown). 1G5 treatment with 10^{-6} M ddC and 2, 4, or 6 mg *S. fusiforme* inhibited cell-to-cell fusion, as measured by luciferase expression in 1G5 cells, by 77, 96, and 98%, respectively (H). Inhibition was similar in cells treated with *S. fusiforme* only, in the absence of ddC, demonstrating low rate of infection by free virus, during the

A) Inhibition kinetics

B) Viability

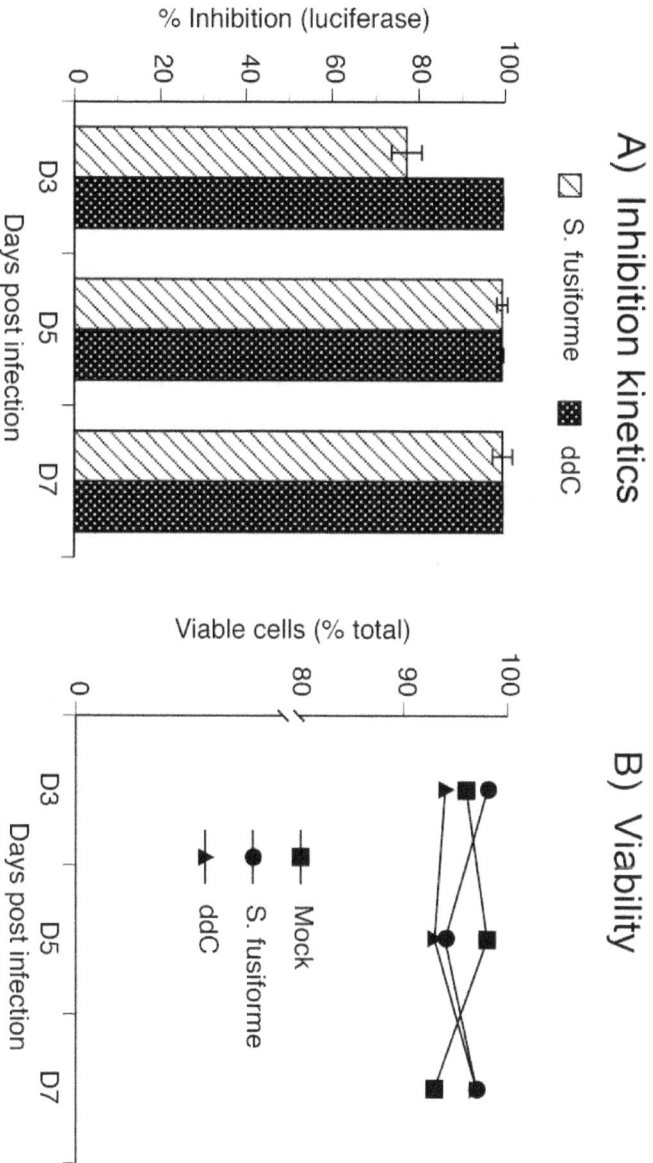

FIGURE 3: Time course of HIV-1 inhibition and viability in T cells. 1G5 T cells were 24 h treated with either 2 mg/ml *S. fusiforme*, or with 10^{-6} M ddC; then infected with NL4-3 at 0.01 moi for 1.5 h, washed 3 times, and returned to culture with same concentration of each treatment for the duration of the experiment. On day 3 post-infection, (A) gene expression of intracellular luciferase was measured from cell lysates adjusted to same number of viable cells, and % inhibition calculated and plotted on the Y-axis. Data are mean +/- SD of triplicates. In parallel, (B) cell viability was determined by trypan blue exclusion assay by counting at least 200 cells each, in three different fields under ×20 magnification using an Olympus BH-2 fluorescence microscope.

24 hours of cocultivation (not shown). In comparison, 1G5 cell treatment with only 10⁻⁶ M ddC, inhibited luciferase expression by 69%.

In the second experiment, we cocultivated HIV infected and untreated 1G5 cells with uninfected and treated HIV-LTR-GFP-expressing GHOST adherent cells [29], and monitored for cell-to-cell fusion by GFP expression from GHOST cells (G). After cocultivation with infected 1G5 cells, mock or only ddC treated GHOST cells can fuse, and form syncytia that emit green florescence, which was detected by phase fluorescence microscopy. GHOST cells that were ddC treated and cocultivated with HIV-1 infected 1G5 cells, resulted in cell-to-cell fusion and fluorescent giant cell formation as is shown by fluorescence micrograph superimposed on the phase contrast black and white image of the same field (G). However, as in CEM-1G5 cocultivation experiment, no giant cells emitting green fluorescence were detected in 1G5 cells cocultivated with GHOST cells that were treated with *S. fusiforme*, with or without ddC (not shown).

Based on the results of these two different experiments, we conclude that *S. fusiforme* blocks HIV-1 infection by cell-to-cell fusion mechanism, which also prevents subsequent multinucleated cell formation and its associated cytophatic effects.

FIGURE 4: Inhibition of cell-to-cell infection and syncytia formation. Uninfected 1G5 T cells were pretreated for 24 h with either (A) mock, (B) 10⁻⁶ M ddC, or with ddC and (B) 2 mg/ml or (C) 4 mg/ml *S. fusiforme*, or with *S. fusiforme* only at (D) 2 mg/ml or (E) 4 mg/ml. 1G5 cells were cocultivated at 1:1 ratio with CEM cells that were infected with NL4-3 at 0.01 moi. 24 h after cocultivation, cells were examined for syncytium formation using Leica DM IL Fluo microscope, ×20 magnification (A-F). Cell cultures were monitored for luciferase expression, and % inhibition was calculated from maximal luciferase expression from untreated 1G5 cells (1.9 × 10⁵ RLU, not shown), which was plotted and is indicated on top of each bar (H). Data are mean +/- SD of triplicates. Uninfected adherent GHOST [29] cells were ddC treated and cocultivated at 1:1 ratio with HIV infected 1G5 cells for 24 h, and examined for syncytia formation by green fluorescence (G). Image shows fluorescence micrograph taken of a green fluorescent giant cell, which was superimposed on the same field phase contrast black and white image.

Cell-to-cell Inhibition

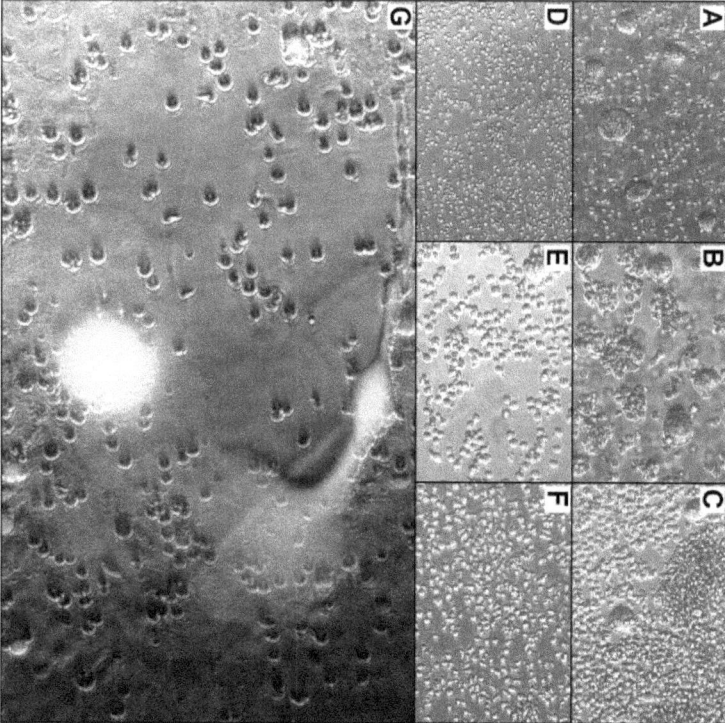

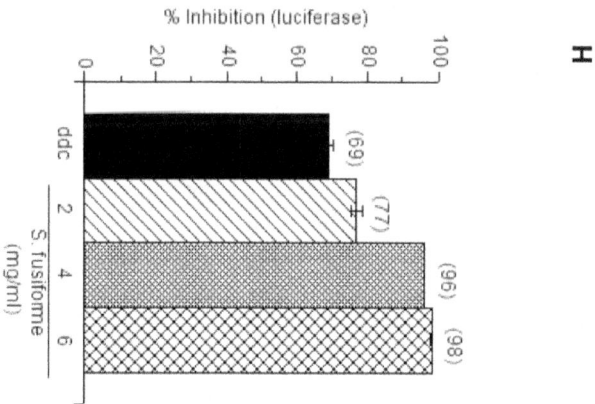

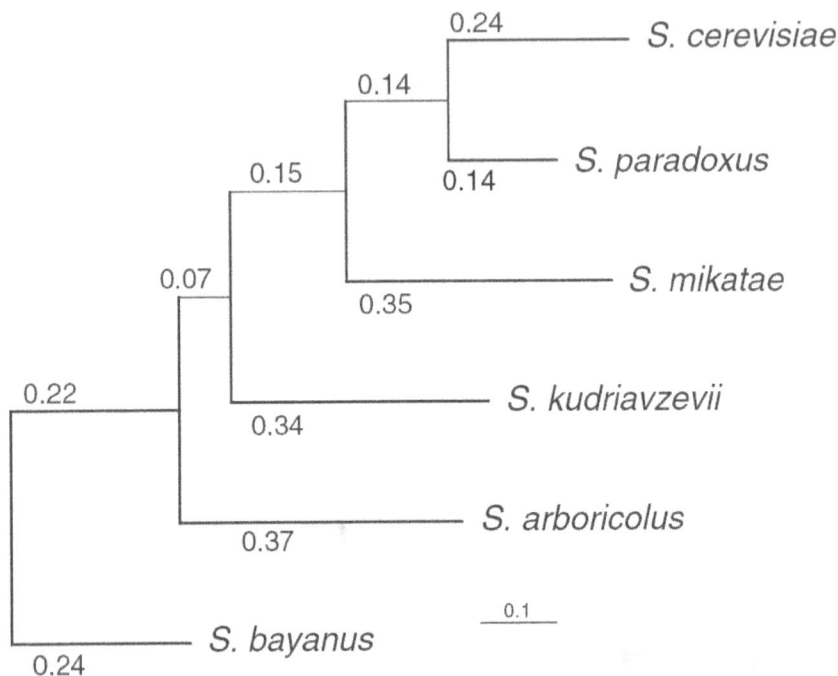

FIGURE 5: Inhibition of HIV-1 expression in human macrophages and microglia. Either, (A) human macrophages or (B) human fetal microglia were 24 h treated with 1 mg/ml *S. fusiforme*, or with 10^{-6} M ddC, infected with primary CCR5-tropic isolate ADA at 0.2 pg of p24/cell for 2 h, washed 3 times, and returned to culture with same concentration of each treatment for the duration of the experiment. At the indicated time points after infection HIV-1 expression was monitored by p24 production in cell-free supernatants by ELISA, % inhibition calculated as described in Methods and plotted on the y-axis. Data are mean +/- SD of triplicates. Representative of 2 experiments.

11.2.5 S. FUSIFORME *INHIBITS HIV-1 INFECTION IN* PRIMARY HUMAN MACROPHAGES AND BRAIN MICROGLIA

Macrophages and brain microglia are productively infected with R5-tropic HIV-1, and are considered to be the primary source of virus replication in the periphery and in the CNS [1]. Because of their importance to HIV infection, we investigated ability of *S. fusiforme* extract to inhibit virus infection in these cells. Primary human macrophages or microglial cell cultures were treated with 1 mg/ml *S. fusiforme* extract and infected with primary R5 isolate ADA [30]. Infection was monitored by measuring viral p24 concentrations in cell-free supernatants, at the indicated time points after infection (Fig. 5).

In infected and untreated macrophage cell cultures, virus levels steadily increased from 19,097 pg of p24/ml on day 4, to a peak of infection on day 14, measuring 163,740 pg of p24/ml, indicating productive HIV-1 infection and *de novo* virus synthesis (not shown). However, treatment with 1 mg/ml *S. fusiforme* extract inhibited ADA replication (dark bars) by over 90% through day 14 after infection, which was comparable to the inhibition with ddC treatment (Fig. 5A).

Next, we treated fetal microglial cell cultures with either 1 mg/ml *S. fusiforme*, or 10^{-6} M ddC, or mock treated, and monitored infection kinetics by p24 production in cell-free supernatants at the indicated time points after infection (Fig. 5B). As in T cells and macrophages, infected and mock treated microglia were productively infected as demonstrated by steadily increasing p24 production that reached a peak on day 14 with 2,313 pg of p24/ml (not shown). Treatment with *S. fusiforme* inhibited this infection by 75% on day 3, by over 90% on day 7 and 10, and by 81% on day 14 after infection. By comparison, virus inhibition by ddC was 72% on day 3, and thereafter remained above 90%.

In parallel to infection kinetics, we monitored cell viability by MTT assay, which remained high and was similar to uninfected cell cultures (not shown). Based on these results we conclude that *S. fusiforme* is a potent inhibitor of R5-tropic HIV-1 infection in primary human macrophages and microglia: inhibition is long lasting, not toxic to cells, and with similar inhibition kinetics to those observed in T cells (Fig. 3A).

11.2.6 S. FUSIFORME *INHIBITS HIV-1 INFECTION DURING ENTRY AND POST-ENTRY EVENTS OF VIRUS LIFE CYCLE*

Collectively, our results demonstrate that *S. fusiforme* extract robustly inhibits HIV-1 infection in a number of cell types, and in a number of infection scenarios. In order to determine how this inhibition works, we tested whether the extract could block infection at a post-entry level of virus replication.

HIV-1 pseudotyped with the vesicular stomatitis virus G-protein (VSV-G) can infect cells without interacting with CD4 and co-receptors. We extended HIV-1 tropism by pseudotyping native HIV-1 (NL4-3) with VSV-G envelope (VSV/NL4-3), which produced native NL4-3 with heterologous envelope glycoproteins that bind to commonly expressed cellular receptors. VSV/NL4-3 virus gains access to the cytoplasm by fusing out of endocytic vesicles [31]. Therefore, any block to VSV/NL4-3 replication would suggest post-entry inhibition. We treated T cells with increasing doses of *S. fusiforme*, infected with NL4-3 or VSV/NL4-3, and monitored infection by luciferase gene expression on day 3 after infection (Fig. 6A). To our surprise, *S. fusiforme* mediated dose dependant inhibition of VSV/NL4-3, inhibiting at 26.6, 32.8, and 62.6% that corresponded to 1, 2, and 3 mg/ml *S. fusiforme* extract treatment, respectively (Fig. 6A, light bars). However, overall inhibition of pseudotyped virus was markedly lower as compared to inhibition of native NL4-3, which was inhibited by 53, 78, and 93% (dark bars). Considering that pseudotyped VSV/NL4-3 has no cell surface entry restrictions, these data suggest that: 1) *S. fusiforme* blocks at a post-entry step of viral replication, and 2) inhibition is also mediated during entry process, as suggested by difference in the levels of inhibition between native NL4-3 and VSV/NL4-3 infections.

To confirm and extend the finding of post-entry inhibition in T cells, we tested for inhibition of VSV/NL4-3 in CD4-negative primary cells. Human astrocytes are CD4-negative cells that are nonproductively infected by HIV-1 in vivo [16], and *in vitro* [32-34]. However, we showed that, *in vitro*, these cells fully support productive virus replication after entry restriction has been bypassed [35]. Infection with VSV/NL4-3 productively infects majority of astrocytes, and serves as model system to study HIV-1 replication in these cells [35]. We infected primary human astrocytes with VSV/NL4-3, and monitored infection kinetics at the indicated time points after infection, by measuring p24 production in cell-free culture supernatants (Fig. 6B). Peak of infection was reached on day 12 with 71,000 pg of p24/ml produced in the infected and untreated cell culture, indicating ongoing virus replication (data not shown). Consistent with post-entry inhibition observed in T cells (Fig. 6A), treatment with 1 mg/ml *S. fusiforme* extract also inhibited post-entry virus replication in primary human astrocytes, by 71, 40, and 54%, on day 3, 6, and 12, respectively (Fig. 6B).

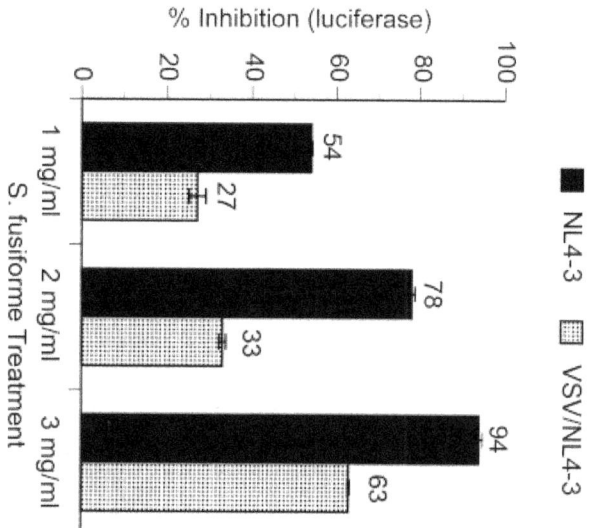

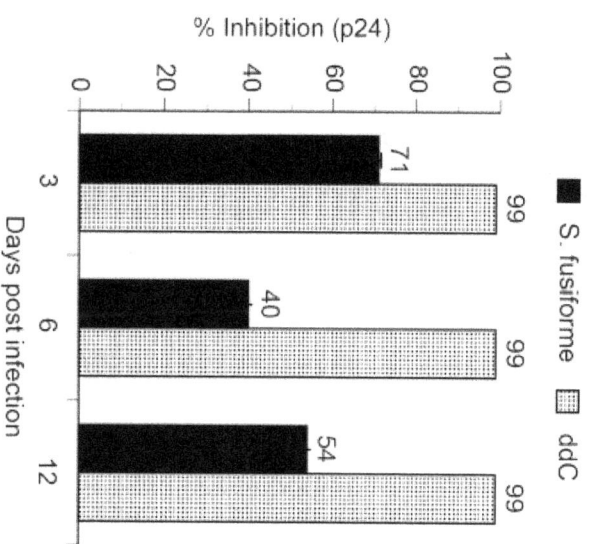

FIGURE 6: Inhibition of infection with pseudotyped HIV-1 in T cells and human astrocytes. (A) 1G5 T cells were treated with increasing concentrations of *S. fusiforme* and infected with either NL4-3 at 0.01 moi or with VSV/NL4-3 at 0.005 moi. 3 days after infection, % inhibition was calculated from luciferase expression from cell lysates adjusted to same number of viable cells by MTT. (B) Human fetal CD4 negative astrocytes were treated with 1 mg/ml *S. fusiforme*, or with 10⁻⁶ M ddC, infected with VSV/NL4-3 at 0.4 moi, and infection kinetics monitored by p24 expression in cell free supernatants at the indicated time points post infection. Data are mean +/- SD of triplicates. Representative of 2 experiments.

These data support our hypothesis that in addition to inhibiting viral entry, *S. fusiforme* extract also blocks viral replication during a post-entry event of the virus life cycle. However, the exact mechanisms of either entry or post-entry inhibition need to be further investigated.

11.3 DISCUSSION

The high rate of HIV-1 mutation and increasing resistance to currently available antiretroviral therapies underscores the need for new antiviral agents. The AIDS pandemic has been especially devastating in the Third world countries that can least afford or have easy access to current therapies, demonstrating a need for affordable treatments aimed at preventing HIV infection [36]. To expand search for novel inhibitors of HIV infection and replication, we studied and identified naturally occurring *S. fusiforme* extract as an efficient inhibitor of HIV-1 replication in T cells, in primary human macrophages, microglia, and astrocytes.

First, we demonstrated that *S. fusiforme* aqueous extract does not inhibit cell growth, is not toxic to cells, and was therefore suitable for further *in vitro* studies of HIV-1 inhibition (Fig. 1). Because it may be easier to block inefficient low level virus replication, we ensured that the observed inhibition was mediated against productive and *de novo* viral synthesis, by monitoring virus replication by either cell free p24 production or intracellular luciferase reporter gene expression. In T cells, *S. fusiforme* extract inhibited HIV-1 replication up to 90%, in a dose dependant manner (Fig. 2). This inhibition was long lasting, up to 7 days of follow-up, and was similar to the levels of inhibition observed with ddC treatment (Fig. 3).

In vivo, one mechanism of HIV-1 infection and viral spread is by a direct cell-to-cell fusion, between infected and uninfected cell [37]. To investigate possible inhibition of this mechanism of infection, in two separate experiments with different cell types, we cocultivated *S. fusiforme* treated cells, with HIV infected cells, and monitored for syncytia formation by microscopy, and for viral replication by luciferase expression (Fig 4). In both experiments, treatment with *S. fusiforme*, with or without ddC control for free virus infection, prevented cell-to-cell fusion and inhibited infection, in a dose dependant manner. These results demonstrate ability of *S. fusiforme* to inhibit physiologically relevant mechanism of spreading infection.

Infected macrophages act as a bridge between the periphery and the CNS, by spreading HIV-1 infection to microglia and astrocytes in the CNS [14]. Treatment with 1 mg/ml *S. fusiforme* extract inhibited active R5-tropic virus replication by 90%, in primary human macrophages and microglial cell cultures (Fig 5). In primary human astrocytes, *S. fusiforme* ihibited VSV/NL4-3 entry independent infection by 71%, which also suggested post entry inhibition of virus replication in these cells (Fig 6B). *S. fusiforme* did not inhibit cell growth or viability in these cells, which was consistent with results in T cells (Fig 1 and 2). These results demonstrate ability of *S. fusiforme* extract to inhibit HIV-1 replication in the two relevant cell types in the CNS, microglia and astrocytes. In this context, it would be of interest to determine whether *S. fusiforme* is capable of crossing the blood-brain barrier (BBB), and be an effective treatment in this important viral reservoir.

Because it was not clear which step of the virus life cycle *S. fusiforme* blocks, we investigated possibility of post entry inhibition. We tested for inhibition of infection with VSV-G pseudotyped HIV-1, which has been used to bypasses any entry restrictions [31,35]. Treatment with increasing doses of *S. fusiforme* inhibited VSV/NL4-3 infection in T cells in a dose dependant manner (Fig. 6A). However, compared to inhibition of native HIV-1, inhibition of VSV/NL4-3 was markedly lower, up to 57% lower, indicating interference with post entry steps of virus life cycle. We extended this finding by infecting CD4-negative human astrocytes with VSV/NL4-3, which was also inhibited by 71% (Fig 6B). Consistent with lower post entry inhibition in T cells, post entry inhibition in astrocytes was also lower, as compared to 99% inhibition with ddC treatment. The reasons for these inhibition differences are not clear, but given that native NL4-3 has entry restrictions and pseudotyped VSV/NL4-3 does not, we interpret these results to mean that *S. fusiforme* mediates HIV-1 inhibition during both entry and post entry steps of virus life cycle. However, the exact mechanisms of this inhibition need to be investigated. Considering *S. fusiforme* inhibition in different cell types, and with different mechanisms of action, we further postulate that this complex aqueous mixture contains more than one biologically active molecule mediating the observed HIV-1 inhibition.

11.4 CONCLUSION

S. fusiforme extract is a potent inhibitor of HIV-1 infection in T cells, in human macrophages, microglia, and astrocytes. Inhibition is mediated during both entry and post entry events of the virus life cycle. Based on these results we propose that *S. fusiforme* is a lead candidate for bioactivity guided isolation and identification of active compounds mediating the observed HIV-1 inhibition. Identification of these compounds will allow investigation of the precise mechanisms of inhibition as well as standardization of the whole extract for potential in vivo use, and for development of novel antiretroviral drugs and microbicides.

11.5 METHODS

11.5.1 GENERATION OF AQUEOUS EXTRACT FROM S. FUSIFORME PLANT MATERIAL

Dried *S. fusiforme* was obtained from the wholesale distributor, South Project LTD. Hong Kong, China. To confirm content and consistency, each separate shipment was first identified botanically, and then incubated at 55°C for 6 hours to eliminate any residual moisture. The dried material was briefly washed in cold water to remove any debris or loose particulate matter, weighed and resuspended to 100 mg/ml H_2O in covered sterile glass beakers, and boiled at 100°C for one hour. Hot water extracts were allowed to cool to room temperature, then filtered three times through a Whatman filter paper #2, and autoclaved for 20 minutes. Each preparation was centrifuged at 100,000 × g for 1 h to remove any additional particulate matter, aliquoted and stored at -20°C until use.

11.5.2 CELLS AND CULTURE TREATMENTS

11.5.2.1 T CELLS

1G5 and CEM T cells were obtained from the NIH AIDS Reagent Repository and cultured in RPMI 1640 suplemented with 10% fetal bovine serum (FBS, HyClone) and penicillin-streptomycin (pen/strep).

11.5.2.2 MONOCYTE-DERIVED HUMAN MACROPHAGES

Monocytes were recovered from peripheral blood mononuclear cells (PBMCs) by countercurrent centrifugal elutriation as previously described [30]. Monocytes were cultured as adherent monolayers (1×10^6 cells/well in 24-well plates), differentiated for 7 days in Dulbecco's modified Eagle's medium (DMEM) supplemented with macrophage colony stimulating factor (M-CSF, a generous gift from Wyeth, Cambridge, MA). Confluent cultures of fully differentiated macrophages were infected with HIV-1 CCR5-tropic ADA primary isolate, as indicated in Figure legends.

11.5.2.3 ISOLATION AND CULTURE OF FETAL MICROGLIAL CELLS

Fetal microglial cells were isolated from second-trimester (gestational age, 17–19 weeks) human fetal brain tissue obtained from elective abortions in full compliance with National Institutes of Health (NIH) guidelines, as previously described [30]. Briefly, the tissue was washed with cold Hanks Balanced Salt Solution (HBSS, MediaTech), then mechanically dissociated and digested with 0.25% trypsin (Gibco) for 30 minutes at 37°C; trypsin was neutralized with FBS (HyClone). Single cell suspensions were plated in DMEM supplemented with 10% FBS, 1000 U/ml M-CSF, and pen/strep. The mixed cultures were maintained at 37°C for 7 days and the media was fully exchanged to remove any cellular debris. The microglial cells, released upon further incubation, were collected and purified by preferential adhesion. Microglia were cultured as adherent monolayers at a density of 0.1×10^6 cells/well in 24-well plates, and were infected as described in Figure legends.

11.5.2.4 HUMAN FETAL ASTROCYTES

Fetal astrocytes were isolated from second-trimester (gestational age, 17–19 weeks) human fetal brains obtained from elective abortions in full compliance with National Institutes of Health (NIH) guidelines, as previously described [35]. Briefly, highly homogenous preparations of astrocytes were obtained using high-density culture conditions in the absence of growth factors in F12 Dulbecco's modified Eagle's medium (GIBCO-BRL, Gaithersburg, Md.) containing 10% FBS, pen/strep, and gentamycin. Cultures were regularly monitored for expression of the astrocytic marker glial fibrillary acidic protein (GFAP) and either HAM56 or CD68 to identify cells of monocyte/macrophage lineage. Only cultures that contained 99% GFAP-positive cells and rare or no detectable HAM56- or CD68-positive cells were used in our experiments [35].

11.4.2.5 CELL CULTURE TREATMENTS

Before infection, cells were grown for 24 h in culture media with the indicated concentration of either *S. fusiforme* extract, or with 10-6 M ddC, washed 3 times with HBSS (GIBCO-BRL), and infected as indicated. After infection cells were washed 3 times, and returned to culture with same concentration of each treatment for the duration of experiment.

11.5.3 HIV-1 MOLECULAR CLONES, ENVELOPE EXPRESSION VECTORS, AND GENERATION OF PSEUDOTYPED HIV-1

T cell tropic HIV-1 molecular clone NL4-3 expresses all known HIV-1 proteins [38], and it was used to infect T cell experimental systems. VSV/NL4-3 viral stocks were prepared by cotransfection of intact NL4-3 DNA (pNL4-3) and VSV envelope expression vector (pL-VSV-G). The VSV-G expression vector pL-VSV-G was obtained from M. Emerman; it contains a VSV-G insert in the pcDNA expression vector modified by replacing the cytomegalovirus promoter with the HIV-1 long terminal repeat [39]. High-titer virus stocks, including pseudotyped virus, were produced in early passage 293T human embryonic kidney cells transfected with the respective DNA by calcium phosphate precipitation [40], as previously described [35]. Cell-free viral stocks were tested for HIV-1 p24 core antigen content by enzyme-linked immunosorbent assay (ELISA) using HIV-1 Ag kit as specified by the manufacturer (Coulter, Hialeah, Fla). Titers of infectious virus were determined by multinuclear activation of β-galactosidase indicator (MAGI) assay [41]. In our hands, a multiplicity of infection of 1 for CD4-positive T cells is equivalent to approximately 1 pg of viral p24 per cell [35]. Macrophage and microglial cells infections were performed using the HIV-1 CCR5-tropic primary isolate ADA, as previously described [30].

11.5.4 INFECTIONS AND ANALYSIS OF HIV-1 EXPRESSION BY LUCIFERASE GENE EXPRESSION AND BY P24 ELISA

T cells, confluent cultures of macrophages, microglial cells, or human fetal astrocytes were infected with native or pseudotyped HIV-1 at the multiplicity of infection (moi) as indicated in the Figure legends, and were washed three times with HBSS (GIBCO-BRL) before being returned to culture. At the indicated times after infection, equal number of viable cells normalized by CellTiter 96 Non-Radioactive Cell proliferation Assay [(3-(4,5-Dimethyl-2-thiazolyl)-2,5-dephenyltetrazolium (MTT)] kit, or by trypan blue exclusion assay, were tested for luciferase expression using Luciferase Assay System kit (Promega) as specified by the manufacturer. Cell-free supernatants were tested for HIV-1 p24 core antigen content by ELISA using the HIV-1 Ag kit as specified by the manufacturer (Coulter, Hialeah, Fla).

Infected T cell cultures were analyzed for syncytium formation at the indicated time points after infection by visualizing cells under an Olympus BH-2 fluorescence microscope, and at least 4 separate wells from a 12-well plate (Costar), from identical experimental systems were analyzed.

11.5.5 CALCULATION OF PERCENT INHIBITION OF INFECTION

Percent (%) inhibition was determined from either luciferase expression or p24 content, utilizing the following formula:

$$Inhibition[\%] = \left[1 - \frac{(Treated\ cells) - (Mock - treated\ cells)}{(Untreated\ cells) - (Mock - treated\ cells)}\right] \times 100$$

REFERENCES

1. Levy JA: HIV and the pathogenesis of AIDS. second edition edition. Washington DC, AMS; 1998.
2. Bushman F, Landau NR, Emini EA: New developments in the biology and treatment of HIV. Proc Natl Acad Sci U S A 1998, 95:11041-11042.
3. Cohen OJ, Fauci AS: Current strategies in the treatment of HIV infection. Adv Intern Med 2001, 46:207-246.
4. Powderly WG: Current approaches to treatment for HIV-1 infection. J Neurovirol 2000, 6 Suppl 1:S8-S13.
5. Volberding PA: Advances in the medical management of patients with HIV-1 infection: an overview. Aids 1999, 13 Suppl 1:S1-9.
6. Graham NM: Metabolic disorders among HIV-infected patients treated with protease inhibitors: a review. J Acquir Immune Defic Syndr 2000, 25 Suppl 1:S4-11.

7. Moyle G: Clinical manifestations and management of antiretroviral nucleoside ana-
    log-related mitochondrial toxicity. Clin Ther 2000, 22:911-36; discussion 898.
8. Perelson AS, Neumann AU, Markowitz M, Leonard JM, Ho DD: HIV-1 dynamics in
    vivo: virion clearance rate, infected cell life-span, and viral generation time. Science
    1996, 271:1582-1586.
9. Chun TWSLMSBELAMJAMBMLALNMAFAS: Presence of an inducible HIV-1
    latent reservoir during highly active antiretroviral therapy. Proc Natl Acad Sci USA
    1997, 94:13193-13197.
10. Chun TW, Carruth L, Finzi D, Shen X, DiGiuseppe JA, Taylor H, Hermankova M,
    Chadwick K, Margolick J, Quinn TC, Kuo YH, Brookmeyer R, Zeiger MA, Bar-
    ditch-Crovo P, Siliciano RF: Quantification of latent tissue reservoirs and total body
    viral load in HIV-1 infection. Nature 1997, 387:183-188.
11. Wong JK, Hezareh M, Gunthard HF, Havlir DV, Ignacio CC, Spina CA, Richman
    DD: Recovery of replication-competent HIV despite prolonged suppression of plas-
    ma viremia. Science 1997, 278:1291-1295.
12. Clements JE, Li M, Gama L, Bullock B, Carruth LM, Mankowski JL, Zink MC:
    The central nervous system is a viral reservoir in simian immunodeficiency virus-
    -infected macaques on combined antiretroviral therapy: a model for human immuno-
    deficiency virus patients on highly active antiretroviral therapy. J Neurovirol 2005,
    11:180-189.
13. Gartner S: HIV infection and dementia. Science 2000, 287:602-604.
14. Gendelman HE, Grant I, Everall I, Lipton AS, Swindells S: The Neurology of AIDS.
    Second Edition edition. Edited by Gendelman HE, Grant I, Everall I, Lipton AS and
    Swindells S. Oxford, Oxford University Press; 2005.
15. Rutka JT, Murakami M, Dirks PB, Hubbard SL, Becker LE, Fukuyama K, Jung S,
    Tsugu A, Matsuzawa K: Role of glial filaments in cells and tumors of glial origin: a
    review. J Neurosurg 1997, 87:420-430.
16. Takahashi K, Wesselingh SL, Griffin DE, McArthur JC, Johnson RT, Glass JD: Lo-
    calization of HIV-1 in human brain using polymerase chain reaction/in situ hybrid-
    ization and immunocytochemistry. Ann Neurol 1996, 39:705-711.
17. McArthur JC, Hoover DR, Bacellar H, Miller EN, Cohen BA, Becker JT, Graham
    NM, McArthur JH, Selnes OA, Jacobson LP, et al.: Dementia in AIDS patients: inci-
    dence and risk factors. Multicenter AIDS Cohort Study. Neurology 1993, 43:2245-
    2252.
18. Kaul M, Garden GA, Lipton SA: Pathways to neuronal injury and apoptosis in HIV-
    associated dementia. Nature 2001, 410:988-994.
19. Enting RH, Hoetelmans RM, Lange JM, Burger DM, Beijnen JH, Portegies P: Anti-
    retroviral drugs and the central nervous system. Aids 1998, 12:1941-1955.
20. Cunningham PH, Smith DG, Satchell C, Cooper DA, Brew B: Evidence for inde-
    pendent development of resistance to HIV-1 reverse transcriptase inhibitors in the
    cerebrospinal fluid. Aids 2000, 14:1949-1954.
21. Wegner SA, Brodine SK, Mascola JR, Tasker SA, Shaffer RA, Starkey MJ, Barile A,
    Martin GJ, Aronson N, Emmons WW, Stephan K, Bloor S, Vingerhoets J, Hertogs
    K, Larder B: Prevalence of genotypic and phenotypic resistance to anti-retroviral
    drugs in a cohort of therapy-naive HIV-1 infected US military personnel. Aids 2000,
    14:1009-1015.

22. Little SJ, Holte S, Routy JP, Daar ES, Markowitz M, Collier AC, Koup RA, Mellors JW, Connick E, Conway B, Kilby M, Wang L, Whitcomb JM, Hellmann NS, Richman DD: Antiretroviral-drug resistance among patients recently infected with HIV. N Engl J Med 2002, 347:385-394.

23. Cowan MM: Plant products as antimicrobial agents. Clin Microbiol Rev 1999, 12:564-582.

24. Yang SS, Cragg GM, Newman DJ, Bader JP: Natural product-based anti-HIV drug discovery and development facilitated by the NCI developmental therapeutics program. J Nat Prod 2001, 64:265-277.

25. Witvrouw M, De Clercq E: Sulfated polysaccharides extracted from sea algae as potential antiviral drugs. Gen Pharmacol 1997, 29:497-511.

26. Hoshino T, Hayashi T, Hayashi K, Hamada J, Lee JB, Sankawa U: An antivirally active sulfated polysaccharide from Sargassum horneri (TURNER) C. AGARDH. Biol Pharm Bull 1998, 21:730-734.

27. Schaeffer DJ, Krylov VS: Anti-HIV activity of extracts and compounds from algae and cyanobacteria. Ecotoxicol Environ Saf 2000, 45:208-227.

28. Aguilar-Cordova E, Chinen J, Donehower L, Lewis DE, Belmont JW: A sensative reporter cell line for HIV-1 tat activity, HIV-1 Inhibitors, and T cell activation effects. Aids research and human retroviruses 1994, 10:295-301.

29. Morner A, Bjorndal A, Albert J, Kewalramani VN, Littman DR, Inoue R, Thorstensson R, Fenyo EM, Bjorling E: Primary human immunodeficiency virus type 2 (HIV-2) isolates, like HIV-1 isolates, frequently use CCR5 but show promiscuity in coreceptor usage. J Virol 1999, 73:2343-2349.

30. Gendelman HE, Orenstein JM, Martin MA, Ferrua C, Mitra R, Phipps T, Wahl LA, Lane HC, Fauci AS, Burke DS, Skillman D, Meltzer MS: Efficient isolation and propagation of human immunodeficiency virus on recombinant colony-stimulating factor-1 treated monocytes. J Exp Med 1988, 167:1428-1441.

31. Matlin KS, Reggio H, Helenius A, Simons K: Pathway of vesicular stomatitis virus entry leading to infection. J Mol Biol 1982, 156:609-631.

32. Tornatore C, Meyers K, Atwood W, Conant K, Major E: Temporal patterns of human immunodeficiency virus type 1 transcripts in human fetal astrocytes. J Virol 1994, 68:93-102.

33. Canki M, Potash MJ, Bentsman G, Chao W, Flynn T, Heinemann M, Gelbard H, Volsky DJ: Isolation and long-term culture of primary ocular human immunodeficiency virus type 1 isolates in primary astrocytes. J Neurovirol 1997, 3:10-15.

34. Bencheikh M, Bentsman G, Sarkissian N, Canki M, Volsky JD: Replication of different clones of human immunodeficiency virus type 1 in primary human fetal astrocytes: enhancment of viral gene expression by Nef. Journal NeuroVirology 1999, 5:115-124.

35. Canki M, Thai JNF, Chao W, Ghorpade A, Potash MJ, Volsky DJ: Highly productive infection with pseudotyped human immunodeficiency virus type 1 (HIV-1) indicates no intracellular restrictions to HIV-1 replication in primary human astrocytes. J Virol 2001, 75:7925-7933.

36. Piot P: AIDS: a global response. Science 1996, 272:1855.

37. Levy JA: Pathogenesis of human immunodeficiency virus infection. Microbiol Rev 1993, 57:183-289.

38. Adachi A, Gendelman HE, koening S, Folks T, Willey R, Rabson A, Martin M: Production of acquired immunodeficiency syndrome-associated retrovirus in human and nonhuman cells transfected with an infectious molecular clone. Journal of Virology 1986, 59:284-291.

39. Bartz RS, Vodicka AM: Production of high-titer human immunodeficiency virus type 1 pseudotyped with vesicular stomatitis virus glycoprotein. y 1997, 12:337-342.

40. Ausubel MF, Brent R, Kingston ER, Moore DD, Seidman GJ, Smith AJ, Struhl K: Current protocols in molecular biology. New York, N.Y., John Wiley & Sons, Inc.; 1995.

41. Kimpton J, Emerman M: Detection of replication-competent and pseudotyped human immunodeficiency virus with a sensitive cell line on the basis of activation of an integrated beta-galactosidase gene. J Virol 1992, 66:2232-2239.

PART III

MOLECULAR BIOLOGY, GENOMICS, AND PROTEOMICS: PLANT CENTERED AND PERSON CENTERED

CHAPTER 12

THE USE OF PHYLOGENY TO INTERPRET CROSS-CULTURAL PATTERNS IN PLANT USE AND GUIDE MEDICINAL PLANT DISCOVERY: AN EXAMPLE FROM *PTEROCARPUS* (LEGUMINOSAE)

C. HARIS SASLIS-LAGOUDAKIS, BENTE B. KLITGAARD, FÉLIX FOREST, LOUISE FRANCIS, VINCENT SAVOLAINEN, ELIZABETH M. WILLIAMSON, AND JULIE A. HAWKINS

12.1 INTRODUCTION

Thousands of plant species are used in traditional medicine around the globe, with almost one in four species on the planet used in traditional medicine in some culture [1]. For decades researchers have worked towards compiling a comprehensive list of medicinal plant species from different regions around the world. The documentation of such knowledge is crucial not only in order to preserve it, but also to understand patterns that shape this knowledge and to direct studies that can lead to the discovery of new medicinal plants. Indeed, in the last decades, the field of bioscreening

This chapter was originally published under the Creative Commons Attribution License. Saslis-Lagoudakis CH, Klitgaard BB, Forest F, Francis L, Savolainen V, Williamson EM, and Hawkins JA. The Use of Phylogeny to Interpret Cross-Cultural Patterns in Plant Use and Guide Medicinal Plant Discovery: An Example from Pterocarpus (Leguminosae). *PLoS ONE 6,7 (2011). doi:10.1371/journal. pone.0022275.*

has been guided by ethnomedicine, the study of traditional medicine, leading to the discovery of several plant-derived pharmaceuticals [2], [3], [4].

Medicinal properties are not randomly distributed in plants. Instead, some plant groups are represented by more medicinal plants than others [5], [6], [7], [8], [9]. Some of these studies suggested than when looking for new medicinal plants, one should sample from the "hot" groups, as they are more likely to deliver [7], [9]. Although this suggests that there is a phylogenetic pattern in medicinal properties, these studies were not explicitly phylogenetic. Phylogenetic conservatism [10], [11] in medicinal properties has been proposed [12], [13]. Lukhoba et al. [14] showed that for the genus *Plectranthus* (Lamiaceae), with 62 of the 300 species used in some sort of ethnomedicinal preparation, most medicinal species were found within the same large phylogenetic clade, suggesting there is a phylogenetic pattern in medicinal properties within the genus. Although this was not quantified, a later study by Forest et al. [15] used a more quantitative approach to show that in the Cape flora of South Africa, ethnomedicinal plants were significantly clumped on the phylogeny. A similar situation is observed in Narcissus species with medicinal properties [13]. The reason for this non-random phylogenetic distribution in medicinal properties might be that closely related plant species share biochemistry [16] and therefore, close relatives are likely to share medicinal properties. The presumption of shared chemistry in close relatives gave rise to the field of chemosystematics [17], [18], [19], [20], [21]. Nowadays taxonomies are no longer proposed based on chemical affinities; instead, phylogeny provides a framework to understand the distribution of chemistry. Combined phylogenetic and phytochemical studies have shown that there is strong phylogenetic signal in the distribution of chemical constituents in plants [22], [23], [24] that can be applied in the research for novel natural products [13], [25], [26], [27]. However, chemical data are unavailable for the majority of species and can be costly to generate. With less than a quarter of plant species screened for bioactivity [28], explicit tools are needed that can predict the phylogenetic position of species with high potential. The emerging field, which we refer to here as "phylogenetic ethnobotany", still lacks quantitative metrics.

Biological phylogenies have proved to be extremely versatile and valuable tools that have been applied in various fields, in order to recover a variety of patterns, including biogeographical [29], [30], ecological [31], [32], [33], developmental [34], chemical [22], [23] and epidemiological [35]. With the exception of consideration of phylogenetic patterns in biodiversity conservation [15], [36], [37] and comparative sequence analyses to identify organisms (DNA barcoding) [38], [39], [40], [41], the potential of phylogenies to more applied fields has been overlooked. Aside from the field of bioscreening, phylogenetic patterns in medicinal plant use can enrich our understanding of traditional ethnobotanical knowledge. The finding that some plant lineages are more heavily used than others [5], [6], [7], [8], [9] and the fact that there is a degree of agreement in those lineages between disparate cultures [9], [42], [43] implies that phylogenetic relationships underlie people's selection of medicinal plants in traditional medicine and in a fashion that overcomes cultural differences. With the exception of some unpublished studies presented at ethnobotanical conferences [44], [45], [46], such findings have not been investigated in an explicitly phylogenetic framework. By superposing medicinal properties on lineages with wide distributions, one can observe cross-cultural phylogenetic patterns in ethnobotany, such as the agreement in usage of closely related lineages in distant cultures [44].

Pterocarpus is a pantropical genus of dalbergioid legumes. It has been the subject of several regional taxonomic treatments [47], [48], [49], [50], [51] and one monographic study by Rojo [52]. In that study, Rojo recognised 20 species (23 taxa), but Lewis [53] estimated this number as 25–30 species, not supporting Rojo's synonymisation of several taxa under the American species *P. rohrii*. The most recent estimate is that of Klitgaard and Lavin [54], where the number of species was estimated as 35–40. The main centre of diversity of *Pterocarpus* is tropical Africa followed by the Neotropics and Indomalaya [52], as shown in Figure 1. Several *Pterocarpus* species are exploited throughout their range as timber as well as in traditional medicine. As Klitgaard and Lavin [54] state, the Indomalayan narra (*P. indicus*) is possibly one of the most important timber legumes globally, and several African species are very important timber trees known as paduak. The genus is used medicinally across its range for a variety of conditions. *Pterocarpus* species have received a lot of attention in recent years in experimental studies that have provided evidence for their bioactivity. Partly due to their extensive use, three species (*P. indicus*, *P.*

santalinus, P. marsupium) are listed under the IUCN Red list of threatened species [55] and *P. santalinus* is also included in CITES Annex II. Because of the wide range of documented ethnomedicinal uses for *Pterocarpus* species, the evidence of bioactivity for some of them, the critical status for some species heavily affected by usage and the distribution of the genus across three regions (Neotropics, tropical Africa and Indomalaya), it is an ideal model group to develop approaches to study phylogenetic patterns in medicinal properties.

12.1.1 OBJECTIVES

The objectives of the present study are to: i) compile information from ethnobotanical sources to produce an ethnomedicinal review of *Pterocarpus* from the literature across its geographic range, ii) provide a phylogenetic hypothesis for the genus based on DNA sequence data, iii) develop methods that allow more explicit use of molecular phylogenetics in bioscreening, iv) highlight taxa that could have medicinal properties and have been overlooked, based on evidence from traditional medicine and the phylogeny and v) explore cross-cultural ethnomedicinal patterns across the range of the genus in light of phylogenetic relationships.

12.2 MATERIALS AND METHODS

12.2.1 ETHNOMEDICINAL INFORMATION

Information on the medicinal uses of *Pterocarpus* species was compiled from extensive literature research from 125 sources, including published articles, online databases and local compendia of traditional medicine. All literature sources are given in Table S1. We collected information on the medicinal applications of *Pterocarpus* species in traditional medicine throughout the range of the genus, as well as pharmacological data from experimental studies. These applications were subsequently organised in

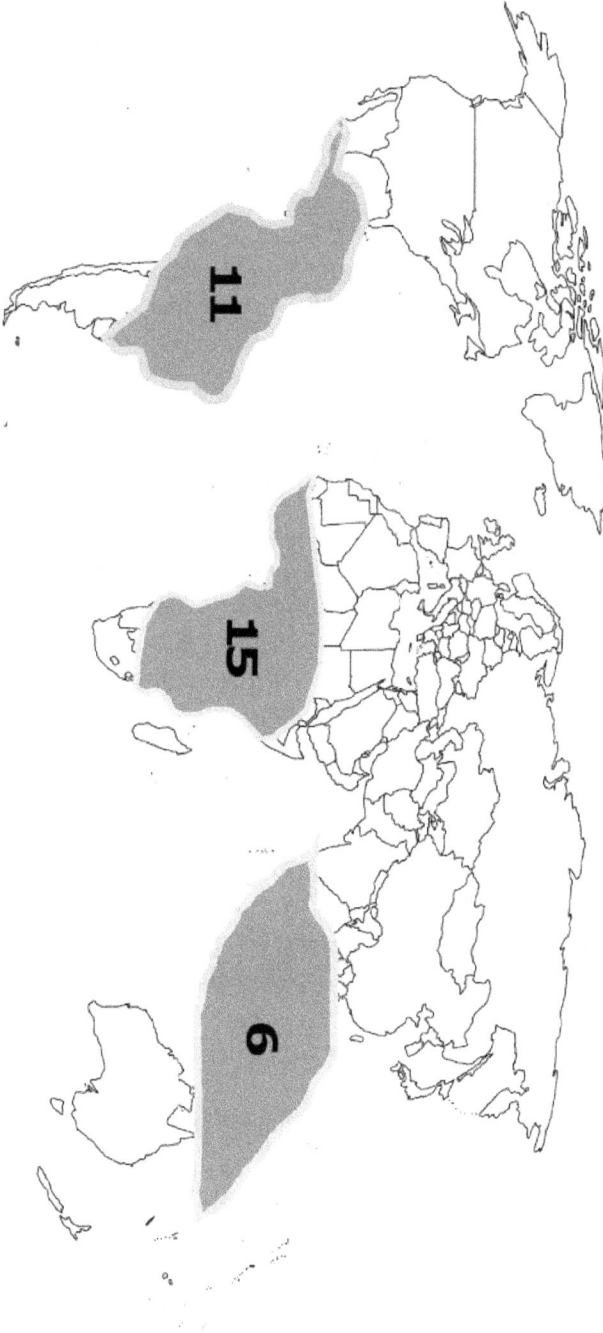

FIGURE 1: The pantropical distribution of *Pterocarpus*. Numbers indicate the numbers of taxa in different geographic regions: Neotropics, Tropical Africa, Indomalaya (Indian Subcontinent and Malay Peninsula/Archipelago).

13 categories of use following [56]: Circulatory/Blood, Gastro-intestinal, Genito-urinary/Fertility, Infections/Fever, Inflammation, Musculo-Skeletal, Nervous, Pain, Poisons treatment, Respiratory, Sensory, Skin and Unspecific.

12.2.2 TAXON SAMPLING

Rojo [52] recognised 23 taxa in 20 species, but Lewis [53] estimated this number to be 25–30 species, not supporting Rojo's synonymisation of several taxa under the American species *P. rohrii*. Specifically, he recognised *P. ternatus*, *P. villosus* and *P. zehntneri* as separate species from *P. rohrii* and we follow this taxonomy here. We included all taxa recognised by Rojo [52] (with the exception of the infraspecific taxon *P. indicus* forma echinatus due to material unavailability), accepting the infraspecific divisions of *P. rotundifolius* [57], [58] and of *P. mildbraedii* [59], and adding two neotropical taxa described after Rojo's monographic work, namely *P. michelianus* [60] and *P. monophyllus* [61]. This brings the total taxa recognised in this study to 30 in 25 species. Finally, we sampled several of the species that have been placed in synonymy under the species complexes *P. rohrii* and *P. tinctorius*. All *Pterocarpus* specimens included in the analyses are shown in Table S2. Outgroups were selected from previous phylogenetic analyses of dalbergioid legumes [62], [63], [64], [65]. We sampled genera closely related to *Pterocarpus*: *Centrolobium*, *Grazielodendron*, *Inocarpus*, *Maraniona*, *Ramorinoa*, *Tipuana*. *Platymisicum* was used as external outgroup taxon for the clade comprising these genera and *Pterocarpus* and defined as such in all analyses. Outgroup accessions are shown in Table S3.

12.2.3 SELECTION OF DNA MARKERS

We selected DNA markers based on amplification efficiency and variability. We used the plastid regions *rbcL* and *matK* that have shown great amplification efficiency across the angiosperms and the legume family [66], [67], [68] and have been successfully amplified and served as barcodes for two species of *Pterocarpus* in the literature [39]. Additionally, we selected the *ndhF-rpL32* intergenic spacer, a plastid marker shown to be potentially one of the most variable within the majority of angiosperm groups in a scan of the plastid genome [69]. Finally, we amplified nrITS2 and the *trnL-F* intergenic spacer, since these regions have provided phylogenetic resolution for closely related genera in previous studies [63], [64], [65], [70].

12.2.4 DNA EXTRACTION AND SEQUENCING

Total DNA was extracted from 0.2 to 0.3 g of leaf and/or flower tissue from herbarium or silica gel dried material using a modification [71] of the Doyle and Doyle method [72]. DNA was purified using QIAquick columns (Qiagen, Crawley, West Sussex, UK) following the manufacturer's protocol.

The internal transcribed spacer 2 (ITS2), including parts of the 5.8S ribosomal RNA gene and the 26S ribosomal RNA gene, was amplified using primers ITS3 and ITS26E [73]. The PCR protocol included a 2 min initial denaturation at 96°C and 32 cycles of 1 min denaturation (96°C), 1 min annealing (48°C), 50 s elongation (72°C), with a final elongation of 7 min at 72°C. The *trnL-F* intergenic spacer was amplified with primers "e" and "f" [74]. The PCR protocol included a 4 min initial denaturation (96°C) and 32 cycles of 1 min denaturation (96°C), 1 min annealing (54°C), 1 min elongation (72°C) and final elongation of 7 min at 72°C. The barcoding fragment of *matK* was amplified with primers X and 3.2 [75]. The PCR protocol included a 1 min initial denaturation (96°C) and 38 cycles of 30 s denaturation (96°C), 40 s annealing (46°C), 1 min elongation (72°C), with a final elongation of 7 min at 72°C. The first half of *rbcL* was amplified with primers *rbcL*1F and *rbcL*724R [76], following a protocol of 4 min initial denaturation (96°C), and 33 cycles of 1 min denaturation (96°C), 1 min annealing (50°C) and 1 min 20s elongation (72°C), with a final elongation of 7 min at 72°C. Finally, the *ndhF-rpL32* intergenic spacer was amplified with primers ndhF and rpL32-R [69]. Due to amplification of non-target product, we modified the PCR conditions given by [69] as follows: one cycle of denaturation (96°C) for 2 min, 30 cycles of 95°C for

40 s, 52°C for 1 min and 65°C for 3 min 20 s with ramp of 0.3/s to 65°C and a final elongation cycle of 65°C for 5 min. All amplifications were performed in 30-μL volume reactions with BioMix (Bioline Ltd. London, UK).

PCR purification and DNA sequencing of both strands were performed by Macrogen Inc. (Seoul, Korea). Complementary strands were assembled and edited with EditSeq (DNASTAR, Madison, WI). Alignments for *rbcL* and *matK* sequences were performed manually in BioEdit v. 7.0. ITS2, and the *trnL-F* and *ndhF-rpL32* intergenic spacer sequences were aligned using CLUSTAL W [77], and adjustments were made manually in BioEdit v. 7.0, following the guidelines of Kelchner [78]. All newly generated sequences have been submitted to GenBank (see Tables S2 and S3) and the data matrix and phylogenetic tree generated here are available on Tree-Base (www.treebase.org) under the accession number 11586.

12.2.5 PHYLOGENETIC ANALYSES AND MANIPULATIONS

Sequence data were analysed under the Maximum Likelihood (ML) criterion, with RAxML [79] using the partitioned model option with the GTR+Γ model and running 1000 bootstrap replicates [80].

We borrowed two metrics from community ecology phylogenetics in order to assess and detect phylogenetic signal in medicinal properties. The first was the "comstruct" option in Phylocom 4.1 [81]. This metric assesses the significance of phylogenetic signal for a community of taxa, which is the subset of a phylogeny. In other words, it calculates how significantly a group of species are clumped on the phylogeny. To do this, the mean phylogenetic distance (MPD) and mean nearest phylogenetic taxon distance (MNTD) for each sample (group of species on the phylogeny) is calculated and they are compared to MPD/MNTD values for randomly generated samples to provide p values for the significance of phylogenetic signal for the given sample (p values are calculated based on the frequency of random samples that were more clumped on the phylogeny than the real sample). For this study, we compiled "communities" of taxa that are used for one of the categories of use. This means that instead of grouping taxa based on which ecological zone or geographical area they are found, we grouped taxa that have similar uses in medicine together under one "community". This way, we are able to assess the phylogenetic signal of each category of use on the phylogeny of *Pterocarpus* and answer the question: Are taxa used for a certain category more significantly related than expected by chance alone?

The second metric used was the command "nodesig" in Phylocom v 4.1 [81]. This option uses the same community sample as described above and tests each node of the phylogeny for overabundance of terminal taxa distal to it. Observed patterns for each sample are compared to those from random samples to provide significance for the observed overabundance. For a node that is identified through this approach, the descendants of this node are significantly more likely to belong to the "community" under consideration that expected by chance alone. As mentioned earlier, a "community" for this study represents the group of species used for a certain category of use. Hence, this technique identifies the exact position of phylogenetic clumping on the phylogeny, namely the "hot" nodes for a category of use. This can help us assess the predictive power of the phylogeny for the discovery of new medicinal species.

The rationale behind using these metric is as follows: If a certain category of use shows strong phylogenetic signal, then closely related species demonstrate similar uses. With the first metric, we can asses which categories of use demonstrate strong phylogenetic signal. For these categories of use, we can subsequently identify which nodes on the phylogeny have more medicinal taxa than expected by chance, using the second tool. Taxa descending from these nodes are the ones that show significant "overabundance" in medicinal properties. Therefore, they deserve further investigation, including those species that are not reported in traditional medicine, as they are likely to share these properties with their relatives, as shown in Figure 2. The matrix showing the samples used for all Phylocom analyses is given in Table S4.

Analyses using these two approaches were carried out for each of the 13 categories of use mentioned above. Additionally, we performed the same analyses for three diseases of particular interest for which there is experimental evidence of bioactivity of *Pterocarpus* species: diabetes, malaria and cancer [82], [83], [84], [85], [86], [87], [88], [89], [90], [91], [92], [93]. This also allowed a test of our methods at different levels of ethnomedicinal specificity (condition versus group of conditions).

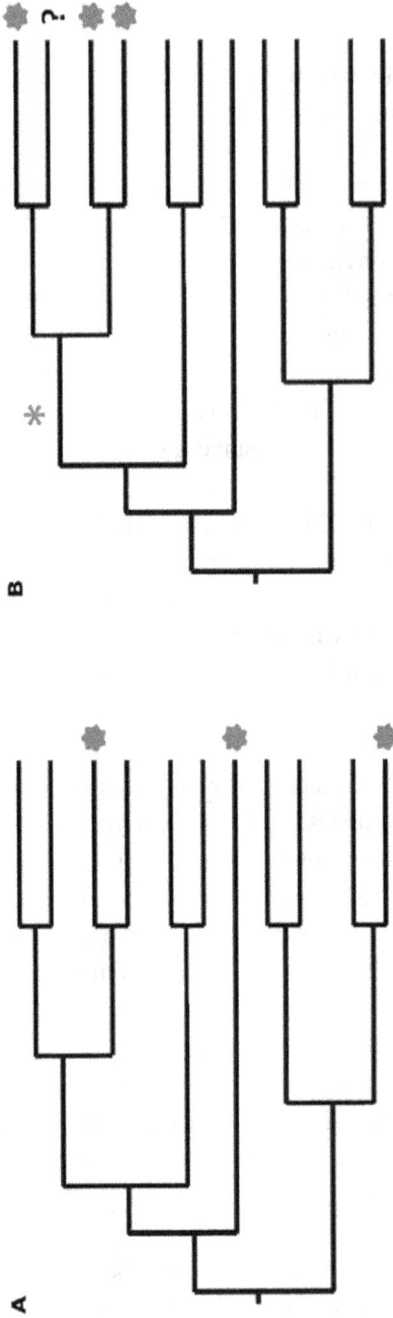

FIGURE 2: Two different scenarios for the distribution of medicinal uses on a hypothetical phylogeny. In both cases there are three medicinal taxa, designated at the tips of the tree. A: There is no significant phylogenetic signal as the taxa are overdispersed. B: The phylogenetic signal is strong as three of the four closely related species are used and the node indicated with "*" shows significant overabundance in medicinal species. In the first case phylogeny cannot act as a guide for discovery of medicinal species. In the second case the species marked with "?" potentially shares medicinal properties with its close relatives.

12.3 RESULTS

12.3.1 ETHNOMEDICINAL REVIEW

Medicinal properties found in the literature for *Pterocarpus* species are shown in Table S1. Nineteen taxa are found with some medicinal applications and the species with the greatest numbers of reported uses are the African *P. erinaceus* (65), *P. angolensis* (56), *P. soyauxii* (37) and the Indomalayan *P. santalinus* (43) and *P. indicus* (32). As shown in Figure 3, *Pterocarpus* species are mainly used for Gastro-intestinal and Skin problems but they also have wide applications for Genito-urinary/Fertility and Respiratory conditions. Anti-inflammatory and poison remedies are the least common. The usage patterns of *Pterocarpus* species are fairly similar across all three regions (Neotropics, Tropical Africa and Indomalaya) of the pantropical range of the genus. For example, Gastro-intestinal and Skin remedies are consistently the most common, while Inflammation Nervous and Pain treatments are the least common in all three regions (Figure 4). One of the most profound differences between the three regions is the heavy use of neotropical taxa to treat Infections/Fever and their low contribution to Genito-urinary treatments, one of the most common uses in tropical Africa and Indomalaya.

12.3.2 PHYLOGENETIC ANALYSES

The matrix included 75 taxa, 68 of which were *Pterocarpus* taxa and seven were closely related genera. The total length of the aligned matrix was 3,592 bp. Phylogenetic reconstruction analysis with RAxML produced the phylogenetic tree shown in Figure 5. *Pterocarpus acapulcensis*, weakly resolved with the outgroup monospecific genus Maraniona, is placed in a sister relationship with the rest of the genus. The rest of the genus is divided into two large clades, one comprising the species complex *P. rohrii* and the rest of the neotropical taxa (BP 100) and the other including all African and Indomalayan taxa (BP 93), the latter nested within the African grade (Figure 5). Several species are not recovered as monophyletic, although most without strong support, except for *P. rohrii*.

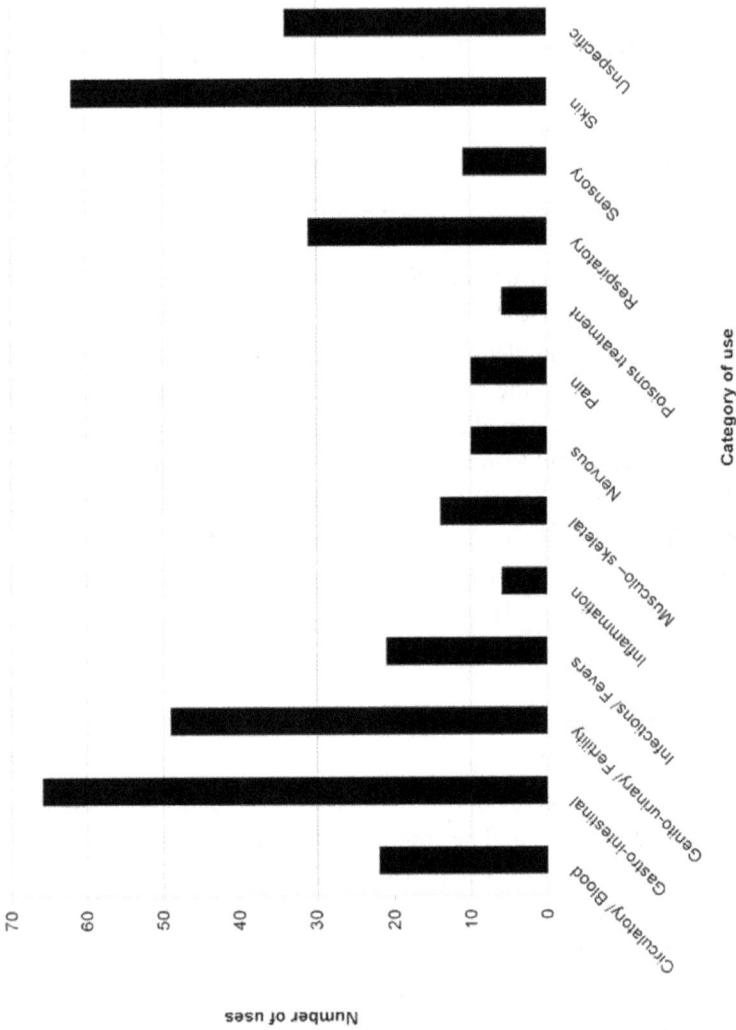

FIGURE 3: Number of uses per category of use for *Pterocarpus* species.

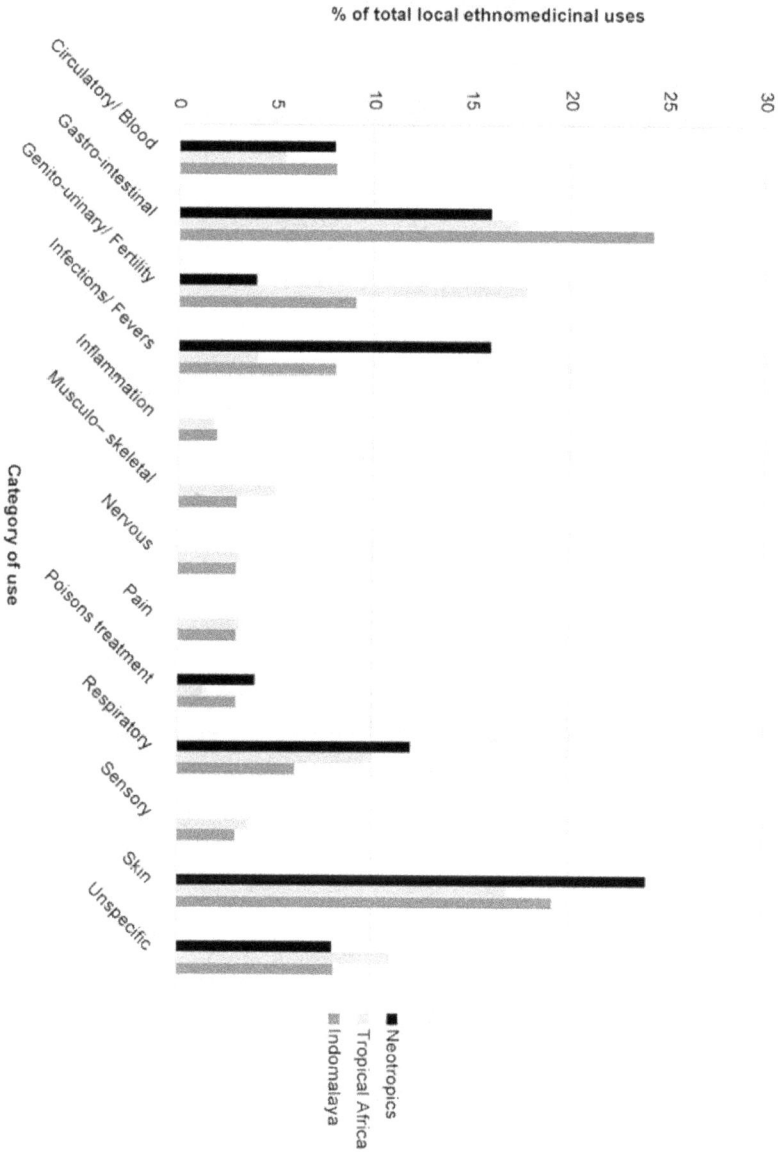

FIGURE 4: Relative usage per category of use for *Pterocarpus* in the Neotropics, Tropical Africa and Indomalaya.

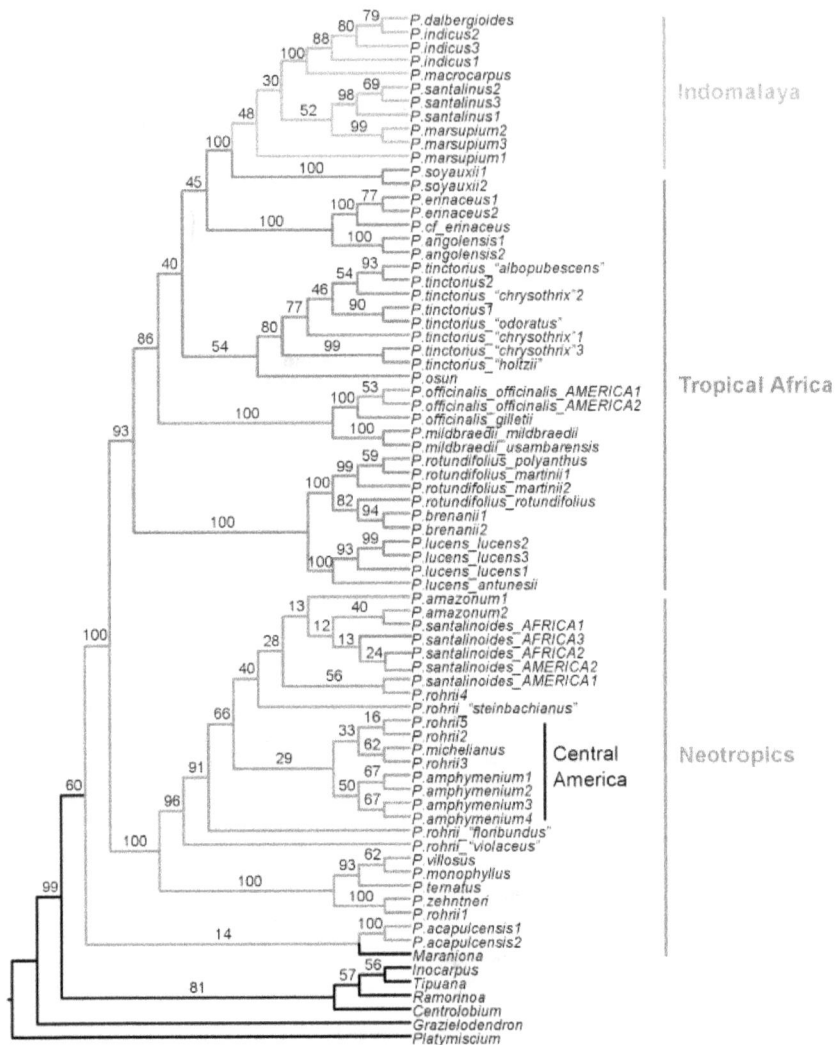

FIGURE 5. ML phylogenetic tree of *Pterocarpus* species and allies. The tree was reconstructed with RAxML and using all DNA markers (nrITS2, *rbcL*, *matK*, trnL and *ndhF-rpL32*). Numbers above branches show bootstrap percentages (BP). Distributions of the main clades are on the right.

12.3.3 PHYLOGENETIC MANIPULATIONS

The assessment of phylogenetic signal, recovered with the "comstruct" tool, is shown in Table 1. Medicinal usage overall was not phylogenetically clumped, meaning that *Pterocarpus* species used medicinally are not found in a certain lineage, but are distributed all over the phylogeny of the genus. However, when the usage was organised in categories we observed some cases of strong phylogenetic signal. The only category of use that showed significant phylogenetic clumping with the MPD was Musculo-skeletal. In contrast, there were six uses (Inflammation, Musculo-Skeletal, Pain, Sensory, Skin and Malaria) that demonstrated significant phylogenetic signal with the MNTD (Table 1).

TABLE 1: Significance (p values) of phylogenetic clumping of medicinal usage of *Pterocarpus* species, assessed with the "comstruct" option in Phylocom v4.1.

Category of use	p value (MPD)	p value (MNTD)
Medicinal uses overall	>0.05	>0.05
Circulatory/Blood	>0.05	>0.05
Gastro-intestinal	>0.05	>0.05
Genito-urinary/Fertility	>0.05	>0.05
Infections/Fevers	>0.05	>0.05
Inflammation	>0.05	**<0.05**
Musculo-skeletal	**<0.05**	**<0.01**
Nervous	>0.05	>0.05
Pain	>0.05	**<0.05**
Poisons treatment	>0.05	>0.05
Respiratory	>0.05	>0.05
Sensory	>0.05	**<0.05**
Skin	>0.05	**<0.05**
Unspecific	>0.05	>0.05
Diabetes	>0.05	>0.05
Malaria	>0.05	**<<0.01**
Cancer	>0.05	>0.05

Numbers in bold indicate cases where significant phylogenetic signal was recovered

The nodes that demonstrated significant overabundance in medicinal species with the "nodesig" command in Phylocom v4.1 for Inflammation, Musculo-Skeletal, Pain, Sensory, Skin and Malaria uses are shown in Table 2. With few exceptions, most of the nodes are located in the clade comprising the African and the Indomalayan species and there is great overlap in the "overabundant" nodes across the uses.

TABLE 2: Nodes recovered as significantly overabundant in medicinal species in the *Pterocarpus* phylogeny, as assessed with the "nodesig" option in Phylocom v4.1.

Category of use	node defined as the MRCA* of
Inflammation	*P.lucens_antunesii-P.dalbergioides*
Inflammation	*P.mildbraedii_usambarensis-P.dalbergioides*
Inflammation	*P.osun-P.dalbergioides*
Inflammation	*P.angolensis2-P.dalbergioides*
Inflammation	*P.angolensis2-P.erinaceus1*
Inflammation	*P.soyauxii2-P.dalbergioides*
Inflammation	*P.marsupium3-P.santalinus2*
Musculo-skeletal	*P.lucens_antunesii-P.dalbergioides*
Musculo-skeletal	*P.mildbraedii_usambarensis-P.dalbergioides*
Musculo-skeletal	*P.osun-P.dalbergioides*
Musculo-skeletal	*P.angolensis2-P.dalbergioides*
Musculo-skeletal	*P.angolensis2-P.erinaceus1*
Musculo-skeletal	*P.soyauxii2-P.dalbergioides*
Musculo-skeletal	*P.marsupium3-P.santalinus2*
Pain	*P.lucens_antunesii-P.dalbergioides*
Pain	*P.mildbraedii_usambarensis-P.dalbergioides*
Pain	*P.osun-P.dalbergioides*
Pain	*P.angolensis2-P.dalbergioides*
Pain	*P.angolensis2-P.erinaceus1*
Pain	*P.soyauxii2-P.dalbergioides*
Pain	*P.marsupium1-P.dalbergioides*
Pain	*P.marsupium3-P.santalinus2*
Sensory	*P.lucens_antunesii-P.dalbergioides*
Sensory	*P.mildbraedii_usambarensis-P.dalbergioides*
Sensory	*P.osun-P.dalbergioides*
Sensory	*P.oson-P.tinctorius_"albopubescens"*

TABLE 2: *Cont.*

Category of use	node defined as the MRCA* of
Sensory	*P.tinctorius_"holtzii"-P.tinctorius_"albopubescens"*
Sensory	*P.angolensis2-P.dalbergioides*
Sensory	*P.angolensis2-P.erinaceus1*
Sensory	*P.marsupium1-P.dalbergioides*
Sensory	*P.marsupium3-P.santalinus2*
Skin	*P.mildbraedii_usambarensis-P.dalbergioides*
Skin	*P.osun-P.dalbergioides*
Skin	*P.osun-P.tinctorius_"albopubescens"*
Skin	*P.tinctorius_"holtzii"-P.tinctorius_"albopubescens"*
Skin	*P.angolensis2-P.dalbergioides*
Malaria	*P.osun-P.dalbergioides*
Malaria	*P.angolensis2-P.dalbergioides*
Malaria	*P.angolensis2-P.erinaceus1*
Malaria	*P.marsupium3-P.dalbergioides*
Malaria	*P.macrocarpus-P.dalbergioides*
Malaria	*P.indicus1-P.dalbergioides*
Malaria	*P.rohrii_"steinbachianus"-P.amazonum1*
Malaria	*P.rohrii4-P.amazonum2*

*Most Recent Common Ancestor

12.4 DISCUSSION

In this study we produced an ethnomedicinal review for the genus *Pterocarpus* (Table S1) and reconstructed the relationships between all *Pterocarpus* species, presenting a well supported molecular multi-locus phylogeny for the genus (Figure 5). Using these tools, we assess the proposed application of phylogenetics to bioscreening and ethnobotany [12], [13], [14], [15] and devise meaningful tools that can predict the phylogenetic position of species with high medicinal potential. Some of the phylogenetic relationships recovered here have been hypothesised based on morphological affinities, adding support to our results. These include the proximity between *Pterocarpus mildbraedii* and *P. officinalis, P. amazonum* and *P. santalinoides*, *P. brenanii* and *P. rotundifolius* [52], *P. monopyllus* and *P. ternatus* [61] and between the five Indomalayan species [52]. As mentioned above it has, however, long been suspected that several *Ptero-carpus* species are paraphyletic - e.g. the Neotropical species *Pterocarpus rohrii* of which the samples included in this study are found in scattered position across the Neotropical clade. Recognising the necessity for well-circumscribed taxonomic entities in useful plants groups, one of us (BBK) is currently undertaking a taxonomic revision of *Pterocarpus*.

In terms of ethnomedicinal uses, our results from an extensive litera-ture review indicate that *Pterocarpus* is a very valuable genus in tradition-al medicine, as almost two thirds of the taxa are used throughout the range of the genus and for multiple uses. Although we found usage under several of the categories suggested by [56], *Pterocarpus* species are mainly used for Gastro-intestinal and Skin afflictions but they also have wide appli-cations for Genito-urinary/fertility and respiratory conditions, as shown in Figure 3. The well supported phylogeny of all species in *Pterocarpus*, along with its richness in medicinal uses, provided a suitable model to test phylogenetic patterns in medicinal properties and allowed us to perform explicit phylogenetic tests.

We detected strong phylogenetic signal in medicinal usage in several cases, indicating that medicinal properties in the genus are not distributed evenly across the phylogeny, but are rather clumped, as was suggested in previous studies of other groups at different hierarchical levels (genus [13], [14] and flora [15]). More specifically, usage for inflammations, musculo-skeletal afflictions, pain, sensory and skin problems, as well as malaria, demonstrated significant clumping on the phylogeny (Table 1). Although most of these categories were the ones with few uses, they also include uses for skin problems, the second most commonly encountered category (Figure 3). As shown in Table 1, phylogenetic signal was recov-ered mainly using the MNTD and not the MPD, where significant signal was found for one category of use only. These two values both measure phylogenetic clumping, however at different hierarchical levels. With the MPD measure, one can detect phylogenetic signal in deep nodes of the phylogeny, whereas with the MNTD clumping is measured towards the tips of the phylogenetic tree [94]. In advising bioscreening schemes, one would like to narrow down selection of putatively useful species to a small number. Therefore, indentifying clumping in deeper nodes of the phylogeny is probably not useful, as deep nodes define clades with numerous species, which means informed and well-defined decisions cannot be made for bioscreening. Thus, clumping toward the tips of the phylogeny (MNTD) is more relevant to bioscreening.

It has been proposed that cross-cultural agreement in plant usage implies bioactivity as independent discovery in disparate cultures should have an empirical basis [9], [95], [96], [97], [98]. Even without taking phylogenetic relationships into account, a degree of agreement among different ethnomedicinal systems is evident. Figure 4 shows that *Pterocarpus* species are used to treat similar conditions in the Neotropics, Tropical Africa and Indomalaya. Given the geographical distance of these three regions and the disparate cultures found there, it is very likely that this parallel usage is the product of independent discoveries, which demonstrates the efficiency of local cultures in identifying plants with relatively similar chemical profiles (the three biogeographical clades within *Pterocarpus*) to treat similar conditions. Undoubtedly, cultural exchange has taken place to a certain degree between these regions. For example, uses of Ocimum species have been recorded in Afro-Brazilian communities, attributed to traditional uses in Africa [99]. Although we acknowledge the possibility that common patterns might be due to cultural exchange, given the large geographic scale of this study, we believe such cases are the exception, rather than the rule. However, we recognise that common ethnobotanical trends, even when independent, might not be the result of underlying bioefficacy in every case. Plant use is often guided by a "doctrine of signatures", the belief that a plant possess medicinal properties due the presence of physical attributes (colour, scent, shape) [100], [101]. The yellow flowers and red sap found in *Pterocarpus* species could be a reason of their applications in urinary and blood disorders. Nevertheless, despite all these possible alternative explanations as to how cross-cultural ethnobotanical patterns arise, we show that phylogenetic interpretation of such patterns allows us to address traditional questions in ethnobotany from novel perspectives.

The two amphiatlantic species (*P. officinalis* and *P. santalinoides*) provide an excellent system to study the use of the same species in notably different medicinal systems, in the light of phylogeny and biogeography.

As Figure 5 shows, *P. officinalis* dispersed from West Africa to the Neo-tropics, as the neotropical subspecies (*P. officinalis* subsp. *officinalis*) is nested in an African clade, while *P. santalinoides* dispersed from the Neo-tropics to West Africa, as the African samples are nested in the neotropical clade. Interestingly, both taxa have more uses in the "new" regions than in their regions of origin and we attribute this pattern to phylogenetic struc-ture. We recorded no uses for *P. officinalis* in Africa and six uses in the Neotropics. Similarly, we found one use for *P. santalinoides* in the Neo-tropics and 22 in Africa. These species, by having no close relatives in the new regions, contribute novel phylogenetic diversity, and hence possibly novel medicinal properties, to these areas. On the contrary, in the region of origin, close relatives with similar phytochemical profiles are available. For example, *P. santalinoides* is used for malaria in West Africa, but not in the Neotropics, where its close relatives *P. amazonum* and *P. rohrii* are used (Table S1). Similarly, *P. officinalis* is used in the Neotropics as an as-tringent, however that use is replaced in Africa, where it is very narrowly distributed, by *P. angolensis* and *P. erinaceus*, the latter being sympatric to *P. officinalis*. Moreover, we found common amphiatlantic use for *P. santa-linoides* as a poison antidote. Such agreement in use has been found to be strongly linked to pharmacological activities at this taxonomic level [97].

Just as knowledge of phylogeny informs the interpretation of ethnobo-tanical use at the species level, confidence in inferences of bioactivity is increased when clades sharing specific ethnomedicinal uses are distributed across regions. For example, Figure 6 shows that the larger of the clades showing use in treating malaria and musculo-skeletal disorders is distrib-uted in Tropical Africa and Indomalaya. As we discuss below, clades which encompass many species for a specific use can become targets for future screening. When these clades are distributed across regions, it seems more probable that selection for ethnomedicinal use reflects underlying activity, and not a preference within a culture for using species which might share particular attributes such as similar overall morphology, because of shared ancestry.

Regarding ethnopharmacology and bioscreening, there are three ways in which our results can be of use. First, as proposed in earlier investiga-tions, close relatives of species with known bioactivity can be prioritised for screening for similar activity [12], [13]. For example, the species *P.*

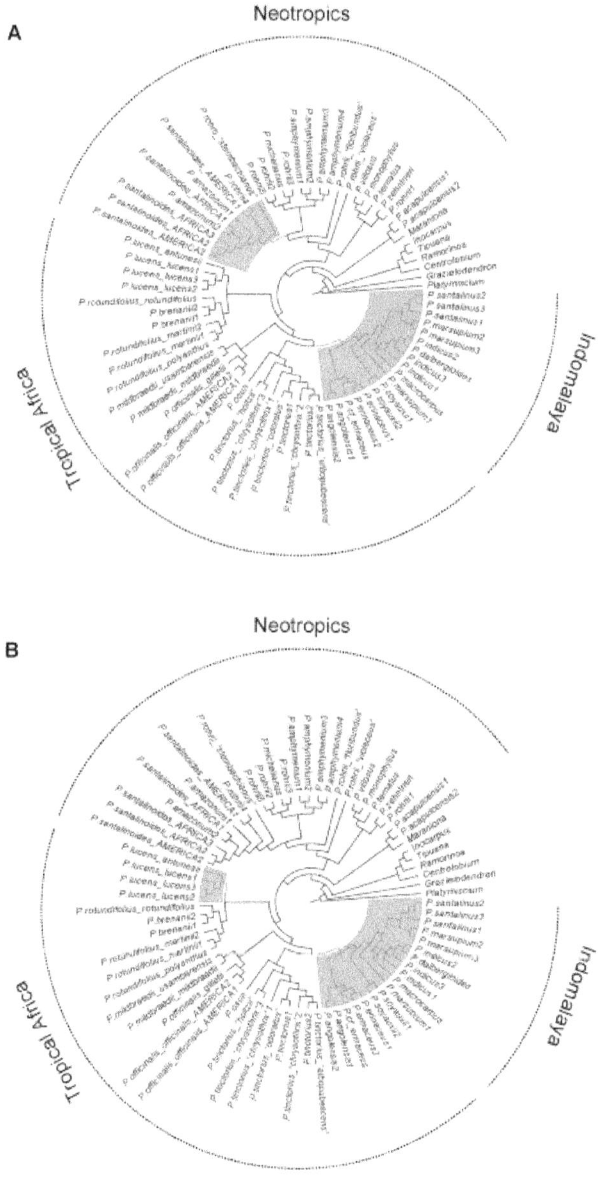

FIGURE 6: Phylogeny of *Pterocarpus* with clades that show significant overabundance in medicinal species highlighted. Results were recovered using the "nodesig" option in Phylocom v 4.1. A: species to treat malaria. B: species to treat musculo-skeletal conditions. Although some clades are used for a variety of conditions, different properties are found in different parts of the phylogeny.

santalinus and *P. marsupium* are very well known species in traditional medicine, especially for their use to treat diabetes [102], [103], [104], [105]. Both species have been studied *in vitro* and have shown notable hypoglycaemic bioactivity [87], [88], [90], [91], [92], [93]. However, *P. santalinus* is listed as endangered and *P. marsupium* as vulnerable on the IUCN Red List [55] and the former is also included in CITES Annex II, therefore their use in medicine is not recommended as overharvesting could pose further threat to their survival. *Pterocarpus dalbergioides*, a stenoendemic of the Andaman Islands, has been shown to possess similar bioactivity [89], however its narrow range would not support sustainable harvesting either. Although the use for diabetes does not demonstrate significant phylogenetic structure on the phylogeny (Table 1), these results suggest that hypoglycaemic bioactivity is shared by all species in the clade defined by the MRCA of *P.marsupium1-P.dalbergioides*, which includes *P. macrocarpus* and *P. indicus* that are widespread in Southeast Asia [52]. We propose that these widespread species be investigated for hypoglycaemic bioactivity to investigate whether they can substitute the use of the more endangered relatives. Should these species prove to share this bioactivity as we predict here, their application will not only provide new medicinal species, but will also assist the conservation of the more restricted and endangered species that are currently used.

Second, in the case of absence of pharmacological data, phylogenetic signal can provide indirect evidence of underlying bioactivity. If closely related species share similar ethnomedicinal properties (which can be interpreted as a case of phylogenetic conservatism [10], [11]), it is very likely that this reflects the underlying bioactivity of these species. For example, the clade comprising species from Africa and Indomalaya is the richest in medicinal properties. The species with the highest numbers of uses, namely *P. erinaceus* (65), *P. angolensis* (56), *P. santalinus* (43), *P. soyauxii* (37) and *P. indicus* (32) are all included in the clade defined by the MRCA of *P.angolensis2-P.dalbergioides* (Figure 5) that is often recovered among the nodes that show significant phylogenetic overabundance for different uses (Table 2). These species and their close relatives are therefore considered to be of high potential for bioprospecting. What is particularly interesting in this clade is that it is distributed in two large biogeographic regions, where very different human cultures are found and it is relatively safe to assume that any common ethnobotanical patterns observed in the two regions were discovered independently and are not due to shared cultural history. Therefore, not only does this clade demonstrate phylogenetic conservatism [10], [11] in medicinal usage, but it also demonstrates cross-cultural agreement in usage (Figure 4 and 6), which has been used as a criterion to imply bioactivity [9], [95], [106], [107]. These two criteria provide multiple lines of evidence pointing towards the bioactivity in this clade, especially for the conditions where significant clumping was observed (inflammations, musculo-skeletal afflictions, pain, sensory and skin problems, as well as malaria; Table 1).

Third, a more sophisticated approach is to identify nodes on the phylogeny that have high potential for bioscreening. We demonstrated that with the tool "nodesig" in Phylocom the exact phylogenetic position of overabundance in medicinal properties can be recovered. For example, several *Pterocarpus* species are being used to treat malaria (Table S1) and our results show that the species used in such applications are significantly clumped on the phylogeny (Table 1), suggesting that phylogenetic proximity is a good proxy for antiplasmodial bioactivity. We can subsequently identify the nodes that are significantly overabundant in "antimalarial" species. These are given in Table 2 and also shown highlighted in Figure 6. As shown, there are two positions in the phylogeny that are overabundant in species with antimalarial activity and they cover all three regions of the range of the genus, again showing both phylogenetic conservatism and cross-cultural usage as evidence for bioactivity.

The first clade is a neotropical clade that includes *P. amazonum*, some *P. rohrii* samples and *P. santalinoides*, the last also found in West Africa. All three species are reported with demonstrable *in vitro* use against malaria [83], [84], [86]. The bioactivity for the amphiatlantic *P. santalinoides* was demonstrated for West African material [84], however as we show here, South American material is extremely likely to share these properties as it falls within this clade and we propose it be further investigated. *Pterocarpus rohrii* is an extremely variable and widespread species, found throughout South and Central America. The results from this study, which has sampled material across the species range, reveal the polyphyly of this species and show that phylogenetic units within the species show geographic structure (Figure 5) suggesting that its taxonomy should be revised. The samples in this "antimalarial" clade are from South America and bioactivity has been demonstrated for South American material only [83]. Based on our results, material of *P. rohrii* from this clade is more valuable as antimalarial, as the other lineages of *P. rohrii* are not recovered significantly overabundant in antimalarial use. Although it is not unlikely that this species possesses bioactivity throughout its range, but it is simply not used across its range due to differences in ethnomedicinal floras in different cultures, it is also possible that antimalarial activity is present in this clade only. Further research in this species on material from different localities is needed to establish whether antimalarial properties are present across its range. Nonetheless, the combination of traditional knowledge and phylogenetic information has already brought to light cryptic diversity demonstrating to be a valid approach to elucidating taxonomy [108] and we believe that such information could be incorporated in a taxonomic revision of *P. rohrii*, as it could clarify which taxonomic units are more valuable in ethnomedicine.

The second antimalarial clade includes all species defined by the MRCA of *P. osun* and *P. dalbergioides* (Table 2). Nevertheless, the only species in this clade that have reported antimalarial uses are *P. angolensis*, *P. erinaceus* (also *in vitro*), *P. indicus* and *P. macrocarpus*. This renders all other species in the clade, namely *P. dalbergioides*, *P. marsupium*, *P. osun*, *P. santalinus*, *P. soyauxii*, *P. tessmanii* and *P. tinctorius* very good candidates for antiplasmodial activity. Out of these, of particular interest are *P. soyauxii* and *P. tinctorius*, as they are widespread in Africa, material availability will be greater and no harvesting pressure will be posed to narrowly distributed or endangered species. The phylogenetic position of the former, which is closely related to *P. angolensis*, *P. erinaceus*, as well as to *P. indicus* and *P. macrocarpus* (Figure 5) makes it a better candidate. Furthermore, we predict that *P. angolensis*, already used traditionally as an antimalarial, will very likely share the *in vitro* activity of its sister species *P. erinaceus*.

12.5 CONCLUSIONS

This, to the best of our knowledge, is the first multidisciplinary study that draws on four different sources (using taxonomic, phylogenetic, biogeographic and ethnobotanical information) to provide new perspectives on bioactivity in plants, based on the criteria of cross-cultural usage and phylogenetic conservatism across different biogeographic regions. Our study demonstrates that phylogeny and biogeography can be used as novel tools in ethnobotany to interpret processes that shape traditional usage and particularly cross-cultural patterns and our community phylogenetic approach demonstrates that similar ethnobotanical uses can arise in parallel in different areas when related plants are available there.The advent of molecular phylogenetics heralded a much deeper understanding of organismal relationships. Phylogenetic tools entered several disciplines to provide explanatory power and recover patterns previously undetected. Molecular data are becoming increasingly available in recent years, especially with the rapid development of next-generation sequencing techniques. At the same time, ethnomedicinal and ethnopharmacological information has also been accumulating over the last decades, providing invaluable insight into the use of nature by humans in traditional medicine. We demonstrated here that the combination of information from these fields using quantitative metrics is particularly meaningful and opens up new opportunities for further biological studies through its potential to direct bioscreening studies, but also enables insights into processes that shape ethnobotanical knowledge. With molecular and ethnomedicinal data publicly available and readily accessible, the potential for them to be combined and reanalysed reciprocally is immense.

These approaches could be developed even further than in this study. For example, ethnomedicinal metrics of confidence in plant use (relative cultural importance index [109], or informant consensus [98]) can be mapped on phylogeny to provide even greater explanatory power. The methods proposed here can be applied to other organisms, at different hierarchical levels (family, infraspecific [110], [111]), sample regions and also for other properties, such as the search for new food plants [112], plants with economical potential [15], or new chemical compounds for medicine or pesticides [25], [26], [27], [113]. Future analyses can include ecological data that can predict in a phylogenetic context which areas harbour medicinal species diversity (medicinal hotspots). Phytochemical and ethnomedicinal data can be combined on phylogenies to test how well they can provide reciprocal illumination. Furthermore, similar studies can further our understanding of cultural processes that shape ethnobotanical knowledge, as phylogenetic similarity can be added as an extra parameter in cross-cultural comparisons of ethnomedicinal systems in order to provide greater insight into usage in different cultures.

Although ethnobotanically directed screening was proposed as a promising way of enhancing rates of bioprospecting schemes and several studies have shown that can lead to more positive hits compared to random sampling [3], [114], there are several reasons why these approaches are not likely to lead directly to new pharmaceutical drugs [115]. However, our study can serve as an example of how understanding patterns of successful traditional medicine can help promote local economic development through trade [116] appreciation of traditional medicine by the scientific community [117] and, most importantly, enhance local community health [118]. We would like to conclude with a reflection upon the ethical questions that arise where phylogenetic ethnobotany results in recovering successful traditional medicines. International legal frameworks, such as the one established by the Convention of Biological Diversity, safeguard the intellectual property of cultures and individuals with specialist knowledge. Profitable results from any such investigations should not only be profitable for both parts (investigators and people with knowledge), but must also focus on alleviating those people's livelihoods and enhance their healthcare [119]. A mechanism of benefit sharing is needed for cases where new medicinal plant discoveries that are not traditionally used in some culture but are based on traditional knowledge of species that are closely related to them.

REFERENCES

1.	Farnsworth NR, Soejarto DD (1991) Global importance of medicinal plants. In: Akerele O, Heywood V, Synge H, editors. The Conservation of Medicinal Plants. Cambridge: Cambridge University Press. pp. 25–52.
2.	Clarkson C, Maharaj VJ, Crouch NR, Grace OM, Pillay P, et al. (2004) *In vitro* antiplasmodial activity of medicinal plants native to or naturalised in South Africa. Journal of Ethnopharmacology 92: 177–191. doi: 10.1016/j.jep.2004.02.011.

3. Fabricant DS, Farnsworth NR (2001) The value of plants used in traditional medicine for drug discovery. Environmental Health Perspectives 109: 69–75. doi: 10.2307/3434847.

4. Wright CI, Van-Buren L, Kroner CI, Koning MMG (2007) Herbal medicines as diuretics: A review of the scientific evidence. Journal of Ethnopharmacology 114: 1–31. doi: 10.1016/j.jep.2007.07.023.

5. Amiguet VT, Arnason JT, Maquin P, Cal V, Sanchez-Vindas P, et al. (2006) A regression analysis of q'eqchi' Maya medicinal plants from southern Belize. Economic Botany 60: 24–38. doi: 10.1016/j.bse.2007.12.010.

6. Bennett BC, Husby CE (2008) Patterns of medicinal plant use: An examination of the Ecuadorian Shuar medicinal flora using contingency table and binomial analyses. Journal of Ethnopharmacology 116: 422–430. doi: 10.1016/j.jep.2007.12.006.

7. Douwes E, Crouch NR, Edwards TJ, Mulholland DA (2008) Regression analyses of southern African ethnomedicinal plants: informing the targeted selection of bioprospecting and pharmacological screening subjects. Journal of Ethnopharmacology 119: 356–364. doi: 10.1016/j.jep.2008.07.040.

8. Moerman DE (1991) The medicinal flora of native North-America - an analysis. Journal of Ethnopharmacology 31: 1–42. doi: 10.1016/0378-8741(91)90141-Y.

9. Saslis-Lagoudakis CH, Williamson EM, Savolainen V, Hawkins JA (2011) Cross-cultural comparison of three medicinal floras and implications for bioprospecting strategies. Journal of Ethnopharmacology 135: 476–487. doi: 10.1016/j.jep.2011.03.044.

10. Crisp MD, Arroyo MTK, Cook LG, Gandolfo MA, Jordan GJ, et al. (2009) Phylogenetic biome conservatism on a global scale. Nature 458: 754–756. doi: 10.1038/nature07764.

11. Prinzing A, Durka W, Klotz S, Brand R (2001) The niche of higher plants: evidence for phylogenetic conservatism. Proceedings of the Royal Society of London Series B: Biological Sciences 268: 2383–2389. doi: 10.1098/rspb.2001.1801.

12. Paton AJ, Springate D, Suddee S, Otieno D, Grayer RJ, et al. (2004) Phylogeny and evolution of basils and allies (Ocimeae, Labiatae) based on three plastid DNA regions. Molecular Phylogenetics and Evolution 31: 277–299. doi: 10.1016/j.ympev.2003.08.002.

13. Rønsted N, Savolainen V, Mølgaard P, Jager AK (2008) Phylogenetic selection of Narcissus species for drug discovery. Biochemical Systematics and Ecology 36: 417–422. doi: 10.1016/j.bse.2007.12.010.

14. Lukhoba CW, Simmonds MSJ, Paton AJ (2006) *Plectranthus*: A review of ethnobotanical uses. Journal of Ethnopharmacology 103: 1–24. doi: 10.1016/j.jep.2005.09.011.

15. Forest F, Grenyer R, Rouget M, Davies TJ, Cowling RM, et al. (2007) Preserving the evolutionary potential of floras in biodiversity hotspots. Nature 445: 757–760. doi: 10.1038/nature05587.

16. Fairbrothers DE, Mabry TJ, Scogin RL, Turner BL (1975) Bases of Angiosperm Phylogeny - Chemotaxonomy. Annals of the Missouri Botanical Garden 62: 765–800. doi: 10.2307/2395273.

17. Gibbs R (1974) Chemotaxonomy of flowering plants. Montreal and London: McGill-Queen's University Press.

18. Harborne J, Turner B (1984) Plant chemosystematics. London: Academic Press. 562 p.

19. Reynolds T (2007) The evolution of chemosystematics. Phytochemistry 68: 2887–2895. doi: 10.1016/j.phytochem.2007.06.027.

20. Harborne JB (1970) Phytochemical Phylogeny. London and New York Academic Press.

21. Bisby FA, Vaughan JG, Wright CA (1980) Chemosystematics: Principles and Practice. London: Academic Press.

22. Wink M (2003) Evolution of secondary metabolites from an ecological and molecular phylogenetic perspective. Phytochemistry 64: 3–19. doi: 10.1016/S0031-9422(03)00300-5.

23. Wink M, Mohamed GIA (2003) Evolution of chemical defense traits in the Leguminosae: mapping of distribution patterns of secondary metabolites on a molecular phylogeny inferred from nucleotide sequences of the *rbcL* gene. Biochemical Systematics and Ecology 31: 897–917. doi: 10.1007/bf02858750.

24. Muellner AN, Samuel R, Chase MW, Pannell CM, Greger H (2005) Aglaia (Meliaceae): An evaluation of taxonomic concepts based on DNA data and secondary metabolites. American Journal of Botany 92: 534–543. doi: 10.3732/ajb.92.3.534.

25. Larsen MM, Adsersen A, Davis AP, Lledó MD, Jäger AK, et al. (2010) Using a phylogenetic approach to selection of target plants in drug discovery of acetylcholinesterase inhibiting alkaloids in Amaryllidaceae tribe Galantheae. Biochemical Systematics and Ecology 38: 1026–1034. doi: 10.1016/j.bse.2010.10.005.

26. Pacharawongsakda E, Yokwai S, Ingsriswang S (2009) Potential natural product discovery from microbes through a diversity-guided computational framework. Applied Microbiology and Biotechnology 82: 579–586. doi: 10.1007/s00253-008-1847-x.

27. Bay-Smidt MGK, Jäger AK, Krydsfeldt K, Meerow AW, Stafford GI, et al. (2011) Phylogenetic selection of target species in Amaryllidaceae tribe Haemantheae for acetylcholinesterase inhibition and affinity to the serotonin reuptake transport protein. South African Journal of Botany 77: 175–183.

28. Soejarto DD, Fong HHS, Tan GT, Zhang HJ, Ma CY, et al. (2005) Ethnobotany/ethnopharmacology and mass bioprospecting: Issues on intellectual property and benefit-sharing. Journal of Ethnopharmacology 100: 15–22. doi: 10.1016/j.jep.2005.05.031.

29. Donoghue MJ (2008) A phylogenetic perspective on the distribution of plant diversity. Proceedings of the National Academy of Sciences 105: 11549–11555. doi: 10.1111/j.1523-1739.1987.tb00050.x.

30. Sanmartin I, Ronquist F (2004) Southern hemisphere biogeography inferred by event-based models: Plant versus animal patterns. Systematic Biology 53: 216–243. doi: 10.1080/10635150490423430.

31. Webb CO (2000) Exploring the phylogenetic structure of ecological communities: An example for rain forest trees. The American Naturalist 156: 145–155.

32. Strauss SY, Webb CO, Salamin N (2006) Exotic taxa less related to native species are more invasive. Proceedings of the National Academy of Sciences 103: 5841–5845. doi: 10.1073/pnas.0508073103.

33. Pennington RT, Richardson JE, Lavin M (2006) Insights into the historical construction of species-rich biomes from dated plant phylogenies, neutral ecological theory and phylogenetic community structure. New Phytologist 172: 605–616. doi: 10.1111/j.1469-8137.2006.01902.x.

34. Arthur W (2002) The emerging conceptual framework of evolutionary developmental biology. Nature 415: 757–764. doi: 10.1038/415757a.

35. Rambaut A, Robertson DL, Pybus OG, Peeters M, Holmes EC (2001) Human immunodeficiency virus: Phylogeny and the origin of HIV-1. Nature 410: 1047–1048. doi: 10.1038/35074179.

36. Purvis A, Gittleman JL, Cowlishaw G, Mace GM (2000) Predicting extinction risk in declining species. Proceedings of the Royal Society of London Series B: Biological Sciences 267: 1947–1952. doi: 10.1663/0013-0001(2003)057[0218:mfotpm]2.0.co;2.

37. Crandall KA, Bininda-Emonds ORP, Mace GM, Wayne RK (2000) Considering evolutionary processes in conservation biology. Trends in ecology & evolution 15: 290–295. doi: 10.1111/j.1523-1739.1987.tb00050.x.

38. Hollingsworth PM, Forrest LL, Spouge JL, Hajibabaei M, Ratnasingham S, et al. (2009) A DNA barcode for land plants. Proceedings of the National Academy of Sciences 106: 12794–12797.

39. Kress WJ, Erickson DL, Jones FA, Swenson NG, Perez R, et al. (2009) Plant DNA barcodes and a community phylogeny of a tropical forest dynamics plot in Panama. Proceedings of the National Academy of Sciences 106: 18621–18626.

40. Lahaye R, van der Bank M, Bogarin D, Warner J, Pupulin F, et al. (2008) DNA barcoding the floras of biodiversity hotspots. Proceedings of the National Academy of Sciences 105: 2923–2928. doi: 10.1016/j.bse.2007.12.010.

41. Chen S, Yao H, Han J, Liu C, Song J, et al. (2010) Validation of the ITS2 region as a novel DNA barcode for identifying medicinal plant species. PLoS ONE 5: e8613. doi: 10.1371/journal.pone.0008613.

42. Leonti M, Ramirez R F, Sticher O, Heinrich M (2003) Medicinal flora of the Popoluca, Mexico: A botanical systematical perspective. Economic Botany 57: 218–230. doi: 10.1663/0013-0001(2003)057[0218:mfotpm]2.0.co;2.

43. Moerman DE, Pemberton RW, Kiefer D, Berlin B (1999) A comparative analysis of five medicinal floras. Journal of Ethnobiology 19: 49–67. doi: 10.1109/tau.1967.1161901.

44. Bletter N (2000) Cross-cultural Phylogenetic Medical Ethnobotany 41st Annual Meeting of the Society for Economic Botany. Colombia, South Carolina, USA.

45. Specht CD (1996) Ethnocladistics: using cladistics to analyze ethnobotanical data. London, UK. Joint meeting of the Society of Economic Botany and the International Society for Ethnopharmacology.

46. Specht CD (1997) Ethnocladistics: A predictive analysis of medicinal properties of plant families based on the ethnopharmacopoeia of the Chacobo, Beni, Bolivia. Meetings of the International Society for Ethnobotany. London, UK.

47. Harms H (1915) Die Pflanzenwelt Afrikas. In: Engler A, editor. Die Vegetation der Erde. 598 p.

48. Bentham G (1860) A synopsis of the Dalbergieae, a tribe of the Leguminosae. Journal of the Proceedings of The Linnean Society IV: 1–134. doi: 10.1111/j.1095-8339.1860.tb02464.x.

49. de Candolle AP (1825) Memoires sur la famille des Legumineuses. Paris: A. Belin.

50. Taubert P (1894) Leguminosae. In: Engler A, Prantl K, editors. Die natürlichen Pflanzenfamilien Leipzig: Engelmann. pp. 70–396.

51. Baker EG (1929) The Leguminosae of tropical Africa. Ostend.

52. Rojo JP (1972) *Pterocarpus* (Leguminosae - Papilionaceae) revised for the world. Lehre, Germany: Verlag Von J. Cramer.

53. Lewis GP (1987) Legumes of Bahia. UK: Royal Botanic Gardens Kew.

54. Klitgaard BB, Lavin M Lewis GP, Schrire B, MacKinder B, Lock M, editors. (2005) Dalbergieae.Legumes of the world. Legumes of the world 307 - 335: UK: Royal Botanic Gardens Kew. doi: 10.1109/tsp.2003.814460.

55. IUCN (2009) IUCN Red List of Threatened Species. Version 2009.2 (www.iucnredlist.org).

56. Cook FEM (1995) Economic Botany Data Collection Standard. International Working Group on Taxonomic Databases for Plant Sciences (TDWG). London: Royal Botanic Gardens, Kew.

57. Lock JM (1999) A change in status for a southern African *Pterocarpus* (Leguminosae: Papilionoideae). Kew Bulletin 54: 208.

58. Mendonça FA, Sousa EP (1968) New and little known species from the flora Zambesiaca area XXI : notes on the genera Lonchocarpus, *Pterocarpus* and Xeroderris Boletim da Sociedade Broteriana 42: 269–270. doi: 10.1600/036364409788606262.

59. Polhill RM (1969) Notes on East African Dalbergieae Bronn (Leguminosae). Kew Bulletin 23: 483–490. doi: 10.2307/4117194.

60. Zamora N (2000) Nuevas especies y combinaciones en Leguminosas de Mesoamerica. Novon 10: 175–180. doi: 10.2307/2399976.

61. Klitgaard BB, de Queiroz LP, Lewis GP (2000) A remarkable new species of *Pterocarpus* (Leguminosae: Papilionoideae: Dalbergieae) from Bahia, Brazil. Kew Bulletin 55: 989–992. doi: 10.3109/13880209109082866.

62. Hughes CE, Lewis GP, Daza Yomona A, Reynel C (2004) Maraniona. A new dalbergioid legume genus (Leguminosae, Papilionoideae) from Peru. Systematic Botany 29: 366–374. doi: 10.1098/rspb.2001.1801.

63. Lavin M, Pennington RT, Klitgaard BB, Sprent JI, de Lima HC, et al. (2001) The dalbergioid legumes (Fabaceae): delimitation of a pantropical monophyletic clade. American Journal of Botany 88: 503–533. doi: 10.2307/2657116.

64. Pirie MD, Klitgaard BB, Pennington RT (2009) Revision and biogeography of Centrolobium (Leguminosae - Papilionoideae). Systematic Botany 34: 345–359. doi: 10.1600/036364409788606262.

65. Saslis-Lagoudakis C, Chase MW, Robinson DN, Russell SJ, Klitgaard BB (2008) Phylogenetics of neotropical Platymiscium (Leguminosae: Dalbergieae): systematics, divergence times, and biogeography inferred from nuclear ribosomal and plastid DNA sequence data. American Journal of Botany 95: 1270–1286. doi: 10.3732/ajb.0800101.

66. Hilu KW, Borsch T, Muller K, Soltis DE, Soltis PS, et al. (2003) Angiosperm phylogeny based on *matK* sequence information. American Journal of Botany 90: 1758–1776. doi: 10.3732/ajb.90.12.1758.

67. Savolainen V, Fay MF, Albach DC, Backlund A, Bank Mvd, et al. (2000) Phylogeny of the Eudicots: A nearly complete familial analysis based on *rbcL* gene sequences. Kew Bulletin 55: 257–309.

68. Wojciechowski MF, Lavin M, Sanderson MJ (2004) A phylogeny of legumes (Leguminosae) based on analysis of the plastid *matK* gene resolves many well-supported subclades within the family. American Journal of Botany 91: 1846–1862. doi: 10.3732/ajb.91.11.1846.

69. Shaw J, Lickey EB, Schilling EE, Small RL (2007) Comparison of whole chloroplast genome sequences to choose noncoding regions for phylogenetic studies in angiosperms: the tortoise and the hare III. American Journal of Botany 94: 275–288. doi: 10.3732/ajb.94.3.275.

70. Ribeiro RAc, Lavin M, Lemos-Filho JP, Filho CVMa, dos Santos FR, et al. (2007) The genus Machaerium (Leguminosae) is more closely related to Aeschynomene Sect. Ochopodium than to Dalbergia: Inferences from combined sequence data. Systematic Botany 32: 762–771.

71. Csiba L, Powell MP (2006) DNA extraction protocols. In: Savolainen V, Powell MP, Davis K, Reeves G, Corthals A, editors. DNA and tissue banking for biodiversity and conservation: theory, practice and uses. Richmond, Surrey, UK: Royal Botanic Gardens, Kew. pp. 114–117.

72. Doyle JJ, Doyle JL (1987) A rapid DNA isolation procedure for small quantities of fresh leaf tissue. Phytochemical Bulletin 19: 11–15. doi: 10.1109/tau.1967.1161901.

73. Sun Y, Skinner DZ, Liang GH, Hulbert SH (1994) Phylogenetic analysis of Sorghum and related taxa using internal transcribed spacers of nuclear ribosomal DNA. Theoretical and Applied Genetics 89: 26–32. doi: 10.3109/13880209109082866.

74. Taberlet P, Gielly L, Pautou G, Bouvet J (1991) Universal primers for amplification of three non-coding regions of chloroplast DNA. Plant Molecular Biology 17: 1105–1109. doi: 10.1007/BF00037152.

75. Ankli A, Sticher O, Heinrich M (1999) Medical ethnobotany of the Yucatec Maya: Healers' consensus as a quantitative criterion. Economic Botany 53: 144–160. doi: 10.3109/13880209109082866.

76. Fay MF, Bayer C, Alverson WS, de Bruijn AY, Chase MW (1998) Plastid *rbcL* sequence data indicate a close affinity between Diegodendron and Bixa. Taxon 47: 43–50. doi: 10.1016/j.bse.2010.10.005.

77. Thompson JD, Higgins DG, Gibson TJ (1994) CLUSTAL W: improving the sensitivity of progressive multiple sequence alignment through sequence weighting, position-specific gap penalties and weight matrix choice. Nucleic Acids Research 22: 4673–4680. doi: 10.1093/nar/22.22.4673.

78. Kelchner SA (2000) The evolution of non-coding chloroplast DNA and its application in plant systematics. Annals of the Missouri Botanical Garden 87: 482–498. doi: 10.1016/j.bse.2010.10.005.

79. Stamatakis A, Hoover P, Rougemont J (2008) A rapid bootstrap algorithm for the RAxML web servers. Systematic Biology 57: 758–771. doi: 10.1080/10635150802429642.

80. Felsenstein J (1985) Confidence limits on phylogenies: An approach using the bootstrap. Evolution 39: 783–791. doi: 10.1016/j.bse.2010.10.005.

81. Webb CO, Ackerly DD, Kembel SW (2008) Phylocom: software for the analysis of phylogenetic community structure and trait evolution. Bioinformatics 24: 2098–2100. doi: 10.1093/bioinformatics/btn358.

82. Chakraborty A, Gupta N, Ghosh K, Roy P (2010) *In vitro* evaluation of the cytotoxic, anti-proliferative and anti-oxidant properties of pterostilbene isolated from *Pterocarpus* marsupium. Toxicology *in Vitro* 24: 1215–1228. doi: 10.1016/j.tiv.2010.02.007.

83. Bertani S, Bourdy G, Landau I, Robinson JC, Esterre P, et al. (2005) Evaluation of French Guiana traditional antimalarial remedies. Journal of Ethnopharmacology 98: 45–54. doi: 10.1016/j.jep.2004.12.020.

84. Valentin A, Mustofa , Benoit-Vical F, Pélissier Y, Koné-Bamba D, et al. (2000) Antiplasmodial activity of plant extracts used in west African traditional medicine. Journal of Ethnopharmacology 73: 145–151. doi: 10.1016/S0378-8741(00)00296-8.

85. Karou D, Dicko MH, Sanon S, Simpore J, Traore AS (2003) Antimalarial activity of Sida acuta Burm. f. (Malvaceae) and *Pterocarpus* erinaceus Poir. (Fabaceae). Journal of Ethnopharmacology 89: 291–294. doi: 10.1016/j.jep.2003.09.010.

86. Muñoz V, Sauvain M, Bourdy G, Callapa J, Bergeron S, et al. (2000) A search for natural bioactive compounds in Bolivia through a multidisciplinary approach: Part I. Evaluation of the antimalarial activity of plants used by the Chacobo Indians. Journal of Ethnopharmacology 69: 127–137. doi: 10.1016/S0378-8741(99)00148-8.

87. Dhanabal SP, Kokate CK, Ramanathan M, Kumar EP, Suresh B (2006) Hypoglycaemic activity of *Pterocarpus* marsupium Roxb. Phytotherapy Research 20: 4–8. doi: 10.1002/ptr.1819.

88. Kar A, Choudhary BK, Bandyopadhyay NG (2003) Comparative evaluation of hypoglycaemic activity of some Indian medicinal plants in alloxan diabetic rats. Journal of Ethnopharmacology 84: 105–108. doi: 10.1016/S0378-8741(02)00144-7.

89. Murthy YLN, Viswanadh GS, Atchuta Ramaiah P, Chandra Sekhar Naidu K (2004) Antidiabetic activity of heartwood extract of *Pterocarpus* dalbergioides. Journal of Tropical Medicinal Plants 4: doi: 10.2307/4117194.

90. Vats V, Grover JK, Rathi SS (2002) Evaluation of anti-hyperglycemic and hypoglycemic effect of Trigonella foenum-graecum Linn, Ocimum sanctum Linn and *Pterocarpus* marsupium Linn in normal and alloxanized diabetic rats. Journal of Ethnopharmacology 79: 95–100. doi: 10.1016/S0378-8741(01)00374-9.

91. Kameswara Rao B, Giri R, Kesavulu MM, Apparao C (2001) Effect of oral administration of bark extracts of *Pterocarpus* santalinus L. on blood glucose level in experimental animals. Journal of Ethnopharmacology 74: 69–74. doi: 10.1016/S0378-8741(00)00344-5.

92. Kondeti VK, Badri KR, Maddirala DR, Thur SKM, Fatima SS, et al. (2010) Effect of *Pterocarpus* santalinus bark, on blood glucose, serum lipids, plasma insulin and hepatic carbohydrate metabolic enzymes in streptozotocin-induced diabetic rats. Food and Chemical Toxicology 48: 1281–1287. doi: 10.1016/j.fct.2010.02.023.

93. Nagaraju N, Prasad M, Gopalakrishna G, Rao KN (1991) Blood sugar lowering effect of *Pterocarpus* santalinus (Red Sanders) wood extract in different rat models. Pharmaceutical Biology 29: 141–144. doi: 10.3109/13880209109082866.

94. Webb CO, Ackerly DD, McPeek MA, Donoghue MJ (2002) Phylogenies and community ecology. Annual Review of Ecology and Systematics 33: 475–505. doi: 10.1146/annurev.ecolsys.33.010802.150448.
95. Bletter N (2007) A quantitative synthesis of the medicinal ethnobotany of the Malinke of Mali and the Ashaninka of Peru, with a new theoretical framework. Journal of Ethnobiology and Ethnomedicine 3: 36. doi: 10.1186/1746-4269-3-36.
96. Moerman DE (2007) Agreement and meaning: Rethinking consensus analysis. Journal of Ethnopharmacology 112: 451–460. doi: 10.1016/j.jep.2007.04.001.
97. Roersch CMFB (2010) Piper umbellatum L.: A comparative cross-cultural analysis of its medicinal uses and an ethnopharmacological evaluation. Journal of Ethnopharmacology 131: 522–537. doi: 10.1016/j.jep.2010.07.045.
98. Trotter RT, Logan MH (1986) Informant consensus: A new approach for identifying potentially effective medicinal plants. In: Etkin NL, editor. Plants in Indigenous Medicine and Diet Biobehavioral Approaches. Bedford Hills, NY: Redgrave Publishing Co. pp. 91–112.
99. de Albuquerque UP, Andrade LdHC (1998) Etnobotánica del género Ocimum L. (Lamiaceae) en las comunidades afrobrasileñas. Anales del Jardín Botánico de Madrid 56: 107–118. doi: 10.1641/b580209.
100. Etkin NL (1988) Ethnopharmocology: Biobehavioral Approaches in the Anthropological Study of Indigenous Medicines. Annual Review of Anthropology 17: 23–42. doi: 10.1111/j.1095-8339.1860.tb02464.x.
101. Bennett B (2007) Doctrine of Signatures: An explanation of medicinal plant discovery or Dissemination of knowledge? Economic Botany 61: 246–255.
102. Grover JK, Yadav S, Vats V (2002) Medicinal plants of India with anti-diabetic potential. Journal of Ethnopharmacology 81: 81–100. doi: 10.1016/S0378-8741(02)00059-4.
103. Jain A, Katewa SS, Galav PK, Sharma P (2005) Medicinal plant diversity of Sitamata wildlife sanctuary, Rajasthan, India. Journal of Ethnopharmacology 102: 143–157. doi: 10.1016/j.jep.2005.05.047.
104. Nadkarni AK, Nadkarni KM (1976) Indian materia medica. Bombay: Popular Prakashan.
105. Nagaraju N, Rao KN (1990) A survey of plant crude drugs of Rayalaseema, Andhra Pradesh, India. Journal of Ethnopharmacology 29: 137–158. doi: 10.1016/0378-8741(90)90051-T.
106. Li RW, Myers SP, Leach DN, Lin GD, Leach G (2003) A cross-cultural study: anti-inflammatory activity of Australian and Chinese plants. Journal of Ethnopharmacology 85: 25–32. doi: 10.1016/S0378-8741(02)00336-7.
107. Lans C (2007) Comparison of plants used for skin and stomach problems in Trinidad and Tobago with Asian ethnomedicine. Journal of Ethnobiology and Ethnomedicine 3: 1–12. doi: 10.1186/1746-4269-3-1.
108. Newmaster S, Ragupathy S (2010) Ethnobotany genomics - discovery and innovation in a new era of exploratory research. Journal of Ethnobiology and Ethnomedicine 6: 2. doi: 10.1186/1746-4269-6-2.
109. Prance GT, Balee W, Boom BM, Carneiro RL (1987) Quantitative ethnobotany and the case for conservation in Ammonia. Conservation Biology 1: 296–310. doi: 10.1111/j.1523-1739.1987.tb00050.x.

110. Baum BR, Mechanda S, Livesey JF, Binns SE, Arnason JT (2001) Predicting quantitative phytochemical markers in single Echinacea plants or clones from their DNA fingerprints. Phytochemistry 56: 543–549. doi: 10.1016/S0031-9422(00)00425-8.
111. Tao J, Luo Z-y, Msangi C, Shu X-s, Wen L, et al. (2009) Relationships among genetic makeup, active ingredient content, and place of origin of the medicinal plant Gastrodia tuber. Biochemical Genetics 47: 8–18. doi: 10.1007/s10528-008-9201-7.
112. Procheş Ş, Wilson JRU, Vamosi JC, Richardson DM (2008) Plant diversity in the human diet: Weak phylogenetic signal indicates breadth. BioScience 58: 151–159. doi: 10.1641/b580209.
113. Weete JD, Abril M, Blackwell M (2010) Phylogenetic distribution of fungal sterols. PLoS ONE 5: e10899. doi: 10.1371/journal.pone.0010899.
114. Lewis WH, Elvin-Lewis MP (1995) Medicinal Plants as Sources of New Therapeutics. Annals of the Missouri Botanical Garden 82: 16–24. doi: 10.2307/2399976.
115. Firn RD (2003) Bioprospecting – why is it so unrewarding? Biodiversity and Conservation 12: 207–216.
116. Uprety Y, Asselin H, Boon E, Yadav S, Shrestha K (2010) Indigenous use and bio-efficacy of medicinal plants in the Rasuwa District, Central Nepal. Journal of Ethnobiology and Ethnomedicine 6: 3. doi: 10.1186/1746-4269-6-3.
117. Taylor JLS, Rabe T, McGaw LJ, Jäger AK, van Staden J (2001) Towards the scientific validation of traditional medicinal plants. Plant Growth Regulation 34: 23–37.
118. McClatchey WC, Mahady GB, Bennett BC, Shiels L, Savo V (2009) Ethnobotany as a pharmacological research tool and recent developments in CNS-active natural products from ethnobotanical sources. Pharmacology & Therapeutics 123: 239–254. doi: 10.1016/j.pharmthera.2009.04.002.
119. Reyes-Garcia V (2010) The relevance of traditional knowledge systems for ethnopharmacological research: theoretical and methodological contributions. Journal of Ethnobiology and Ethnomedicine 6: 32. doi: 10.1186/1746-4269-6-32.

This article has supplemental information that is not featured in this version of the text. To view these files, please visit the original version of the article as cited in the beginning of this chapter.

CHAPTER 13

ETHNOBOTANY GENOMICS: DISCOVERY AND INNOVATION IN A NEW ERA OF EXPLORATORY RESEARCH

STEVEN G. NEWMASTER AND SUBRAMANYAM RAGUPATHY

13.1 INTRODUCTION

Ethnobotany genomics is a novel approach that is poised to lead botanical discoveries and innovations in a new era of exploratory research. The concept for this new approach is founded on the concept of 'assemblage' of biodiversity knowledge, which includes a coming together of different ways of knowing and valorizing species variation in a novel approach seeking to add value to both traditional knowledge (TK) and scientific knowledge (SK). Ethnobotany genomics draws on an ancient body of knowledge concerning the variation in the biological diversity that surrounds different cultures; combined with modern genomic tools such as DNA barcoding it also explores the natural genetic variation found among

This chapter was originally published under the Creative Commons Attribution License. Newmaster SG and Ragupathy S. Ethnobotany Genomics: Discovery and Innovation in a New Era of Exploratory Research. Journal of Ethnobiology and Ethnomedicine *6,2 (2010). doi:10.1186/1746-4269-6-2.*

organisms. This genomic variation is explored along a gradient of variation in which any organism inhabits. We present here the first introduction to ethnobotany genomics including some background and several case studies in our lab, which define an approach to this new discipline that may evolve quickly with new ideas and technology. The motivation for this new approach is a quest to understand how the diversity of life that surrounds us can serve society-at-large with nutrition, medicine and more.

Ethnobotany implicitly embodies the concept of interdisciplinary research. The term "ethnobotany" is derived from ethnology (study of culture) and botany (study of plants); it is the scientific study of the relationships that exist between people and plants. Historically, ethnobotanists documented, described and explained the complex relationships between cultures and their utility of plants. This often included how plants are used, managed and perceived across human societies as foods, medicines, cosmetics, dyes, textiles, building materials, tools, clothing or within cultural divination, rituals and religion. Much of this research assumes that TK can be imposed upon a SK classification of living things. We suggest that this is a biased approach and call for a more unified approach that includes concept of 'assemblage' [1] a coming together of different ways of knowing and valorizing biological variation. This novel approach seeks to add value to both aboriginal knowledge and modern science such as biodiversity genomics (DNA barcoding) to understanding diversity as they work together to potentially create new knowledge. Exploring the ways in which these different knowledge practices are worked together as 'useful knowledge' [2] will show how such inquiries contribute to the common aim of the protection of cultural and biological diversity [3]. An interdisciplinary approach such as this will respond to the increasing urgent global imperatives to conserve both cultural and biological diversity as urged by the Convention of Biological Diversity [4], UNESCO's 'Man and Biosphere Programme' and the Declaration on the Rights of Indigenous People (2007).

There is a global effort to expedite the documentation and understanding of the planet's natural diversity and the scientific underpinnings of different biological classification systems [5,6]. This includes studies that have documented aboriginal classification systems for plants and animals [7-10]. Our understanding of ethnobiological classification has recently advanced and is more complex that originally thought. TK often includes multiple mechanisms of classification [11,12] that goes beyond morphology and includes sensory perception, ecology and utilitarian characters [5,13-18]. This presents an impediment to utilizing these ancient classification systems for interpreting biodiversity because they are very complicated, which requires a great deal of time to fully comprehend, reconstruct and utilize.

Ethnobotany genomics engages modern tools that can overcome taxonomic impediments to exploring biodiversity. Contemporary Biodiversity Genomics includes intense sampling of organisms at different taxonomic levels for the same genomic region (DNA barcode) [19]. This provides a link between variation in taxa, sequence evolution and genomic structure and function, providing a good estimate of the evolutionary process. The approach integrates "Genomic Thinking" (high-volume, high-throughput) with the natural variation encountered in ecosystems to explore biological diversity. The recent development and application of DNA-based approaches enables biodiversity genomics and the development of new areas of research such as ethnobotany genomics.

DNA barcoding is a critical technique employed in biodiversity genomics. Hebert et al. [19] developed DNA barcoding as a method of species identification and recognition in animals using specific regions of DNA sequence data [20]. He has developed barcoding in animals, which is well documented and can be reviewed online via the Canadian Barcode of Life [21] and the Consortium for the Barcode of Life [22]. Although the difficulties of plant barcoding have been debated [23-26], detailed studies [27-37] have demonstrated the utility of barcoding as an effective tool for plant identification. Recently DNA barcoding has been used as a modern genomics tool for identifying cryptic plant species [28-30,33,34]. The applications to Ethnobiology are discussed for the first time in the literature in this paper.

The goal of this paper is to introduce a unified approach to exploring biodiversity that draws on different knowledge systems. These systems include both traditional knowledge (TK) and scientific knowledge (SK). The later utilizes DNA barcoding, as a modern identification technique to assess inter/intraspecific genetic variation among taxa, all of which is intrenched in alpha taxonomy. We use two case studies (Ethnobotany genomics of *Biophytum* and *Tripogon*) to present this approach as examples that other research labs might model, contributing to the assemblage of a larger body biodiversity knowledge, which includes TK and SK and perhaps creates new knowledge in the process.

13.2 MATERIALS AND METHODS

13.2.1 STUDY AREA

The study site (longitude 6° 40' to 7° 10' E and latitude 10° 55' to 11° 10' N) is located within the Velliangiri holy hills, which forms a major range in the Western Ghats in the Nilgiri Biosphere Reserve. The research was conducted among seven hills with altitudes ranging from 520 m - 1840 m, which is bordered by the Palghat district of Kerala on the western boundary, the plains of Coimbatore district to the east, the Nilgiri mountains to the north, and the Siruvani hills on the southern boundary.

13.2.2 ETHNOBOTANY SURVEYS

Floristic explorations were made within respective study areas within India [18,29,33,38-41]. Collections were made from April 2004-January 2009 and included all seasons in order to collect any ephemerals or specialized phenotypes. Six collections or "specimens" from each population were collected, labelled with locations and collection numbers for of 19 *Biophytum* species (Figure 1) and 12 *Tripogon* species (Figure 2). Corresponding field data included details of the specimens (habit, flower colour, phenology and presence or absence of latex) and environmental variables (habitat, latitude, longitude, altitude, soil type and plant associations). Multiple populations were sampled along transects separated by 2 km in order to insure that we were collecting distinct populations and not vegetative colonies. This also accounted for local morphological variants within the different ecosites. The survey used is that of earlier methodologies

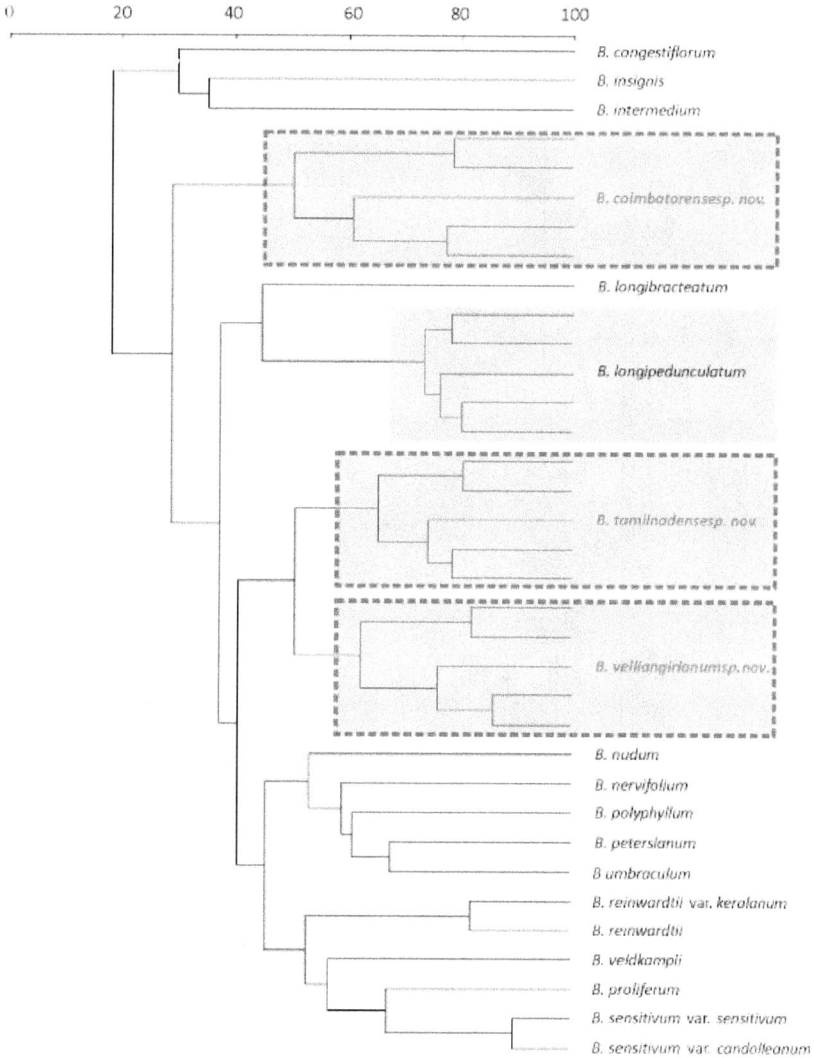

FIGURE 1: Classification tree from DNA barcoding sequence data (rbcL, matK and trnH-psbA + 41 quantitative variables) of 19 Biophytum species and varieties including three new species (dotted boxes; grey boxes outlines intraspecific variation recognized as ethnotaxa).

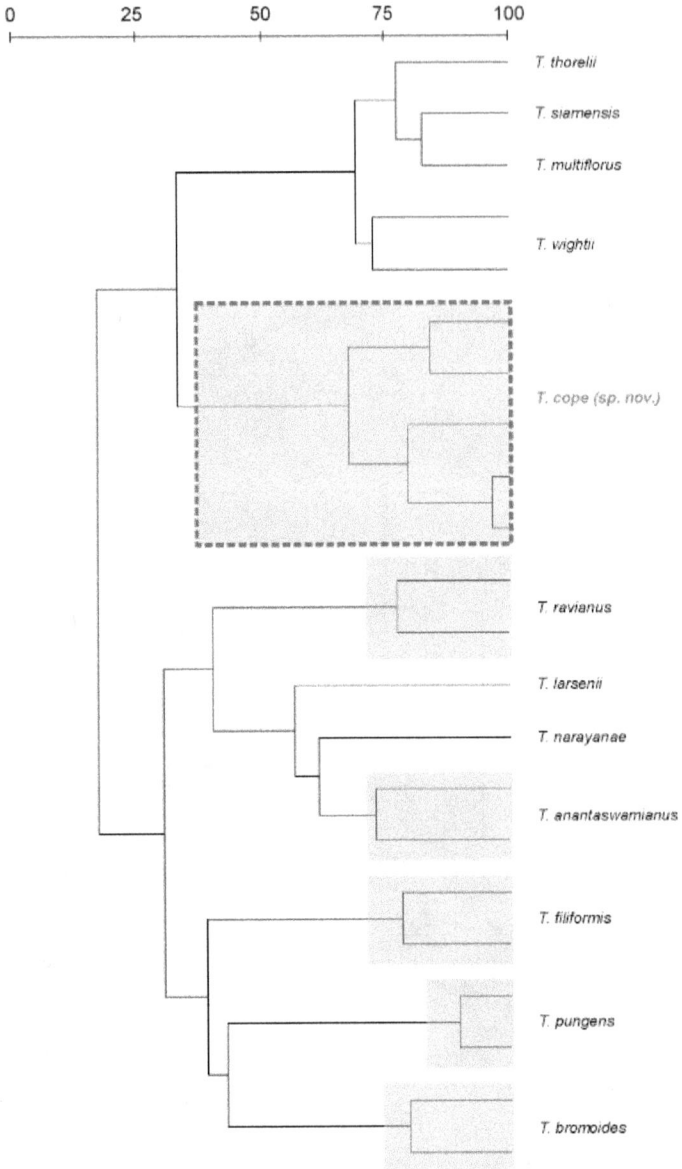

FIGURE 2: Classification tree from DNA barcoding sequence data (rbcL, matK and trnH-psbA) of 12 *Tripogon* species one new species (dotted boxes; grey boxes outlines intraspecific variation recognized as ethnotaxa).

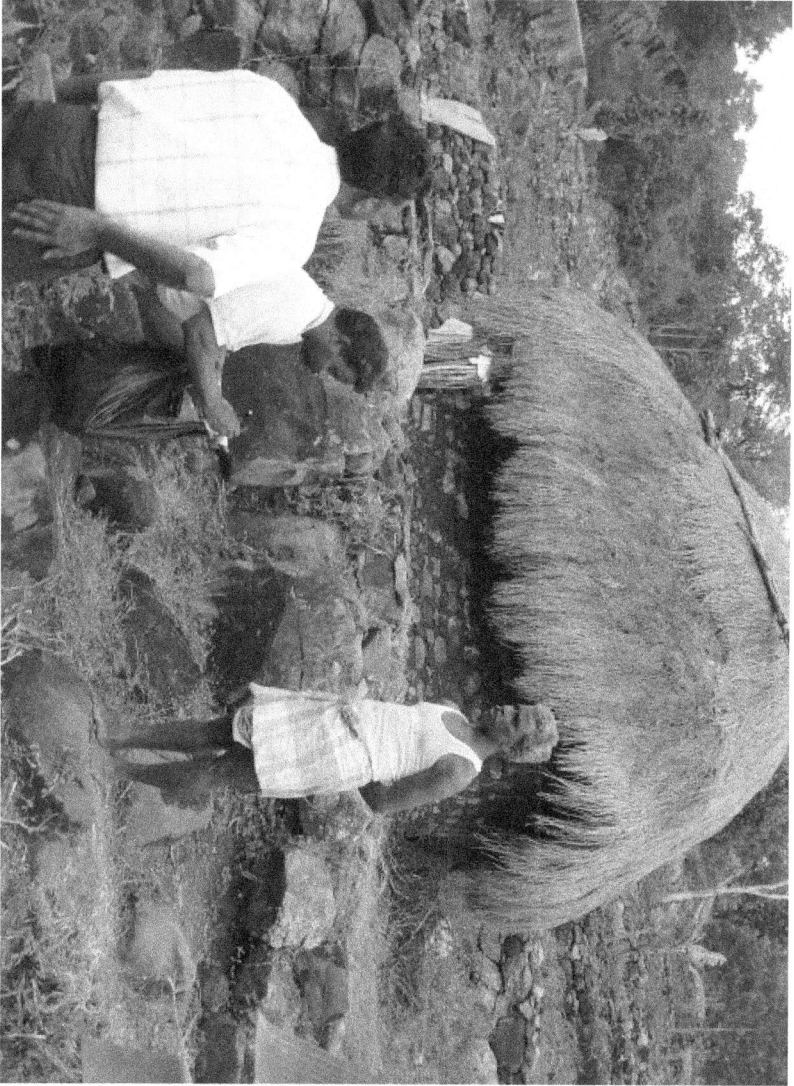

FIGURE 3: Conducting survey with informant, Vadaman Chakkan Palanisamy.

[12,18,33,41] to identify local experts in traditional botanical knowledge. We interviewed over 120 informants from which we selected 80 informants. Vouchers were collected and labelled for all taxa identified (Figure 3). The data were gathered in a series of structured, semi-structured and unstructured interviews, and participatory approach regarding plant uses, identification, and nomenclature. To elucidate cultural domains and determine differences in knowledge or taxonomy among aboriginals, a cross check was made with other aboriginal respondents by using various research protocols such as free recall lists, pile sorts, and consensus analysis.

13.2.3 PLANT VOUCHERS

Plant samples were collected from the aboriginal community and preserved for both herbaria and DNA barcode analysis (Figure 4). Leaf, stem and flower parts collected in situ were fixed in silica gel, FAA (50% ethanol, 5% acetic acid, 10% formalin, 35% water) and stored in 70% ethanol for morphological study ex situ. Herbarium specimens were prepared as per Jain and Rao's [42] manual and deposited in the herbarium of Kongunadu Arts and Science College, Coimbatore. The isotypes of new taxa and other taxonomically significant plant species were deposited at Madras Herbarium (MH), Southern Circle, Botanical Survey of India, Coimbatore and Ontario Agricultural College (OAC) Herbarium, Biodiversity Institute of Ontario, University of Guelph, Canada.

13.2.4 IDENTIFICATION ANALYSIS

Calculation of a Consensus Factor (Fic), and pile sorting relative frequency (RF) was used to test homogeneity of knowledge (SK & TK) in identifying specimens, revealing cryptic taxa or limitations of the classification without the use of molecular data. Voucher samples collected from five collection sites were systematically identified by the taxonomists and aboriginal informants. The relative frequency (RF) of each specimen from the interviews were calculated to determine a quantitative value for choosing a plant name (latin binomial or aboriginal ethno-taxon) from the pool

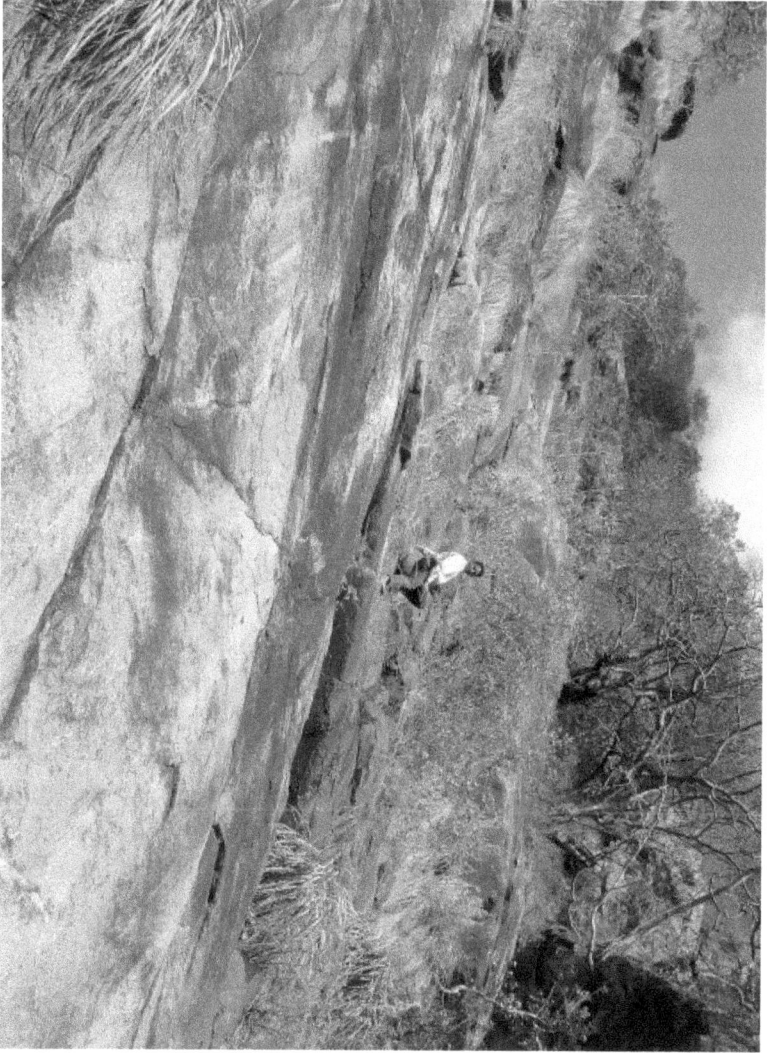

FIGURE 4: Collecting Bare foot in the Velliangiri holy hills.

of collected vouchers and placing it in a species concept [12]. RF is the simple calculation of the percentage of specimens associated with a taxon when taxonomists or aboriginal informants are presented with a pool of vouchers and asked to perform "pile sort". Trotter and Logan [43] provide the calculation of a Consensus Factor [Fic = Nur-Nt/(Nur-1)], which is adopted to evaluate the degree of partition into categories [44]. We have adopted this to include 'aboriginal utility' by the aboriginal informants [33,18,39,41], where Nur is the number of use-reports of informants for particular category (TK plant use) factor, where a use-report is a single record for use of a plant mentioned by an individual, and Nt refers to the number of species used for that particular category for all informants [18].

13.2.5 DNA BARCODING

Three DNA regions (*rbcL, matK* and *trnL-F*) were selected based on the previous plant barcoding studies [27,30,35,36]. We isolated total genomic DNA from approximately 10 mg of dried leaf material from each sample using the kit, NucleoSpin® 96 Plant II (MACHEREY-NAGEL). Extracted DNA was stored in sterile microcentifuge tubes at -20°C. The selected loci were amplified by PCR on a PTC-100 thermocycler (Bio-Rad). DNA was amplified in 20 μl reaction mixtures containing 1 U AmpliTaq Gold Polymerase with GeneAmp 106PCR Buffer II (100 mM Tris-HCl pH 8.3, 500 mM KCl) and 2.5 mM $MgCl_2$ (Applied Biosystems, Foster City, CA), 0.2 mM dNTPs, 0.1 mM of each primer (0.5 mM for matK), and 20 ng template DNA. Amplified products were sequenced in both directions with the primers used for amplification, following the protocols of the University of Guelph Genomics facility. Products from each specimen were cleaned using Sephadex columns and run on an ABI 3730 sequencer (Applied Biosystems, Foster City, CA). Bidirectional sequence reads were obtained for all the PCR products. Sequences were assembled using Sequencher 4.5 (Gene Codes Corp, Ann Arbor, MI), and aligned manually using Bioedit version 7.0.9. The sequences were used in combination with the morphometric analysis to produce classification trees.

13.2.6 MORPHOMETRIC DATA COLLECTION AND ANALYSES

Morphological data variables, were recorded for all specimen collections. A matrix of specimens and morphological characters were used in a multivariate phenetic analysis. Canonical ordination was used to detect groups of specimens and to estimate the contribution of each variable to the analysis. A cluster analysis was used to classify the specimens because it is better at representing distances among similar specimens [45]. Cluster analysis was carried out using NTSYS [46]. A distance matrix was generated from the specimens and characters using an arithmetic average (UPGMA) clustering algorithm and standardized data based on average taxonomic distance subjected to the unweighted pair-group method. The resulting distance matrix from the cluster analysis used in combination with the sequence data above to produce classification trees.

13.3 RESULTS AND DISCUSSION

13.3.1 BIOPHYTUM *ETHNOBOTANY GENOMICS*

The genus *Biophytum* DC. (ca. 80 species, *Oxalidaceae*) is predominantly pantropical to subtropical in distribution [47]. *Biophytum* is one of only eight genera in three families of flowering plants (*Lythraceae, Oxalidaceae,* and *Potederiaceae*) that are tristylous [48]. The genus is poorly studied with limited floristic treatment in Knuth's [49] monograph of *Oxalidaceae*, which was later revised by Veldkamp [50]. The genus has been confused with that of *Oxalis*. Linnaeus described *Oxalis sensitiva* [51], from a neotype later classified as *Biophytum sensitivum* (L.) DC. Veldkamp [52] noted that the genus *Biophytum* appears to be first described in a treatise by Acosta [53], which later appeared with a plate in Clusius' treatment (1605) of *Herba viva*. A brief narrative of the historical nomenclature on *Biophytum* of the old world is provided by Veldkamp [52]. Veldkamp [52] states that there is no comprehensive treatment of the genus, which contains many undescribed species.

The contribution of the local aboriginal knowledge concerning variation in *Biophytum* within India is considerable. India has a high diversity of *Biophytum*; the *Biophytum* flora of India is currently represented by 17 species and two varieties of which four species are endemic, representing taxa that are in need of conservation status and protection [54]. Recent floristic surveys are reporting considerable diversity within protected religious areas in India, some of which preserve a significant portion of the *Biophytum* flora [55,18,33]. All 19 species and varieties of *Biophytum* in this study are found in the Western Ghats, which is part of Nilgiri Biosphere Reserve (NBR) in Tamil Nadu. The Velliangiri hills of India are also known for their rich anthropogenic diversity. The aboriginals living in the Velliangiri hills are the "Malasars, Mudhuvars and Irulas" [11,12,18,33,41]. They have accumulated extensive ethnobotanical knowledge by their long association with their diverse, local flora [38]. In our floristic study within the Velliangiri hills we recorded 177 plants, which are used by the local people for various purposes [12,18]. These aboriginals recognize plants of the genus *Biophytum* ("thottal sinungi", trnsl. 'touch me not') naming and identifying many ethnotaxa including an ecological knowledge of them [11,12,38]. It is this TK that provided clues to the identity of several new species [29,55] while working with the aboriginals in the Velliangiri hills. The respective classifications of the genus *Biophytum* using both SK and TK are not homogeneous. Taxonomists identified taxa with 84% (RF) accuracy, while the Aboriginal informants identified the same specimens with 97% (RF) accuracy [38]. Consensus factors were high (Fic = 0.94 - 0.99) and not partitioned among the Aboriginal informants. The TK classification recognizes considerable fine scale variation among *Biophytum* samples (Figure 1). The TK classification of *Biophytum* is hierarchical, employing several TK classification characters; morphology, ecology, experience, gestalt and utility including 4 secondary classification mechanisms (e.g., nutritional, medicinal, technical or ritual). Interestingly these new species corresponded to unique aboriginal taxa with respective nomenclature and medicinal use [29,30,12,33,18,41].

DNA barcoding validated three new cryptic species to science that were previously recognized by TK classifications of the Irulas and Malasars. These species include 1) 'Vishamuruchi' (translation—detoxification of the poison; *Biophytum coimbatorense* sp. nov.), which is used as an antidote for poisonous scorpion bites, 2) 'Thear chedi' (translation —Chariot umbrella; *Biophytum tamilnadense* sp. nov) is used as a bait plant for fish and crab and 3) 'Idduki poondu' (translation—between the rock; *Biophytum velliangirianum* sp. nov.) is used for curing ear aches. A Classification tree from DNA barcoding sequence data (rbcL, matK and trnH-psbA + 41 quantitative variables) resolved 19 *Biophytum* species and varieties including the three new species (Figure 1). DNA barcoding discriminated the cryptic ethnotaxa *Biophytum coimbatorense* sp. nov. ('Vishamuruchi') from the morphologically similar species of *B. longipedunculatum* Govind. ('Thotal sinungi'). Amplifications were highly specific with a clear background in the agarose gel. Although there were no differences in the rbcL or atpF sequences for these two cryptic species, the matK and more variable non-coding spacer regions such as trnH-psbA sequences were consistently different. Several segregating sites in the matK sequences are found consistently among the five distant populations. Several other studies [30,36] have also found that closely related species are not distinguished by several plastid regions like rbcL or atpF.

Ethnobotany genomics is currently being used to determine the distribution of rare species and their ecological requirements, including traditional ecological knowledge so that conservation strategies can be implemented. We are currently conducting further research on more species in the genus *Biophytum* in collaboration with several other aboriginal cultures in order to resolve species concepts within the world distribution and provide a phylogeny for the genus. Combined with a further biological and ecological data this information will contribute to conservation initiatives at a global scale.

13.3.2 TRIPOGON *ETHNOBOTANY GENOMICS*

The genus *Tripogon* Roem. & Schult. consists of nearly 40 species in tropical and subtropical regions [56-58]. The diversity of this genus of grass has been described thoroughly within the catalogue of world grasses by Peterson et al. [59], a revision of African species of *Tripogon* [60,61], the description of new species of *Tripogon* from Africa [62], a summary of grass genera worldwide [56], an online world grass flora by [58], and nomenclature changes by Veldkamp [63]. Rúgolo de Agrasar & Vega [64] reported that Indo-Asia constitutes the centre of diversity for this genus, with 23 species of which 16 species are native to China and 21 species including eight endemics are native to India [29]. Most of what has been published within the Indian flora and includes three new species of *Tripogon*[65-67,29].

We recently discovered a new species of *Tripogon* (T. cope Newm.) during an ethnobotany genomics study in the Nilgiri Biosphere Reserve, Western Ghats, India [29]. We worked with aboriginal informants who are members of the local hill tribes (Irulas and Malasars). The informants revealed ethno taxa that we later confirmed to be a new species. The ability of our field taxonomists and the Hill Tribe informants to identify species in the genus *Tripogon* was high, but the respective classifications of SK and TK are not homogeneous. Our taxonomists identified seven taxa from the 40 specimens with 96% (RF) accuracy among individuals. Aboriginal informants identified eight taxa from the same 40 specimens with 98% RF among the informants. A closer investigation of the voucher samples revealed that what we called T. wightii the informants split into two distinct ethnotaxa; 'Sunai pul' and 'Kattai pul'. The TK classification of *Tripogon* is hierarchical, employing several TK classification characters; ecology, experience, gestalt and utility including 4 secondary classification mechanisms (e.g., nutritional, medicinal, technical or ritual). An additional TK character used to distinguish 'Sunai pull' was that it is a 'hot' plant (see discussion below).

The cryptic ethnotaxa 'Sunai pul' and 'Kattai pul' have utility in the local hill tribes. Our ethnobotany surveys concluded that there was no partition of Fic among the 'Malasars and Irulas'. High consensus factors (0.95-0.99) confirmed that seven of the ethnotaxa are commonly used for a variety of purpose: snake hunting, fodder for domesticated animals and thatching. The new cryptic ethnotaxa 'Sunai pul' is a unique grass which is very important to both cultures with ritualistic and economic utility. 'Sunai pul' was not distinguished by the SK classification with vouchers lumped within the taxonomy of *Tripogon wightii*, which was labelled as 'Kattai pul' within the TK classification.

Further research validated that the cryptic ethnotaxa 'Sunai pul' was indeed a new species. Morphometric [29] and genetic studies [33] confirmed that the cryptic ethnotaxa 'Sunai pul' (*Tripogon cope* Newm.) was distinct from the morphologically similar species of *Tripogon wightii* ('Kattai pul'). We looked at herbarium vouchers and found that the close resemblance of *T. cope* to *T. wightii* has resulted in misidentifications by taxonomists during previous botanical surveys. Although the hill tribes can easily identify these species, these cryptic species are only differentiated by minor floral characters; slight variation (1 mm) in the rachilla internodes and the number (1-3) of awns at the lemma apex. The local aboriginal classification systems species are clearly discriminated by different life cycles. We grew the plants in the greenhouse and found that 'Sunai pul' (*T. cope*) is an annual and 'Kattai pul' (*T. wightii*) is a perennial. We also used DNA barcoding to discriminate the new species (Fig 2). Our classification tree from DNA barcoding sequence data (*rbcL, matK* and *trnH-psbA*) clearly distinguished the 12 *Tripogon* known species from T. cope (Fig. 2). Intraspecific variation within the classification tree are recognized by the hill tribes as ethnotaxa of which 'Sunai pul' (*T. cope*) and 'Kattai pul' (*T. wightii*) are clearly differentiated. The DNA amplifications were highly specific with a clear background in the agarose gel. The *matK* and *trnH-psbA* sequences had several segregating sites in sequences that were found consistently among the distant populations. There is a gross interspecific variation (p-distance 0.00234) and no intraspecific variation among T. cope and T. wightii. Interspecific variation among all eight species ranged from (p-distance 0.002-0.003). Intraspecific p-distance was 0.00 for all regions within all eight species.

13.4 CONCLUSION

Although there are many descriptive qualitative surveys of TK, few studies consider aboriginal classifications with respect to TK [12,33,18,41]. These studies have revealed novel ethnomedicine such as in Ragupathy et al. [39] whom discovered that cryptic ethnotaxa such as 'Modakathon' (*Cardiospermum halicacabum*—balloon vine) is part of the daily healthy life style used by several aboriginal cultures to control joint pain. In many cultures *Cardiospermum halicacabum* is harvested in backyards for both medicinal and food value. In fact, it provides an income supplement for some families from impoverished communities of third world countries. The paradox is that weed scientists have described balloon vine as a poisonous, noxious weed, which should be eradicated from the globe. Ragupathy et al. [18] identified several ethnotaxa of which one is a traditional cure to a common ailment, rheumatoid arthritis.

In both of the case studies we presented there is considerable TK associated with the new species to science, which are traditional ethnotaxa. 'Vishamuruchi' (*Biophytum coimbatorense* sp. nov.) is a detoxification for poisonous scorpion bites. The juice or extract of roots and rhizosphere is made into fine powder that is applied to a scorpion bite. A closely related cryptic species not differentiated by the taxonomist, 'Thotal sinungi' (translation—touch me not; *B. longipedunculatum*) is used to alleviate a soar throat; the leaves are squashed in the palms of their hands to extract the juice, which is dropped into the ear three times a day for three days with immediate results within in a few hours. 'Thear chedi' (*Biophytum tamilnadense* sp. nov) is bait plant for fish and crab. The Irulas collect fresh plants from the forest and tie them in bundles weighing about 1 kg. They bring 2-3 bundles to the pond and throw them into the water and wait. As soon as they see that fish are gathering near the bundle they throw their fishing net and harvest the catch. Later, crabs will inhabit the area around the bundle and can be gathered for food. 'Idduki poondu' (*Biophytum velliangirianum* sp. nov.) grows in small pockets at high elevations and is a remedy for ear aches. The preparation is similar to that of 'Thotal sinungi' (*B. longipedunculatum*).

The new grass species in our study has considerable utility to the hill tribes. In our study we found that the 'Malasars and Irulas' classified *Tripogon* taxa into eight ethnotaxa of which seven are used for similar utility; cattle and goat feed or thatching. However, the aboriginal informants recognized a common grass as 'Sunai pul' (*T. cope*) that is clearly differentiated by them from another grass 'Kattai pul' (*T. wightii*). The etymology for 'Kattai pul' refers to a cold, hard and stout grass that lives for many seasons and is used for cattle and goat feed as many other common grasses. 'Sunai pull' is a very special species to these cultures. The etymology for 'Sunai pull' refers to the hot, bushy, hairy snake grass that lives for only one monsoon season. While working in the field, the Irulas informants first introduced us to 'Sunai pull' with a warning. "Do not step near 'Sunai pull' because this is where the cobra seeks shelter. In fact, the local Irulas snake catchers come into the hills to catch cobras among the patches of 'Sunai pull'. They told us that 'Sunai pull' is hot, or gives of heat and that the snakes like to sleep there. Snake catching is viable part of the economy of several local villages because the demand for snake venom and skins. The extracted venom is purified, frozen and then freeze-dried to make the pure venom powder that is used by government laboratories for the production of anti-venom serum. To produce just one gram of pure cobra venom, 10 snakes are needed, while to produce the same amount of the saw-scaled viper venom the Irulas have to catch 750 snakes. A gram of the venom can cost up to $1,500 (USD) for some species of vipers. The snake skin is used to make cosmetics and industry representatives (often from export companies) come to the remote villages to buy skins from the Irulas. The importance to theses aboriginal cultures is apparent; the recognition by modern science is lagging behind because of taxonomic impediments.

DNA barcoding may provide an important tool for identifying cryptic species and validating ethnotaxa. One of the greatest utilities of barcoding is its use in overcoming taxonomic impediments; identifying cryptic materials such as unknown leaves, roots, etc. Barcoding was used in the study of nutmeg [29] to identify species in the *Myristicaceae* that are primarily separated by androecium characters in small, short-lived flowers that are only available for two weeks of the year. This study identified several crytic taxa including population level differences in Compsoneura associated with ecotypic differences and vicariance, suggesting several new cryptic species. DNA barcoding is a tool that ethnobiologists can employ to 1) validating ethnotaxa, 2) help overcoming hurdles of ambiguity, 3) gain credibility in science, and 4) stimulate new theory on understanding, preserving biological and cultural diversity.

We have initiated further ethnobotany genomic studies in other cultures to develop theoretically sophisticated insights concerning the encounter between 'local' and 'scientific' approaches to biodiversity knowledge. These will further contribute to a body of research on the social, cultural and political underpinnings biodiversity science; our understanding of the natural variation that surrounds us. Furthermore, the research will add to a unifying global effort to speed up the documentation (via DNA barcoding) and understanding of the planet's biodiversity, while concurrently respecting cultural heterogeneity as a vital component of biological diversity. This is aligned with the Convention on Biological Diversity [4] that was signed by over 150 nations, and thus the world's complex array of human-natural-technological relationships has effectively been re-organized.

REFERENCES

1. Watson-Verran H, Turnbull D: Science and other indigenous knowledge systems. In Handbook of Science and Technology Studies. Edited by Jasanoff S, Markle G, Petersen J, Pinch T. London and New Delhi: Sage Publications; 1995.
2. Strathern M: Useful Knowledge. The Isiah Berlin Lecture. University of Manchester, Brunswick, UK Sunil CN, Pradeep AK (2001) Another new species of *Tripogon* (Poaceae) from India. Sida 2005, 19:803-806.
3. Biber-Klemm S, Cottier T: Rights to plant genetic resources and Traditional knowledge: Basic issues and prospective. Oxfordshire: Nosworthy Way; 2006.
4. CBD: Sustainable use is defined under Article 2 of the Convention on Biological Diversity. 31 International Legal Materials; Rio de Janeiro 1992, :818.
5. Ellen R: Indigenous Environmental Knowledge and its Transformations: Critical Anthropological Perspectives. Edited by Parkes P, Bicker A. Amsterdam and Routledge, London: Harwood Academic; 2000.
6. Sillitoe P, Bicker A, Pottier J: Participating in Development: Approaches to Indigenous Knowledge. London: Routledge; 2002.
7. Berlin B: The relation of folk systematics to biological classification and nomenclature. Annual Review of Ecological and Systematics 1973, 4:259-271.
8. Ellen R: The Cultural Relations of Classification: An Analysis of Nuaulu Animal Categories from Central Seram. Cambridge, Massachusetts: Cambridge University Press; 1993.
9. Atran S: Itzaj Maya folk biological taxonomy. In Folk Biology. Edited by Medin DL, Atran S. Cambridge, Massachusetts: The MIT Press; 1999::119-204.
10. Brown CH: Folk classification: An introduction. In Ethnobotany: A Reader. Edited by Minnis PE. Norman, Oklahoma: University of Oklahoma Press; 2005::65-68.
11. Newmaster SG, Ragupathy S, Ivanoff RF, Nirmala CB: Mechanisms of Ethnobiological Classification. Ethnobotany 2006, 18(1,2):4-26.
12. Newmaster SG, Ragupathy S, Balasubramaniam NC, Ivanoff RF: The Multi-mechanistic Taxonomy of The Irulas In Tamil Nadu, South India. Journal of Ethnobiology 2007, 27:31-44.
13. Begossi A, Clauzet M, Guarano L: Are biological species and high-ranking groups real? The ethnotaxonomy of fish on the Atlantic Forest coast of Brazil. In 20th Meeting of the Society for Human Ecology. Salt Lake City, Utah; 2005.
14. Ellen R: A test of the applicability of general principles of ethnobiological classification to fungi: a nuau [abstract]. The Tenth International Congress of Ethnobiology, Chiang Rai, Thailand 2006.

15. Mourão JS, Araújo HFP, Almeida FS: Ethnotaxonomy of mastofauna as practiced by hunters of the municipality of Paulista, state of Paraíba-Brazil. Journal of Ethnobiology and Ethnomedicine 2006, 2(19):1-7.
16. Lampman AM: General principles of Ethnomycological classification among the Tzeltal Maya of Chiapas, Mexico. Journal of Ethnobiology 2007, 27(1):11-27.
17. Souza PS, Begossi A: Whales, dolphins or fishes? The ethnotaxonomy of cetaceans in São Sebastião, Brazil. Journal of Ethnobiology and Ethnomedicine 2007, 3:9.
18. Ragupathy S, Newmaster SG, Murugesan M, Velusamy B, Huda M: Consensus of the 'Malasars' traditional aboriginal knowledge of medicinal plants in the Velliangiri holy hills, India. Journal of Ethnobiology and Ethnomedicine 2008, 4(8):1-14.
19. Hebert PDN, Cywinska A, Ball SL, DeWaard JR: Biological identification through DNA barcodes. Proceedings of the Royal Society B: Biological Sciences 2003, 270:313-321.
20. Ratnasingham S, Hebert PDN: BOLD: the Barcode of Life Data System. Molecular Ecology Notes 2007, 7:355-364.
21. Canadian Barcode of Life [http://www.bolnet.ca]
22. Consortium for the Barcode of Life CBOL [http://www.barcoding.si.edu]
23. Chase MW, Salamin N, Wilkinson M, Dunwell JM, Kesanakurthi RP, Haidar N, Savolainen V: Land plants and DNA barcodes: short-term and long-term goals. Philosophical Transactions of the Royal Society B: Biological Sciences 2005, 360:1889-1895.
24. Kress WJ, Wurdack KJ, Zimmer EA, Weigt LA, Janzen DH: Use of DNA barcodes to identify flowering plants. Proceedings of the National Academy of Sciences, USA 2005, 102:8369-8374.
25. Cowan RS, Chase MW, Kress WJ, Savolainen V: 300 000 species to identify: problems, progress, and prospects in DNA barcoding of land plants. Taxon 2006, 55:611-616.
26. Pennisi E: Wanted: a barcode for plants. Science 2007, 318:190-191.
27. Newmaster SG, Fazekas AJ, Ragupathy S: DNA barcoding in the land plants: evaluation of rbcL in a multigene tiered approach.
28. Canadian Journal of Botany 2006, 84:335-341.
29. Newmaster SG, Ragupathy S, Janovec J: A Botanical Renaissance: State-of-the-art DNA Barcoding Facilitates an Automated Identification Technology (AIT) System for Plants. International Journal of Computer Applications in Technology 2009, in press.
30. Newmaster SG, Velusamy B, Murugesan M, Ragupathy S: *Tripogon* cope, a new species of *Tripogon* (Poaceae: Chloridoideae) in India with a Morphometric analysis and synopsis of *Tripogon* in India. Systematic Botany 2008, 33(4):695-701.
31. Newmaster SG, Fazekas AJ, Steeves R, Janovec J: Testing Candidate Plant Barcode Regions in the Myristicaceae. Molecular Ecology Resources 2008, 8:480-490.
32. CBOL Plant Working Group: A DNA barcode for land plants. Proceedings of the National Academy of Sciences USA 2009, 106(31):12794-12797.
33. Kress J, Erickson DL: Plant DNA barcodes and a community phylogeny of a tropical forest dynamics plot in Panama. Proceeding of the National Academy of Sciences, USA 2009, 106:18621-18626.

34. Ragupathy S, Newmaster SG, Velusamy B, Murugesan M: DNA barcoding discriminates a new cryptic grass species revealed in an ethnobotany study by the hill tribes of the Western Ghats in southern India. Molecular Ecological Resources 2009, 9(Supp l):172-180.

35. Newmaster SG, Ragupathy S: Testing Plant Barcoding in a Sister Species Complex of Pantropical Acacias (Mimosoideae, Fabaceae). Molecular Ecological Resources 2009, 9(Suppl 1):172-180.

36. Fazekas AJ, Kesanakurti PR, Burgess KS, Percy DM, Graham SW, Barrett SCH, Newmaster SG, Hajibabaei M, Husband BC: Are plant species inherently harder to discriminate than animal species using DNA barcoding markers? Molecular Ecological Resources 2009, 9:130-139.

37. Fazekas AJ, Burgess KS, Kesanakurti PR, Percy DM, Hajibabaei M, Graham SW, Husband BC, Barrett SCH, Newmaster SG: Assessing the utility of coding and noncoding genomic regions for plant DNA barcoding. PLOS ONE 2008, 3:1-12.

38. Lahaye R, Bank M, Bogarin D, Warner J, Pupulin F, Gigot G, Maurin O, Duthoit S, Barraclough TG, Savolainen V: DNA barcoding the floras of biodiversity hotspots. Proceedings of the National Academy of Sciences USA 2008, 105:2923-2928.

39. Newmaster SG, Murugesan M, Ragupathy S, Nagaraj N, Velusamy B: Ethnobotany Genomics study reveals three new species from the Velliangiri Hills in the Nilgiri Biosphere Reserve, Western Ghats, India. Ethnobotany 2009, 21:1-28.

40. Ragupathy S, Newmaster SG, Gopinadhan P, Newmaster C: Exploring Ethnobiological Classifications for Novel Alternative Medicine: a case study of Cardiospermum halicacabum L. (Modakathon, Balloon Vine) as a traditional herb for treating rheumatoid arthritis. Ethnobotany 2008, 19:1-20.

41. Newmaster GS, Ragupathy S: Ethnobotany Genomics - Use of DNA Barcoding to Explore Cryptic Diversity in Economically Important Plants. Indian Journal of Science and Technology 2009, 2(5):2-8.

42. Ragupathy S, Newmaster SG: Valorizing the 'Irulas' traditional knowledge of medicinal plants in the Kodiakkarai Reserve Forest, India. Journal of Ethnobiology and Ethnomedicine 2009, 5(10):1-13.

43. Jain SK, Rao RR: A Handbook of field and Herbarium Methods. New Delhi: Today and Tomorrow's Printers & Publishers; 1977.

44. Trotter R, Logan M: Informant consensus: a new approach for identifying potentially effective medicinal plants. In Plants in indigenous medicine and diet: biobehavioural approaches. Edited by Etkin NL. New York: Redgrave Publishers; 1986::91-112.

45. Heinrich M: Ethnobotany and its role in drug development. Phytotherapy Research 2000, 14:479-488.

46. Sneath P, Sokal R: Numerical taxonomy. San Francisco, California: W.H. Freeman; 1973.

47. Rohlf F: NTSYS: Numerical Taxonomy and Multivariate Analysis System, Version 2.1. New York: Exeter Software; 2000.

48. Lourteig A: Flora of Panama. Part IV. Family 84. Oxalidaceae. Annals of the Missouri Botanical Garden 1980, 67:823-850.

49. Weller SG: Evolutionary modifications of tristylous breeding systems. In Evolution and Function of Heterostyly. Edited by Barrett SCH. Berlin: Springer-Verlag; 1992::247-272. Monogr. Theor. Appl. Genet. 15

50. Knuth R: Oxalidaceae. In Das Pflanzenreich Regni vegetalis conspectus IV. Edited by Engler HGA. Verlag von. HR Engelmann, Berlin IV; 1930::391-417.
51. Veldkamp JF: Oxalidaceae. In Flora Malesiana. Volume 1. Edited by Leiden Ser. van Steenis CGGJ; 1971::162-164.
52. Linnaeus C: Species plantarum.Stockholm 1753, :1.434
53. Veldkamp JF: Notes on *Biophytum* (Oxalidaceae) of the Old World. Taxon 1989, 38(1):110-116.
54. Acosta C: Tractado de las drogas, y medicinas de las Indias Orientales Burgos. In Portuguese Edition Edited by Walter J. 1964, 1578:147-148.
55. Manna MK: Oxalidaceae (*Biophytum* DC.). In Flora of India, (Malpighiaceae-Dichapetalaceae). Volume 4. Edited by Hajra PK, Nair VJ, Daniel P. Calcutta, India: Botanical Survey of India; 1997::231-255.
56. Murugesan M, Ragupathy S, Balasubramaniam V, Nagarajan N, Newmaster SG: Three new species of the genus *Biophytum* DC. (Oxalidaceae-Geraniales) from Velliangiri hills in the Nilgiri Biosphere Reserve, Western Ghats, India. Journal of Economic Taxonomic Botany 2009, :10-26.
57. Watson L, Dallwitz MJ: The grass genera of the world: descriptions, illustrations, identification, and information retrieval; including synonyms, morphology, anatomy, physiology, phytochemistry, cytology, classification, pathogens, world and local distribution, and references. [http://delta-intkey.com] 1992.(Revised version: 28th November 2005
58. Peterson PM, Webster RD, Valdes Reyna J: Genera of new world eragrostideae (Poaceae: Chloridoideae). Smithsonian Contributions to Botany 1997, 87:1-50.
59. Clayton WD, Harman KT, Williamson H: Grassbase - the Online World Grass Flora. [http://www.kew.org/data/grasses-db] 2006.
60. Peterson PM, Soreng RJ, Davidse G: Catalogue of new world grasses (Poaceae): II. Subfamily Chloridoideae (*Tripogon* p. 231). Contributions from the United States National Herbarium 2001, 41:1-255.
61. Phillips SM, Launert E: A revision of the African species of *Tripogon* Roem. and Schult. Kew Bulletin 1971, 25:301-322.
62. Phillips SM: Flora of Tropical East Africa, Gramineae (Part 2). Edited by Clayton WD, et al. London: Crown Agents; 1974::288-294.
63. Cope TA: Some new Arabian grasses II. Kew Bulletin 1992, 4:655-664.
64. Veldkamp JF: Name changes in Agrostis, Arundinella, Deyeuxia, Helictotrichon, *Tripogon* (Gramineae). Blumea 1996, 41:407-411.
65. Rúgolo de Agrasar ZE, Vega AS: *Tripogon* nicorae, a new species and synopsis of *Tripogon* (Poaceae: Chloridoideae) in America. Systematic Botany 2004, 29(4):874-882.
66. Naik VN, Patunkar WB: Two new grasses from Marathwada. Bulletin of the Botanical Survey of India 1973, 15(1-2):157-158.
67. Sreekumar PV, Nair VJ, Nair NC: *Tripogon* anantaswamianus - a new grass from Kerala, India. Bulletin of the Botanical Survey of India 1983, 25:185-187.
68. Sunil CN, Pradeep AK: Another new species of *Tripogon* (Poaceae) from India. Sida 2001, 19:803-806.

CHAPTER 14

PRESCRIPTIONS OF TRADITIONAL CHINESE MEDICINE ARE SPECIFIC TO CANCER TYPES AND ADJUSTABLE TO TEMPERATURE CHANGES

PEI-HSUN CHIU, HSIN-YING HSIEH, AND SUN-CHONG WANG

14.1 INTRODUCTION

According to the World Health Organization (WHO), cancer is the number one cause of mortality worldwide, accounting for 7.6 million deaths, or 13% of all deaths, across the globe in 2008 [1]. The toll is expected to rise continuously to over 11 million in 2030. Environmental factors are believed to be a primary contributor to the pathogenesis. The hazards range from physical agents such as ionizing and ultraviolet radiations, chemical agents such as dioxins and arsenic, to biological agents such as human papillomavirus and hepatitis B virus. Other risk factors include smoking, alcoholism/diet, obesity, ageing and genetics. Cancer cells, with mutated genomes, share three characteristics: uncontrolled cell multiplication, invasion of adjacent tissues, and migration to non-adjacent sites [2]. Metastasis of cancer, usually via bloodstream or lymphatics, to other vital organs

This chapter was originally published under the Creative Commons Attribution License. Chiu P-H, Hsieh HY, and Wang SC. Prescriptions of Traditional Chinese Medicine are Specific to Cancer Types and Adjustable to Temperature Changes. PLoS ONE 7,2 (2012), doi:10.1371/journal.pone.0031648.

such as lungs, liver, brain and bones adds to the malignancy and worsens the prognosis of the disease.

Treatment of cancer in modern western medicine includes surgery, radiotherapy and chemotherapy. Treatment modality depends on the site of cancer origin and stage of cancer progression, and typically involves a combination of modalities, for example a surgical removal followed by radiation or chemotherapy. Radiotherapy kills cells by breaking the DNA with X-, gamma-rays or charged particles and the free radicals generated in the radiation. Cytotoxic chemotherapy tames cells by stopping their division with small molecules that stop cell cycle or DNA synthesis. The two therapies seldom eliminate all cancer cells as, at increasing dosages, more nearby healthy and normal fast growing cells are compromised. A new and encouraging development in the last 15 years is targeted therapy which employs small molecules or monoclonal antibodies that bind and block the functions of the overly expressed genes in cancer cells [3], [4]. Examples of the inhibited targets are tyrosine kinases, vascular endothelial growth factors (VEGF) and histone deacetylases (HDAC) that are involved in growth signaling, angiogenesis and epigenetic regulation, respectively, of the cancer cells.

The outcome of the "war on cancer," initiated 40 years ago by the United States administration, has been debated in public media. According to a latest analysis by the American Cancer Society, the overall age-adjusted death rate of all cancers in men (women) dropped by 11% (6%) to 2.2 (1.5) per 1000 in the United States in 2006, compared to that in 1970 [5]. The declines were however largely attributed to better prevention and early detection including reduced smoking and increased mammogram and Pap tests, suggesting room for further development of new, complementary and alternative (CAM), as well as integrative cancer therapies. Targeted therapy may illustrate the trend of development. The effectiveness of targeted therapy was found to vary from patient to patient, depending on the carried cancer subtypes [6], [7]. Furthermore, combining a drug targeting cell proliferation and a drug targeting angiogenesis may enhance the effect of the treatment and ameliorates the issue of drug resistance [8]. Neither the concept of personalized medicine nor the prescription of drug mixtures is new to traditional Chinese medicine (TCM) [9], [10], a CAM that originated in China two thousand years ago and still thrives in far east Asia today.

What cancers are in TCM is best revealed from TCM prescriptions to cancers. Toward a systematic and scientific investigation of TCM treatment of cancers, the elements in TCM prescriptions have to be established and standardized, similar to the consideration of genes as the fundamental elements in genomics. In a typical TCM prescription to a patient can be found, for example, two TCM formulas and four TCM herbs. TCM formulas are believed to evolve from synergistic combinations of multiple TCM herbs. Many TCM formulas from authoritative TCM classics [11], with specified ingredient herbs and relative weights, stand the test of time and are still highly received today. The chemical composition within an herb can change depending on the harvest times/regions and processing methods. Minimizing the variability in the chemical profiles of the herbs/formulas can be relegated to certified manufacturers of TCM medicinals. A certification system involving government, for example, mandatory GMP compliance, also helps eliminate the concern of herbal toxicity due to heavy metal, pesticide and microbiological contaminations [12]. A TCM prescription p is then represented by $p = a_1 m_1 + a_2 m_2 + \ldots + a_N m_N$, where mi can be either a TCM herb or a classical TCM formula, ai a numeric value between 0 and 1 for the percentage weight of mi in the prescription, and N the number of mi in the prescription so that $a_1 + a_2 + \ldots + a_N = 1$. The representation is simple yet practical as prescriptions by a TCM doctor to patients of the same western, molecularly diagnosed, disease can contain exactly the same herbs/formulas mi's and N but different weights ai's, one of the manifestations of personalized medicine in TCM

TCM has developed its own system of diagnostics or TCM syndrome differentiation via for example tongue and pulse readings. Outcomes of TCM diagnoses in TCM terms could lack of consistency among TCM doctors [13], [14]. As modern western medicine has become an integral part of the core curriculum of the TCM education in Taiwan, diagnosis made in western terms, i.e., the International Classification of Diseases codes (ICD-9), has been enforced for the reimbursement of TCM prescriptions to the public health insurance program in Taiwan. With a large quantity of diagnosis and prescription data, we are then able to statistically associate an ICD-9 coded cancer to a TCM prescription: $p(\text{cancer ICD9 code}) = a_1 m_1 + a_2 m_2 + \ldots + a_N m_N$. ICD-9 codes on one side of the association and ai's on the other side can also be regarded as a bridge between modern western medicine and traditional Chinese medicine.

A mapping from TCM prescriptions to cancers sheds light on cancer therapy as TCM, as well as many other ancient medicines, is believed to be holistic [15]. On the other hand, mapping cancers to TCM prescriptions allows a better understanding of TCM as cancer biology has been extensively and rigorously investigated at the molecular and cellular levels. Specifically, with a year's worth of collection of 187,230 TCM prescriptions to over 30 cancer types in Taiwan in 2007, the questions we would address include: what are the most common TCM formulas and herbs for all and individual cancers? How are the relative weights of the individual formulas and herbs in a prescription distributed? Are the TCM prescriptions different for different cancers? How cancer type-specific are they? What are the possible mechanisms of actions, at cellular level, of harmonizing TCM formulas in comparison to tonifying TCM formulas? What diet is potentially beneficial for cancer patients? Do TCM cancer prescriptions change with seasons? If so, what cancer patients are susceptible to which meteorological variables?

14.2 MATERIALS AND METHODS

14.2.1 ETHICS STATEMENT

No informed consent was required because the data were analyzed anonymously.

14.2.2 NATIONAL HEALTH INSURANCE RESEARCH DATABASE (TAIWAN)

Every citizen of Taiwan is under the National Health Insurance program, which is a public, single-payer insurance plan covering many treatments including outpatient TCM treatment. When registered healthcare providers file a reimbursement to the Bureau of National Health Insurance (BNHI), the original claim including diagnosis and prescription is submitted. We applied for and obtained from BNHI [16] the complete TCM claims made throughout Taiwan in 2007. Note that information on personal identification in the data was scrambled before its release to researchers so that patient privacy is protected. From the number of distinct individuals (= 6,609,872) in the TCM data and population of Taiwan in 2007, we estimated that 28.8% of the Taiwan population patronized TCM in 2007. Note that if we include self-pay TCM treatments which are not in the reimbursement data, the prevalence should rise. From the total number of claims, we estimated the average number of visits per patient per year to be 5.3. The diagnosis column in the data can have up to three ICD-9 codes, for the primary, secondary and tertiary diagnosis of the patient during that clinic visit. We focus on cancers by limiting the primary ICD-9 codes to be within 140 and 239, which are the codes allocated for neoplasms by the International Classification of Diseases published by the WHO. The resulting 187,230 cancer diagnoses and the corresponding TCM prescriptions are the object of current study.

14.2.3 DATA ANALYSIS

14.2.3.1 CANCER-HERB DATA MATRIX.

A repertoire of classical TCM formulas and single TCM herbs in various forms (e.g. powder, pill) derived from concentrated herbal extracts manufactured by certified, GMP-compliant TCM suppliers were approved and used in Taiwan. Potency changes with forms according to TCM [17] and we found the numbers of formulas and herbs including their different forms to be 336 classical formulas and 410 single herbs as of 2007. A numeric matrix of dimensions 746 by 100 was created, where 746, the number of rows, comes from the number of reimbursable TCM formulas (i.e. 336) plus the number of reimbursable TCM herbs (i.e. 410), and the number of columns 100 is the number of cancers from the 3-digit ICD-9 codes from 140 to 239 designated for neoplasms. The cancer-herb matrix was initialized to zero. For every claim, the percentage weight ai of each TCM formula or herb in the prescription was calculated and added to the corresponding cell of the cancer-herb matrix. The procedure iterated over the 187,230 claims. We then divided the column by the frequency of the cancer to adjust for the effect of different cancer occurrences. Note that in the preparation for such matrices, we had two scenarios: i) the prescriptions for those which have only primary but have neither secondary nor tertiary diagnosis (No. of claims = 100,679); and ii) those which have primary cancer and any secondary but none tertiary diagnosis (No. of claims = 51,275). The purpose of the second scenario was to study prescription changes due to a secondary morbidity.

A TCM formula delivers one of the 21 categories of TCM therapeutic effects according to TCM [18]. We show in Table S1 the TCM categories and numbers of formulas in each of the categories. In the study of TCM category and cancer, a 21 by 100 cancer-category data matrix was created from the 187,230 claims in the same way described above for the cancer-herb data matrix. A cancer-nature matrix and a cancer-flavour matrix were also prepared the same way for the studies of TCM natures and TCM flavours and cancers. Information and assignment of TCM categories to formulas and TCM natures and flavours to herbs were as previously described [19]. The numbers of reimbursable herbs in each of the TCM natures and flavours are shown in Tables S2, S3.

14.2.3.2 HIERARCHICAL CLUSTERING.

A technique in statistical data analysis and bioinformatics that identifies i) subsets of observations called clusters; and ii) the hierarchical relations among the clusters [20]. The result of the hierarchy of clusters is usually presented in a tree-like diagram. The observations in the current application are the cancer-herb data matrix prepared above. Specifically, when the weight distributions of the 746 TCM formulas and herbs to two cancers are similar, the two cancers are considered to be in a cluster. Similarly, if the weight distributions of two formulas (two herbs, or one formula and one herb) across the 100 cancers are similar, the two formulas (two herbs, one formula and one herb) are said to be clustered. The algorithm runs bottom-up to grow the cluster and build the hierarchy of the clusters along the way. We used the heatmap function in R [21] with the default parameter setting for the hierarchical clustering analysis.

14.2.3.3 PRINCIPAL COMPONENT ANALYSIS.

A method of exploratory data analysis that transforms the original high dimensional data into a low dimensional space while preserving most of the information, i.e. variance, in the data [20]. In the present case, a cancer is characterized by 746 formulas and herbs. Two herbs may be correlated because their weight distributions across the 100 cancers are identical or nearly identical. We may then replace the two herbs by using the mean of the two without losing much information. The dimension of the data, i.e. 746, is then reduced by one. Principal component analysis (PCA) is a procedure that identifies and constructs the uncorrelated axes, called principal components (PCs), using linear combinations of the original and usually highly correlated axes, in achieving dimension reduction. Note that we order PCs so that cancers spread out in the space of the first few, usually 2 or 3, PCs. We used the prcomp function in R [21] with the default parameter setting for the PCA analysis.

14.3 RESULTS

We start with cancers which are not accompanied with any secondary morbidities, the number of such cases totalling 100,679 in 2007. The female and male proportions are 69% and 31% while the distributions of ages (at diagnosis) are 47 ± 13 and 56 ± 16 years old as shown in Figure S1. The age distributions for both sexes slightly tilt to the old age as age is known to be a risk factor for the disease. Cancers differ by their occurrences. As shown in the cancer frequency distribution of Figure S2, uterine leiomyoma ranks number one, followed by female breast cancer, liver cancer and nasopharyngeal cancer. The top four cancers account, respectively, for 21%, 15%, 6% and 4% of all the cancer diagnoses. The top two cancer types explain the predominance of female TCM patients in Taiwan. The high frequency of nasopharyngeal cancer mirrors the known epidemiology of high nasopharyngeal carcinoma occurrence in the regions of southern China and Taiwan [22]. In the rest of the study, we focus on the top 30 cancers of Figure S2, which account for 90% of all the cancer diagnoses in the data.

14.3.1 ZIPF-LIKE DISTRIBUTION OF THE TCM FORMULAS AND HERBS TO CANCERS

The average percentage weight ai of a formula or herb in a prescription, normalized for the cancer frequency, was obtained as described in Material and Methods. We rank the formulas and herbs according to the weights ai's and plot weights against ranks in Figure 1A. For the top ranking formulas and herbs, we observe a power-law decrease of weight with rank: weight $\sim$rank$^{-\beta}$, where $\beta = 0.61$. In many other disciplines of sciences, including natural, social, economical and biological sciences, similar behaviours were found with β close to 1 and the distribution is called Zipf's law [23]. Prominent examples include the frequencies of words and phrases in a book [24] and the sizes of firms in the United States [25]. The analysis was also done on individual cancers as shown in Figure 1B. We found that benign neoplasms have a statistically significantly larger Zipf exponent $\beta = 0.80$ than malignant cancers $\beta = 0.54$ (t-test P-value = 0.002 and Figure S3). For $\beta = 0.80$ (0.54), the relative weights of the top 5 formulas/herbs go like: 1.00 (1.00), 0.57 (0.69), 0.42 (0.55), 0.33 (0.47) and 0.28 (0.42). A smaller β may therefore indicate a less consensus, as a consequence of the complexity of the disease, among the TCM doctors on the treatment of malignant cancers.

14.3.2 SPECIFICITY OF TCM PRESCRIPTIONS TO CANCER SITES

Benign neoplasms do not metastasize, distinguishing themselves from malignant ones. A different Zipf exponent of the formulas/herbs is intriguing. To look for further differences, we performed a hierarchical clustering of the cancer-herb data matrix. The results, on the top dendrograms of

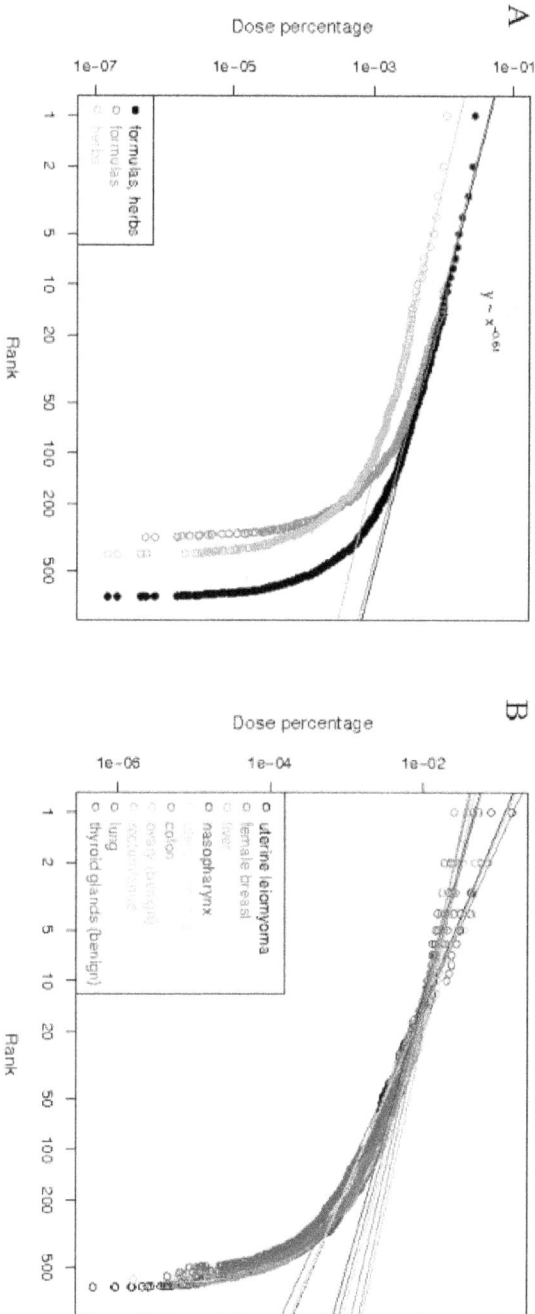

FIGURE 1: Zipf distributions of TCM formulas and herbs to cancers. The percentage weight of a formula or herb in a prescription is calculated. The weights are averaged over individual cancers, and then over the 30 cancer types. Formulas and herbs are ranked according to the averaged weights. (A) Weights averaged over the 30 cancers are plotted against their ranks. Note of the log scale of the axes. Lines are linear regressions to their top 50 formulas and/or herbs. The slopes of the lines give the Zipf exponents. (B) Weights over individual cancers are plotted against their ranks. Lines are linear regression fits to their top 20 formulas and herbs.

Figures 2 and S4, show that benign neoplasms, based on similarity in the prescribed formulas and herbs, were grouped together into clusters by the algorithm, reconfirming the result of Zipf analysis. Moreover, malignant cancers which are proximal in their anatomical positions (e.g. mouth, tongue and nasopharynx) or similar in the physiological functions (e.g. esophagus, stomach, colon and rectum) cluster together. Since the clustering of cancers was based on the profiles of percentage weights, the result indicates that, through weighted combinations of TCM formulas and herbs, TCM cancer prescriptions are specific to anatomical sites and physiological functions.

On the left dendrograms of Figures 2 and S4 show the clustering of the formulas and herbs based on their weights across the different cancers. The result indicates that TCM formulas play a more significant role than single herbs in a prescription as they weigh relatively heavier than single herbs in the prescription. Further analysis shows that a TCM cancer prescription consists on average of 2.2 ± 1.2 formulas and 4.0 ± 2.8 herbs and that the average (median) weight of a formula is 2.4 ± 0.4 (1.2 ± 0.8) times the average (median) weight of an herb in the prescription. The practice of combining formulas and herbs echoes the reported pattern of TCM co-prescriptions to acute nasopharyngitis in Taiwan [26].

14.3.3 TCM CANCER PRESCRIPTIONS ARE TONIFYING, HARMONIZING AND FIRE-PURGING

It is interesting to learn more about cancer care from TCM perspectives. A TCM formula is traditionally classified into one of 21 TCM therapeutic categories [18]. Given that TCM formulas are important players in TCM cancer prescriptions, we ranked the TCM categories of the TCM cancer formulas. The top five most common categories for malignant cancers were found to be tonifying, mediating (or harmonizing), dryness-treating, fire-purging, and peptic. Furthermore, the clustering result in Figure 3A reveals TCM treatments combining tonifying, mediating and fire-purging formulas to most of the malignant cancers while dryness-treating formulas to nasopharyngeal and mouth cancers and peptic formulas to esophagus, rectum and stomach cancers. For benign neoplasms, the top five categories were carbuncle-treating, blood-regulating, tonifying, mediating and fire-purging.

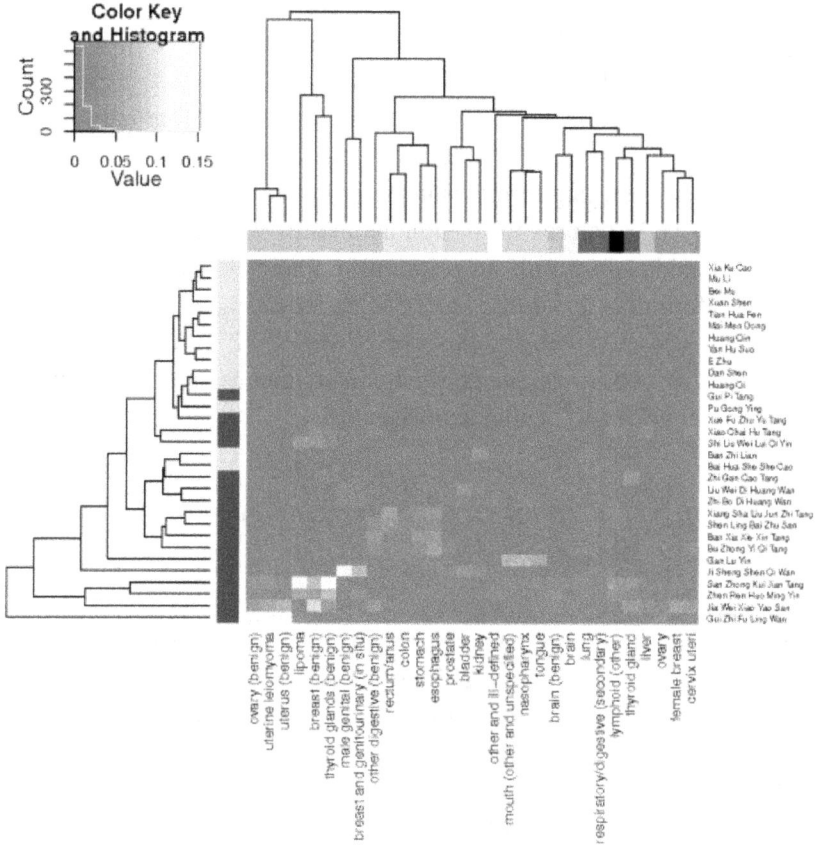

FIGURE 2: Heatmap and hierarchical clustering of cancers and TCM formulas/herbs. Cancers similar in terms of the prescribed TCM formulas and herbs are clustered and shown within the branches of the tree on the top. Horizontal color stripes encode cancer types. For example, benign neoplasms are in gray. Formulas and herbs that are similar in terms their usage across the cancers are clustered and shown on the left tree. Blue color in the vertical color bar indicates formulas while green indicates herbs. The heatmap shows only the 30 heaviest formulas/herbs. Color key and histogram show the value and distribution of the percentage weights. Figure S4 is the heatmap with all the 746 formulas and herbs.

Carbuncle-treating formulas were common to lipoma and blood-regulating formulas to uterus and ovary neoplasms, as shown in the figure.

Single herbs in a TCM prescription play supporting roles according to TCM principles, which our weight analysis above also corroborates. Herbs spread out under the prism of TCM cold-hot nature [19], [27]. We ranked and clustered the TCM natures of the herbs in TCM cancer prescriptions as shown in Figure 3B. For malignant cancers, the top four natures were found to be cold, warm, mild-cold and neutral, suggesting that cold herbs enhance the fire-purging formulas in the prescriptions. On the other hand, the top four TCM natures for benign neoplasms were found to be warm, mild-cold, cold and neutral, suggesting warm herbs to enhance the blood-regulating formulas. In addition to TCM natures, singles herbs carry their TCM flavors based on the principles of TCM [19], [27]. A similar analysis in Figure 3C shows sweet, pungent-bitter and bitter as the top three flavors for both malignant and benign neoplasms.

14.3.4 ADJUSTMENT OF TCM PRESCRIPTIONS TO SECONDARY DIAGNOSES

The analysis has so far been on prescriptions to cancer patients without other complications. We identified 51,275 diagnoses which have a secondary ICD-9 in addition to their primary cancer ICD-9. The sex and age distributions of these patients are 62% (female), 38% (male) and 51±13 (female), 58±15 (male) years old as shown in Figure S5. The most common secondary morbidities are found to be stomach functional disorder, ICD-9 = 5369, and sleep disturbance, ICD-9 = 7805, as shown in the secondary ICD-9 distribution in Figure S6. We performed clustering analysis on the data derived from the 51,275 claims to find that peptic formulas become the third common formulas after tonifying and mediating for the treatment of all the primary cancer diagnoses with stomach functional disorder as the accompanying secondary diagnosis as shown in Figure 4A. Similarly, the top three TCM categories for the cancers with sleep disturbance as the secondary diagnosis are found, in Figure 4B, to be tonifying, tranquilizing (or sedative) and mediating formulas. We conclude that TCM prescriptions to cancers with secondary mobility are adjusted by the incorporation of relevant TCM formulas.

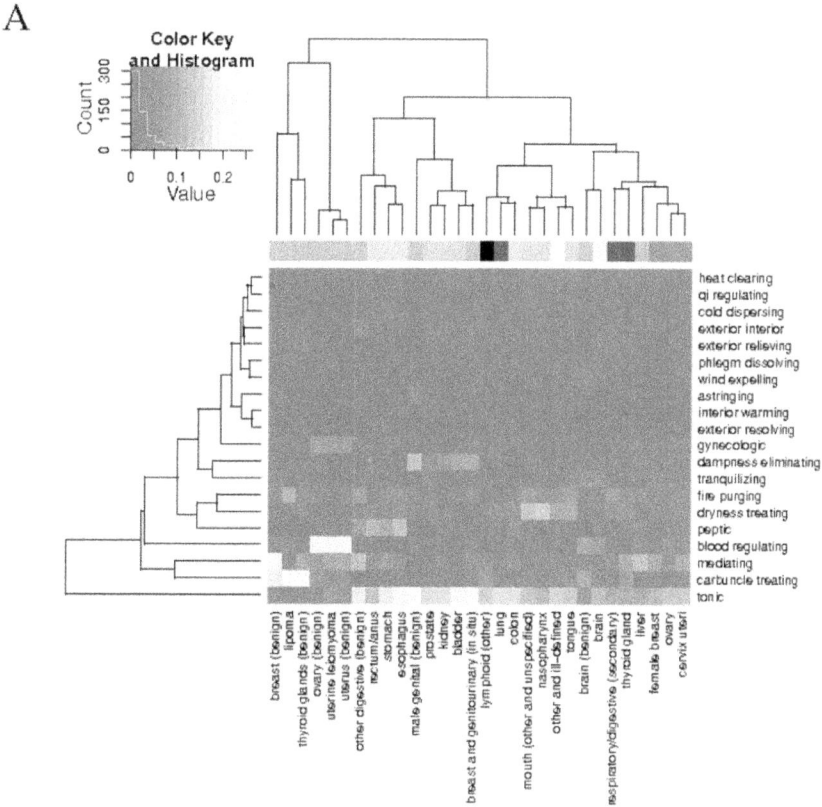

FIGURE 3: Heatmap and hierarchical clustering of cancers and TCM categories, natures, and flavors. The effect of a TCM formula is classified into one of the 21 TCM categories. The average percentage weight of a category in the prescriptions to each cancer is calculated. In (A) shows the heatmap of the cancer by category weights. Similarly, an herb is designated its TCM nature and TCM flavor. The heatmaps of the cancer by nature and cancer by flavor weight matrices are shown in (B) and (C).

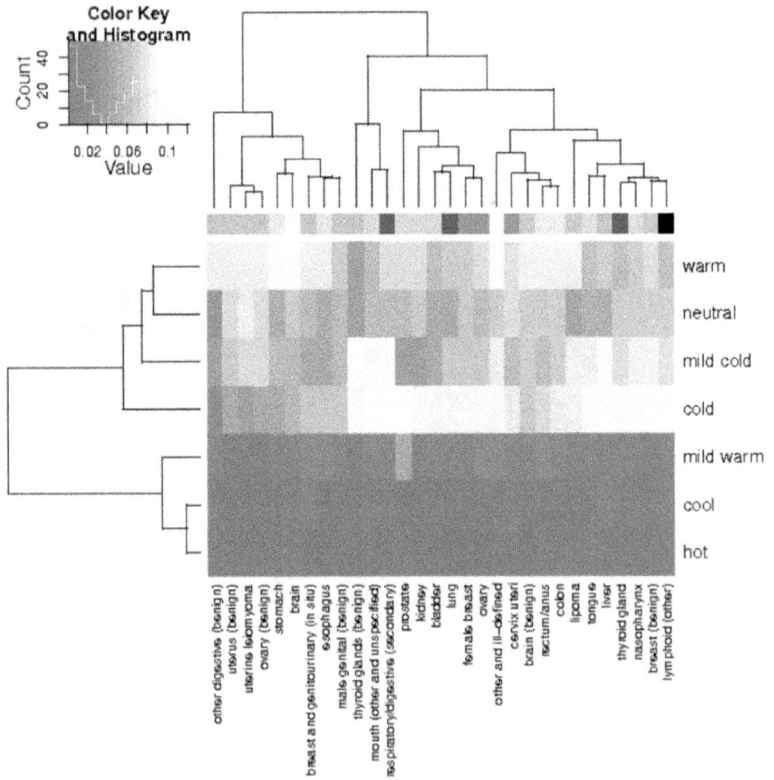

FIGURE 3: *Cont.*

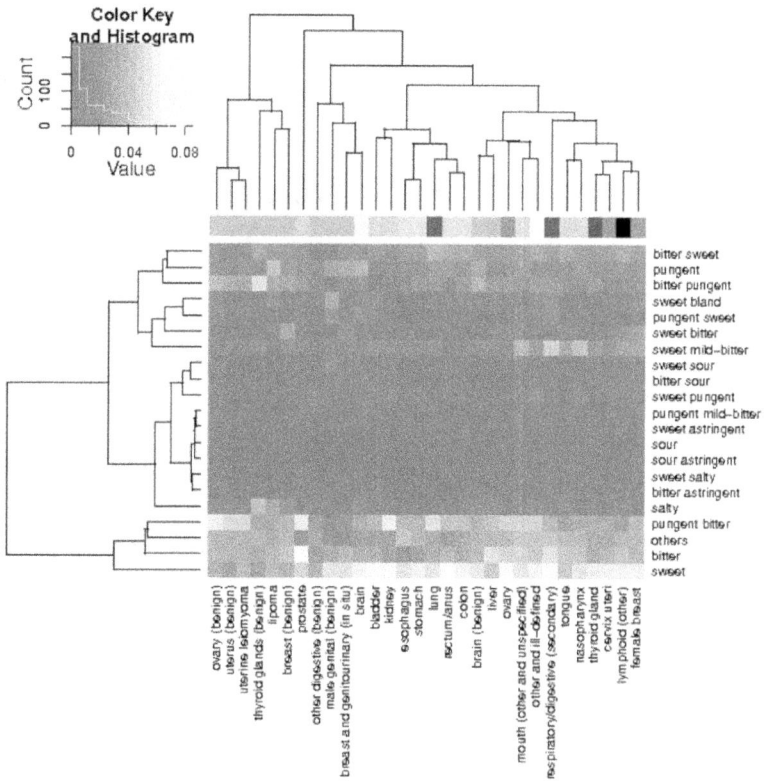

FIGURE 3: *Cont.*

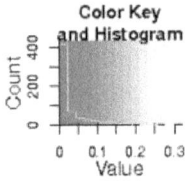

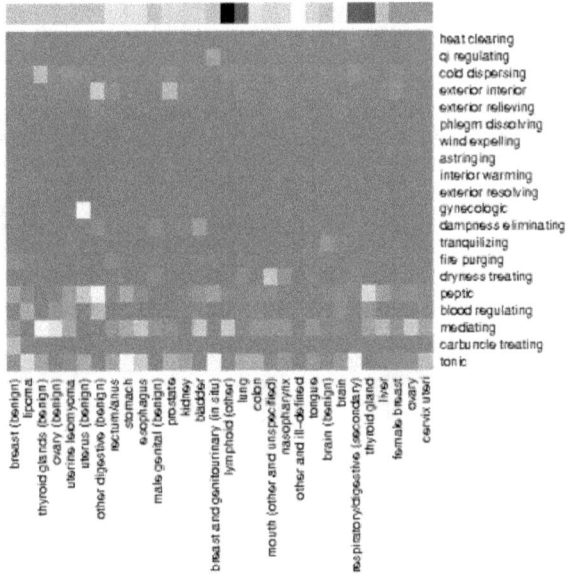

FIGURE 4: Heatmap of TCM categories and cancers with a secondary morbidity. Orderings of cancers and categories follow those of Figure 3A for easy comparison. (A) The secondary diagnosis is stomach disorder, ICD-9 = 5369. (B) The secondary diagnosis is sleep disturbance, ICD-9 = 7805.

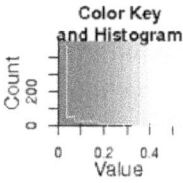

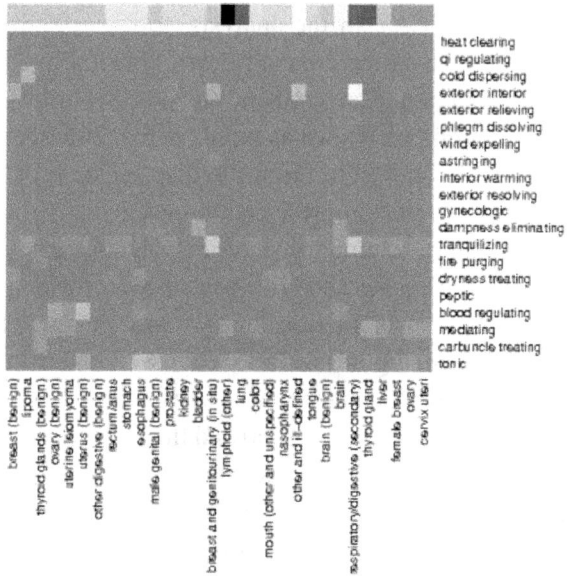

FIGURE 4: *Cont.*

14.3.5 ADJUSTMENT OF TCM PRESCRIPTIONS TO CANCERS OF THE LUNGS, GI TRACT AND FEMALE REPRODUCTIVE SYSTEMS IN TAIWAN IN WINTER

We divided the raw data into four parts: spring (March, April, May), summer (June, July, August), autumn (September, October, November) and winter (December, January, February) based on the dates when the diagnoses and prescriptions were made. Variability in treatment can be due to patient genotypes, TCM doctors, and/or seasons. To remove minor fluctuations (due, e.g., to different TCM clinics) while retaining most of the variances (due, e.g., to different cancer types and seasonal effects) in the data, we employed PCA on the 746 by 746 covariance matrix of the 746 by 120 herb-cancer-season weight matrix (see Material and Methods for details on PCA). In the analysis, formulas/herbs prescribed to a cancer diagnosed in spring are considered potentially different from those to the cancer diagnosed in summer, etc. The season-wise cancer-specific TCM prescriptions are shown as points in the first three PC space in Figures 5A and S8, and S9, and S10. From the displacement of points between seasons, the between-season prescription changes were calculated in Figure S11, showing that autumn to winter displays the most changes in the prescriptions. On the other hand, the season-wise mean temperatures, relative humidities and precipitations of Taiwan, available from the government [28] and shown in Figures S12, S13, and S14, indicate that the largest temperature change in Taiwan happens between autumn (= 25 degree Celsius) and winter (= 18 degree Celsius) and that both relative humidities and precipitations dramatically change from summer to autumn. The autumn-winter prescription changes are stratified over the cancer types in Figure 5B. We conclude that TCM treatments for cancers of the lungs, gastrointestinal tract and female reproductive system are subject to adjustment in Taiwan in winter when the average temperatures drop.

14.4 DISCUSSION

Environmental changes induce physiological responses. Therapies that take into account interactions between the environment and the individual are conceived to be more productive. Among changes in the three meteorological variables, only drop in temperatures was found to correlate temporally with the changes in prescription. According to Figures S12, S13, and S14, Taiwan summer is both hottest and dampest while Taiwan winter is coldest but not necessarily driest. If prescriptions were adjusted to drop in temperatures in winter, it would be expected that they be adjusted to rise in temperatures and humidities in summer too. One explanation is that most Taiwan households are equipped with air-conditioners. Indoor conditions in summer are therefore not as hot and humid as the records show. On the other hand, Taiwan winter is cold both indoor and outdoor as typical Taiwan households are not equipped with heaters. Lungs could be affected as they take in cold airs. The digestive and female reproductive systems might need to adjust as the body needs more energy and blood in cold days. Our analysis of the TCM prescriptions to cancers in Taiwan therefore identifies the relevant environmental factor, organs and patients for better care.

TCM theories hold that imbalance or disharmony in the interactions among the functional elements in the body or in the interaction between the body and the environment lead to disease. TCM is allopathic like modern western medicine. It is therefore interesting to learn, from the prescription data, what cancers are in TCM perspective. Peptic and tranquilizing formulas are relatively few in the repertoire of reimbursable TCM formulas, ranking, respectively, 11th and 16th in the 21 TCM categories (see Table S1). However, in TCM prescriptions to cancer patients with stomach and sleep secondary disorders, the percentage weights of peptic and tranquilizing formulas were among the top three along with tonifying and mediating formulas. A sensible mapping between ICD-9 and TCM therapeutic categories seems to be established, helping dialogue between the two medicines. Furthermore, in the prescriptions to single, primary malignant cancers without comorbidities, mediating formulas rose to 2nd heaviest from their 7th position in the TCM categories of Table S1, in contrast to tonifying formulas, which, although the heaviest, are the most common (cf Table S1). Tonifying formulas, unlike mediating, are thus probably not peculiar in cancer treatment. According to TCM theories, mediating formulas are for the so-called Shao Yang syndromes which are neither exterior nor interior, and neither cold nor warm. The indeterministic nature of

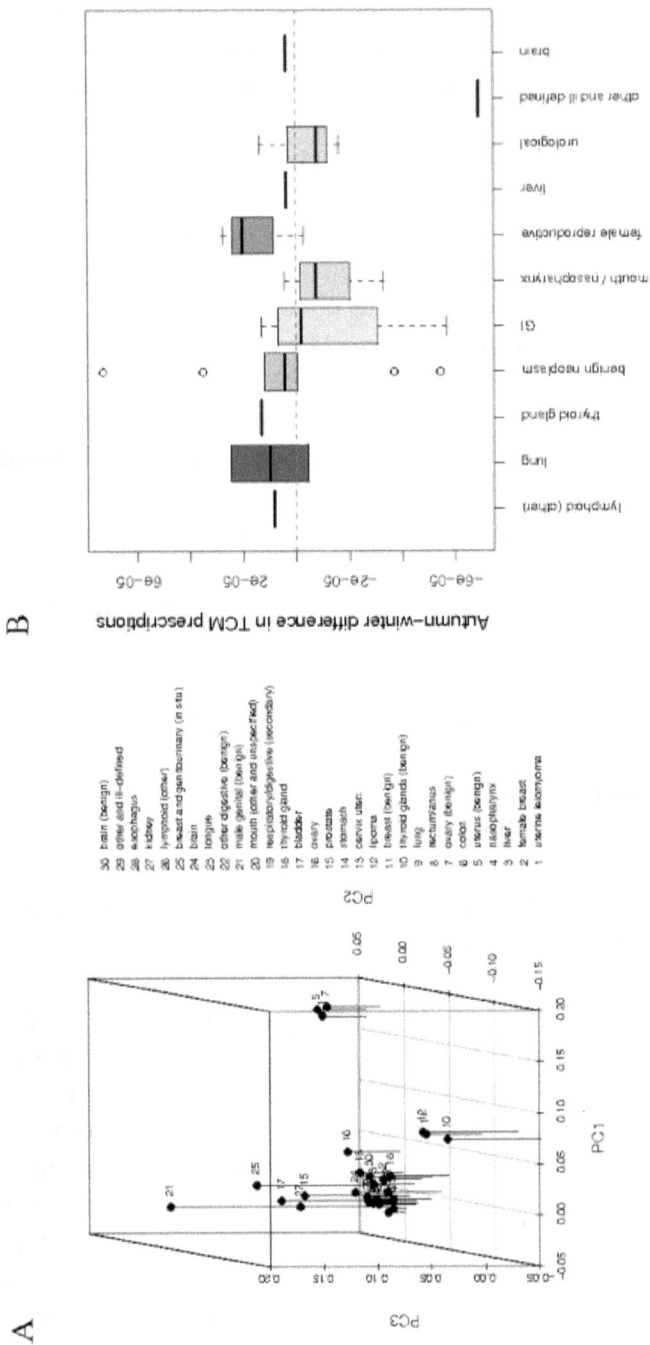

FIGURE 5: Variations in TCM prescriptions between seasons. (A) A cancer prescription is represented by a point in the three dimensional space spanned by the first three PCs, that together account for 55% of the data variation as shown in Figure S7. The points come from prescriptions made in spring. Figures S8, S9, and S10 show the prescriptions made in summer, autumn and winter, in the space defined by the same three PCs. (B) Differences between autumn- and winter-prescriptions are plotted against cancers. Cancer color codes follow those of Figure 2.

the TCM syndrome in regard to malignant cancers may be recapitulating the transformability and/or metastasizing of the disease.

Likewise, comparing TCM natures' weights in the cancer prescriptions with the natures' relative frequencies in the arsenal of the reimbursable herbs (warm, cold, neutral, mild-cold, cool, mild-warm, hot, in the order of their frequencies as shown in Table S2), we found predominance of cold or mild-cold TCM natures to neoplasms. The same comparison of Figure 3C and Table S3 leads to pungent-bitter TCM herbs in the TCM cancer prescriptions. Since, in TCM theories, cold herbs antagonize warm syndromes and pungent herbs move and disperse, the analysis may suggest that TCM views neoplasms as a warm and stagnant syndrome. As warmth and swelling are two of the features of inflammation, anti-inflammatory regimens such as exercise and toxin-free diets/environment may help prevent cancers. Indeed, the chemopreventive effect of non-steroidal anti-inflammatory drugs on colorectal and probably other cancers has been recognized and clinical trials for the evaluation of risks and benefits have been underway [29].

The ICD-9 codes in the study share a common denominator, that is, they are cancers with the same hallmarks at the cellular level. They differ otherwise, originating from different anatomical organs of different physiological functions. The design of the study helps address the issue of tissue-specificity of TCM prescriptions. Provided that the TCM treatments of cancers were efficacious, the result supports tissue-specificity of TCM prescriptions via weighted combinations of formulas and herbs. In western pharmaceutics, a targeted therapy drug which was approved for a cancer was later approved for other indications. The knowledge of TCM combinations may help inspire further indication expansion of targeted cancer drugs.

In linguistics, less specific words have higher frequencies. Use of low (high) specificity words, although appealing to speakers (hearers), incurs decoding (memory) cost of the hearers (speakers). A trade-off in the efforts between both parties was shown to lead to Zipf's distribution of words [30]. Abundances of expressed genes in human normal and cancer tissues were found to be Zipf-distributed [31]. In the chemical world, a recent study shows that the distributions of such features as rigid segments, ring systems and circular substructures of small, organic molecules follow power law [32]. The Zipf distribution of the weights of the TCM formulas and herbs may therefore suggest TCM treatment as a dialect, with herbs as words and formulas as phrases, in the communications to the human body. Note that Zipf distributions are considered a necessary but not sufficient condition for a language as 'words' in random texts were also found to exhibit Zipf distributions [33]. The Zipf-like distribution however may have implications in the dosage optimization of targeted cancer drug cocktails.

Modern western medicine is the major treatment modality in Taiwan. TCM patients might have received prior western cancer therapy or be under concomitant therapies. The information is not available in the dataset, nor is the information about prognosis of the TCM treatment. Interpretation can become diverse. For example, the most prescribed tonifying formulas and sweet herbs in TCM prescriptions could be aiming at fatigue, which is the most common side effect of radiation and chemotherapy. Despite the limitations, the systematic and exploratory analysis of the current study sheds light on TCM treatment of cancer, providing a fertile ground for the development of an integrated cancer management.

REFERENCES

1. WHO website. Available: http://www.who.int/mediacentre/factsheets/fs297/en/index.html. Accessed 2011 Sep 17.
2. Hanahan D, Weinberg RA (2011) Hallmarks of Cancer: the Next Generation. Cell 144: 646–674. doi: 10.1016/j.cell.2011.02.013.
3. Gerber DE (2008) Targeted Therapies: a New Generation of Cancer Treatments. Am Fam Physician 77: 311–319.
4. Aggarwal S (2010) Targeted cancer therapies. Nat Rev Drug Discovery 9: 427–428.
5. Jemal A, Ward E, Thun M (2010) Declining Death Rates Reflect Progress against Cancer. PLoS ONE 5: e9584. doi: 10.1371/journal.pone.0009584.
6. Miller VA, Kris MG, Shah N, Patel J, Azzoli C, et al. (2004) Bronchioloalveolar Pathologic Subtype and Smoking History Predict Sensitivity to Gefitinib in Advanced Non-Small-Cell Lung Cancer. J Clin Oncol 22: 1103–1109. doi: 10.1200/JCO.2004.08.158.
7. Liu CC, Prior J, Piwnica-Worms D, Bu G (2010) LRP6 overexpression defines a class of breast cancer subtype and is a target for therapy. Proc Natl Acad Sci U S A 107: 5136–5141. doi: 10.1073/pnas.0911220107.
8. Sawyers CL (2007) Cancer: mixing cocktails. Nature 449: 993–996. doi: 10.1038/449993a.

9. Unschuld PU (2003) Huang Di Nei Jing Su Wen: Nature, Knowledge, Imagery in an Ancient Chinese Medical Text. University of California Press. 536 p.

10. Zhang Z, Ye F, Wiseman N, Mitchell C, Feng Y (1999) Shang Han Lun: On Cold Damage, Translation and Commentaries. Paradigm Publications. 746 p.

11. Wiseman N, Willms S, Ye F (2009) Jin Gui Yao Lue – Essential Prescriptions of the Golden Coffer. Paradigm Publications. Summer 2009 (in press).

12. Harris ES, Cao S, Littlefield BA, Craycroft JA, Scholten R, et al. (2011) Heavy metal and pesticide content in commonly prescribed individual raw Chinese Herbal Medicines. Sci Total Environ 409: 4297–4305. doi: 10.1016/j.scitotenv.2011.07.032.

13. Sung JJ, Leung WK, Ching JYL, Lao L, Zhang G, et al. (2004) Agreements among traditional Chinese medicine practitioners in the diagnosis and treatment of irritable bowel syndrome. Aliment Pharmacol Ther 20: 1205–1210. doi: 10.1111/j.1365-2036.2004.02242.x.

14. Zhang GG, Lee WL, Lao L, Bausell B, Berman B, et al. (2004) The variability of TCM pattern diagnosis and herbal prescription on rheumatoid arthritis patients. Altern Ther Health Med 10: 58–63. doi: 10.2307/2700127.

15. Patwardhan B, Warude D, Pushpangadan P, Bhatt N (2005) Ayurveda and traditional Chinese medicine: A comparative overview. Evid Based Complement Alternat Med 2: 465–473. doi: 10.1093/ecam/neh140.

16. NHRI website. Available: http://w3.nhri.org.tw/nhird/en/index.htm. Accessed 2011 Sep 17.

17. Yang S-Z (1998) The Divine Farmer's Materia Medica: A Translation of the Shen Nong Ben Cao. Blue Poppy Press. 205 p.

18. Wu FM, Hsieh MH (2001) Collected Exegesis of Recipes, Wang Ang (1682). ACME Publishing, (in Chinese).

19. Hsieh HY, Chiu PH, Wang SC (2011) Epigenetics in traditional Chinese pharmacy: a bioinformatic study at pharmacopoeia scale. Evid Based Complement Alternat Med 2011: 816714. doi: 10.1093/ecam/neq050.

20. Wang S-C, Petronis A (2008) DNA Methylation Microarrays: Experimental Design and Statistical Analysis. CRC Press. 256 p.

21. R Development Core Team (2009) R: A language and environment for statistical computing. (Vienna, Austria): R Foundation for Statistical Computing. ISBN 3-900051-07-0.

22. Yu MC, Yuan JM (2002) Epidemiology of nasopharyngeal carcinoma. Seminars in Cancer Biol 12: 421–429. doi: 10.1201/9781420067286.

23. Adamic L (2011) Complex systems: Unzipping Zipf's law. Nature 474: 164–165. doi: 10.1038/474164a.

24. Ha LQ, Sicilia-Garcia EI, Ming J, Smith FJ (2003) Extension of Zipf's law to words and phrases. Proc 19th Intl Conf Comput Linguistics 2003: 315–320. doi: 10.1201/9781420067286.

25. Axtell RL (2001) Zipf Distribution of U.S. Firm Sizes. Science 293: 1818–1820. doi: 10.1126/science.1062081.

26. Hsieh SC, Lai JN, Lee CF, Hu FC, Tseng WL, et al. (2008) The prescribing of Chinese herbal products in Taiwan: a cross-sectional analysis of the national health insurance reimbursement database. Pharmacoepidemiol Drug Saf 17: 609–619. doi: 10.1002/pds.1611.

27. Li Shizhen (1578) Ben Cao Gang Mu. Beijing: People Hygiene Publishing House, 1982.
28. Central Weather Bureau website. Available: http://www.cwb.gov.tw/V7/climate/monthlyMean/Taiwan_tx.htm. Accessed 2011 Sep 1.
29. Cuzick J, Otto F, Baron JA, Brown PH, Burn J, et al. (2009) Aspirin and non-steroidal anti-inflammatory drugs for cancer prevention: an international consensus statement. Lancet Oncol 10: 501–507. doi: 10.1016/S1470-2045(09)70035-X.
30. Ferrer-i-Cancho R, Sole RV (2003) Least effort and the origins of scaling in human language. Proc Natl Acad Sci U S A 100: 788–791. doi: 10.1073/pnas.0335980100.
31. Furusawa C, Kaneko K (2003) Zipf's law in gene expression. Phys Rev Lett 90: 088102. doi: 10.1103/PhysRevLett.90.088102.
32. Benz RW, Swamidass J, Baldi P (2008) Discovery of Power-Laws in Chemical Space. J Chem Inf Model 48: 1138–1151. doi: 10.1021/ci700353m.
33. Li W (1992) Random Texts Exhibit Zipf's-Law-Like Word Frequency Distribution. IEEE Transactions on Information Theory 38: 1842–1845. doi: 10.1109/18.165464.

This article has supplemental information that is not featured in this version of the text. To view these files, please visit the original version of the article as cited in the beginning of this chapter.

PART IV

PERSONALIZED OR
PERSON-CENTERED MEDICINE

CHAPTER 15

TRADITIONAL, COMPLEMENTARY, AND ALTERNATIVE MEDICAL SYSTEMS AND THEIR CONTRIBUTION TO PERSONALIZATION, PREDICTION, AND PREVENTION IN MEDICINE: PERSON-CENTERED MEDICINE

PAOLO ROBERTI DI SARSINA, MAURO ALIVIA, AND PAOLA GUADAGNI

15.1 REVIEW

15.1.1 THE NEED FOR PERSON-CENTRED MEDICINE

Patients themselves demand an improvement in the quality of medical interventions with greater humanisation, personalisation of treatments and adequate information received in a safe environment to be able to make choices about their therapeutic process freely [1]. They want a doctor who

This chapter was originally published under the Creative Commons Attribution License. di Sarsina PR, Alivia M, and Guadagni P. Traditional, Complementary, and Alternative Medical Systems and Their Contribution to Personalization, Prediction, and Prevention in Medicine: Person-Centered Medicine. EPMA Journal 3,15 (2012), doi:10.1186/1878-5085-3-15.

will talk to them, listen to what they say and give them advice about how to get better and protect their health in the future. They want to be given the time and the space to express during the consultation, and once a therapeutic relationship is established, they wish to continue seeing the same person to give continuity to the process of healing. In many cases, the wish for a prescription is secondary to the wish of being cared for [2].

Many doctors and caregivers already practise person-centred medicine (PCM) with growing interest from colleagues and institutions. There is a perceived need to create a more satisfying therapeutic relationship, individualising treatments beyond clinical guidelines to suit the whole person in the context of his or her bio-psycho-spiritual biography [3]. PCM takes on the task to rebuild an effective therapeutic relationship based on trust, empathy, compassion and responsiveness to individual needs and values. To become individualised, diagnosis and treatment need to take into consideration the human being in his or her full expression [4]. The central question in PCM is: how can we restore the integrity, the dignity and the sacred and ethical value of the human being as a bio-psycho-spiritual entity? This raises the further question: how can we develop a concept of the 'whole' if only the physico-chemical forces acting in the organism are considered real and amenable to investigation by scientific research? How can we investigate the psychological and spiritual realities of the human being? How can we go beyond a dualistic view? PCM is a concept that is becoming increasingly used in medical education, in primary care and in other fields of health care where there is a need to reintegrate the analytical and fragmented image of the human being provided by specialism [4,5].

Biomedicine, the dominant western medical approach, is based on a mechanistic model of the human being, which stems from Virchow's theory of the cell as the unit of life. Life is considered to be no more than cellular activity ruled by physico-chemical laws. 'Living organisms appeared to me like moved bodies, their only difference from inorganic bodies being their tendency to form cells, but always with mechanical movements.' 'If up until now it has been impossible to produce the origin of life starting from purely physical and chemical laws, it seems to me that every reasonable physiologist who admits to an origin before life, cannot look for it in anything other than the combined action of physico-chemical forces' [6].

Virchow's thinking erased the traditional philosophy from which Hippocratic and Galenic medicine had developed in Europe and were continued by the medieval monastic tradition and further developed by Paracelsus. This was based on a holistic, sacred view of the human being based on principles which we now call salutogenesis, resilience, sense of coherence, internal and external sustainability, personal responsibility, self-regard and individual value, in other words, person-centred medicine. The Greek concept of the four humours was the result of a profound reflection more than of rational investigation [7].

However, the time came to move away from this, towards a 'scientific vision [that] no longer consists of religious faith and philosophical transcendence'. 'The knowledge of laws is quite sufficient; investigating the foundations of the law is a form of transcendent conceit' [8]. This has allowed the development of analytical thinking but in the main, only what is demonstrable and reproducible, linked by a mechanical cause-and-effect model, is considered truthful and scientific. There is no science outside this. Current biomedicine, which has developed from this model, is responsible for undeniable advances. Cells, organelles, physiological and chemical reactions, pathophysiological and biochemical processes, DNA and genetic codes, and more recently systems biology are studied in great detail, giving us a huge body of knowledge and therapeutic interventions developed as a consequence of these discoveries, but this is no longer enough. Life is more than the result of measurable biochemical reactions [9]. Thoughts, feelings and cognitively based actions are more than the result of physico-chemical processes. How can we not lose the human being? How can we broaden our concepts of science and medicine to investigate and heal the human being as a whole in a scientific way?

15.1.2 TRADITIONAL, COMPLEMENTARY AND ALTERNATIVE MEDICINE AND PERSONALISATION, PREVENTION AND PREDICTION IN MEDICINE

We can find answers to these questions in traditional, complementary and alternative medical (TCAM) systems which are used by 80% of people in the so-called developing world, by 360 million people in China and by around 150 million citizens and 300,000 registered health-care professionals in Europe [7,10].

What is traditional, alternative and complementary medicine?

- TCAM is a term used to represent a variety of different medical systems and health care methods that stem from European culture and from other philosophical backgrounds and traditions.
- They are based on the knowledge, skills and practices used to protect and restore health.
- They aim to prevent, diagnose and treat physical or mental illness and include medication and non-medication therapies.
- They share a vision of the human being as a unique physical, psychological and spiritual entity where, as Aristotle put it, 'the whole is more than the sum of its parts'.
- Within this holistic view, it is the physiological or pathological interaction between these aspects that determines health or illness. The genesis of health or illness also depends on the interaction between the human being, nature and the cosmos.
- TCAM systems are based on salutogenetic principles. Patients perceive this generation of health as a growing feeling of wellbeing, consequent to the stimulation of innate self-healing abilities through the adoption of a healthier lifestyle and the medication and non-medication therapies specific to each TCAM system [11].

Traditional Chinese medicine (TCM) is founded on the principles that preserving health is the best approach to disease prevention, it is better to reinforce our body's health before the insurgence of illness rather than having to cure it once it has developed and it is better to regulate lifestyles and nutrition regimes before the development of disease rather than having to prescribe treatments once problems have arisen. The integration between mind and body is essential. The body (Xing) is seen as the material substrate of mental activity, and the mind (Shen) is the governor of the body. One cannot do without the other.

In traditional Tibetan medicine (TTM), the human being is seen as body, mind and energy. The mind and the three great mental poisons of anger, attachment and mental obtuseness are essential both for wellbeing and health. The mind and the five elements are represented by three humours that are the quintessence of the energy that constantly flows into the human body and maintains health and mental alertness. Both TCM and TTM have a complex therapeutic system that includes plant-based remedies, forms of physical therapies such as massage and acupuncture, baths, forms of meditation and ritual movement (Yoga or Tai Chi). They are examples of a multifaceted therapeutic system that can address the human being as a bio-psycho-spiritual whole, with an intrinsically salutogenetic approach to disease prevention and healing [12].

In Ayurvedic medicine, life is seen as the continuous interaction between the body, sense organs, mind, soul and a living being in continuous interaction and adaptation between sensory perception, mental elaboration and adaptive response towards the environment. The core aim of Ayurveda is to prevent illness, look after health, maintain health and promote longevity. To this aim, topical and systemic therapeutic options are individualised according to the three Ayurvedic principles (Dosha): Kapha, Pitta and Vata, the articulated expressions of matter which govern the bio-psycho-spiritual functions of the human being. The individual human being is characterised by the unique combination of the three Dosha that make up his or her individual constitution which influences not only the bio-psycho-spiritual characteristics of a person, but also the predisposition towards certain diseases and states of imbalance. A constitutional assessment can guide primary prevention and also give the diagnostic and therapeutic tools to identify a pathological tendency in its initial stages, before it becomes established with symptoms or overt organic pathology [13].

Other TCAM systems also allow these forms of personalisation, prediction and prevention, each from their point of view. All TCAM systems are holistic; they relate physical symptoms to all other aspects of the human being, his or her natural and social environment; they share the common element of being person-centred. These systems are based on an understanding of health that is intrinsically and ontologically connected to the person in its entirety, as an individual, inseparable in body, psyche and spirit, which includes all behavioural, psychological, spiritual, environmental and cultural aspects. With the danger of being simplistic, we could say that biomedicine has developed a militaristic vision based on focusing on disease in various parts of the body, localising it and eliminating it using technologies and treatments that can be necessary and life-saving but unfortunately economically inaccessible to a large proportion of the world's population. TCAM systems have developed a therapeutic continuum with concepts of prevention, philosophically and ecologically developed on maintaining health, on the local ecosystem as a source of medicines, on food as medicine, on the importance of the caregiver-patient relationship as a therapeutic tool, on 'taking care of the person' in the long term in a more sustainable way, not only from an economical point of view. Emergencies need a biomedical approach; complex illnesses and the huge burden of chronic diseases need a complex approach that needs to be broadened with the person-centred vision of TCAM systems for a social and epistemological reformulation of medicine.

15.1.3 BROADENING HEALTH AND HEALING

In a person-centred, salutogenetic context, the concept of health needs to be broadened. Health is more than the absence of illness. It has been described as a complete state of physical, mental and social wellbeing [14]. However, this definition brings a static and even utopic element to the concept of health that can appear abstract and far away from the daily realities of human life. Challenges are a part of life and illness is a challenge to our bio-psycho-spiritual integrity. We live in the constant pursuit of a subtle and mobile equilibrium between health, illness and healing. According to salutogenetic principles, it is not the absence of hardship or illness that determines health, but our ability to deal with them positively, with the confidence to face them, with the knowledge that we can rely on ourselves to overcome them and with the trust that these difficult events hold meaning for our lives. A dynamic concept that reflects what we live through daily in different forms is introduced to the concept of health. Health becomes the ability to adjust and self-manage. The pursuit of health and the process of healing become an active process of continuous adjustment between our physiological, psychological and spiritual integrity, and the outer or inner influences that can strengthen or undermine this [15].

Healing is a broader concept than curing. According to Jonas, 'healing is the process of recovery, repair and the return to wholeness, in contrast with "curing" which focuses on the eradication of disease. While mainstream health care has traditionally operated from a "cure" model, the time has come to create a new model of health care delivery that makes room for both healing and cure' [16]. Returning to 'wholeness' implies a process that concerns not only physical aspects, but also psychological and spiritual ones. It is a process that takes time. It requires active involvement on the part of the whole person with the help and guidance of the caregiver. The element of change over time has an evolutionary quality: going through experiences that challenge the essence of our being and finding ourselves again, or 'returning to wholeness'; we are not the same as we were before we started.

This attempt to unite healing and cure is central to the future development of medicine. At the core of this are people: patients, doctors and health-care professionals in general. It is interesting to note how, in policy and research terminology, we are far away from this. 'Physicians' become 'providers', and 'patients' become 'consumers' or 'clients' [17]. This is not just a question of nominalism but is symptomatic of a deeper change. We understand the need for objective research, for parameters that will allow the rational distribution of limited resources and for guidelines to inform clinical decisions and ensure a basic and uniform standard of care. In this attempt, however, evidence-based medicine (EBM) has become too rigid and impersonal. When randomised controlled trials (RCTs), the most impersonal research method available, are considered the only form of evidence that can influence regulatory decision-making, this shows a progressive change away from the core of the medical act which is a meeting between people: the physician (and other caregivers, each with their competencies) and the patient. 'Healing' and 'disease alleviation' are the tasks of medicine; they are not 'primary outcome measures'. The risk of having an impersonal research method to guide and evaluate care is that the abilities of the art of treatment and of empathic engagement continue to wither away [18,19]. 'Doctors lose the ability to heal'. By applying guidelines, they become reliant on controlling disease processes with drug progressions or repeating the same tests sequentially to detect when another medication may be needed [10]. The medical act needs to be placed at the centre of medicine. The key to a successful and satisfying therapeutic process centres on the meeting between human beings: a physician, or other caregivers, and a patient, who work together towards healing. Establishing participatory medicine [20] is important to end paternalism in the doctor-patient relationships [21]. Patients are increasingly informed and need to be informed about their care. The consultation needs to be based on the encounter between individuals as equals, each with their competencies. Physicians and health-care professionals bring their professional, technical and caring skills; patients bring knowledge of their illness, the experience of their discomfort and their life.

Patient-centered medicine is, above all, a metaphor. "Patient centred" contrasts with "doctor centred" and replaces a Ptolemaic universe revolving around the physician with a Copernican galaxy revolving around the patient. The flaw in the metaphor is that the patient and the doctor must co-exist in a therapeutic, social, and economic relation of mutual and highly interwoven prerogatives. Neither is the king, and neither is the sun. Health relies on collaboration between the patient and the doctor, with many others serving as interested third parties. Patient and physician must therefore meet as equals, bringing different knowledge, needs, concerns, and gravitational pull but neither claiming a position of centrality. A better metaphor might be a pair of binary stars orbiting a common centre of gravity, or perhaps the double helix, whose two strands encircle each other, or—to return to medicine's roots—the caduceus, whose two serpents intertwine forever' [22].

15.1.4 DECISION-MAKING AND EVALUATION IN PERSON-CENTRED HEALTH CARE

There are many studies and papers that underline the importance of patient experiences, patient preferences and patient-based outcomes to guide therapeutic choice. The concept of goal-oriented care complements a disease outcome-based paradigm of care where managing diseases as well as possible, according to guidelines and population goals, is valued more than asking what patients want. Doing what is right for the patient takes on a central role in the future of medicine. Any evaluation of success in complex, chronic situations must, above all, consider patients' preferred outcomes.

In goal-oriented care, the most important signs and symptoms to evaluate conditions like heart failure or COPD are those connected with carrying out daily activities that are important and meaningful to the patient.

This can be dyspnoea in walking their grandchild to school, rather than in the context of a generalised list of symptoms benchmarked against disease-specific outcomes. An elderly patient with hypertension and postural hypotension may decide not to take blood pressure-lowering medication in order to be able to walk with less fear of falling [23]. Together with our patients, after having explained the meaning and the implications of a choice, we may decide that an improvement in being able to carry out daily life activities is more important than lowering blood pressure to prevent a potential stroke. For another patient, the reverse may be true.

PCM needs to be founded on sound clinical judgment. A cluster RCT looked at patients with type 2 diabetes and hypertension. One group was treated according to guidelines, the other at the physician's discretion. They noticed that there was no difference in blood pressure control after 1 year. However, the guideline group was more likely to receive higher doses of antihypertensive drugs and had consulted the physicians significantly more often [24]. This brings evidence towards the importance of clinical judgment in individualising treatments that are suited to a particular person. This can reduce the amount of drugs prescribed and the dose required with a consequent reduction in costs and a better quality of life for the patient. Clinical judgment needs to be developed alongside a good understanding of EBM during training and needs to form an important part of continued professional development. The method of cognition-based medicine [25] can give additional research tools for the scientific evaluation of individualised interventions. To investigate complex interventions in all their aspects and their context, a circular model of evidence can be used (Figure 1) [26]. The hierarchical model of EBM holds good internal validity, but this does not necessarily correlate with external validity. It is also difficult to translate it to practical clinical life when evaluating complex clinical situations or complex medical systems like TCAM systems. A circular model of evidence relies on the complementarity of the research methods that balance respective strengths and weaknesses. There is no privileged vantage point from which to define truth. This is a strategy to evaluate complex interventions that can add investigative tools to PCM and to the pluralism of thorough but open-minded scientific research [26].

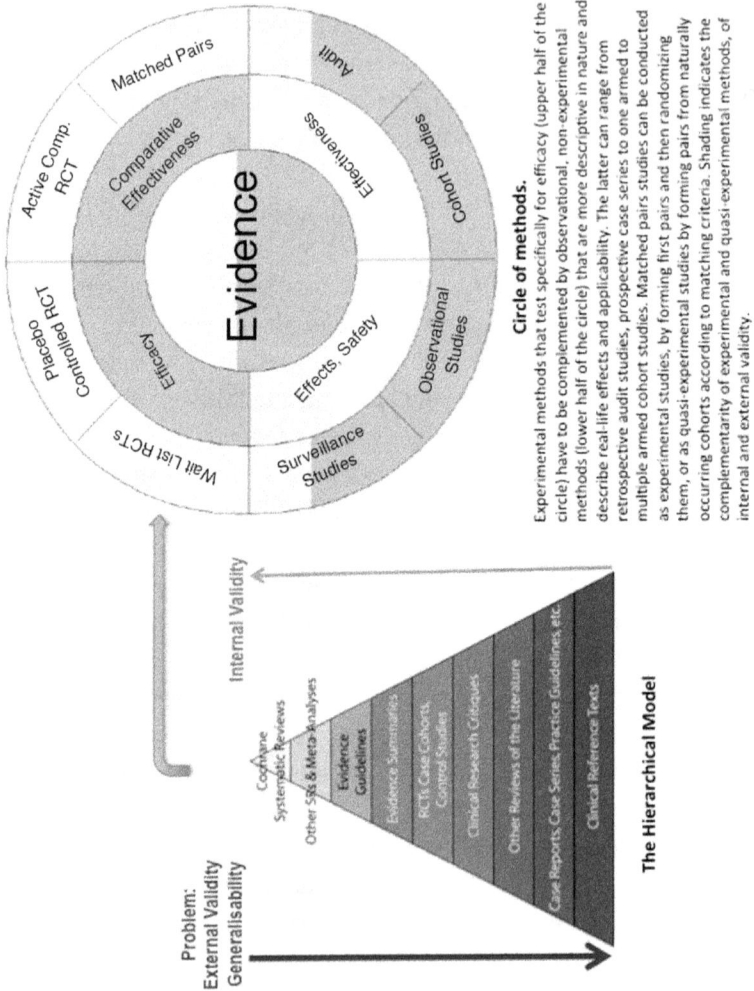

Circle of methods.

Experimental methods that test specifically for efficacy (upper half of the circle) have to be complemented by observational, non-experimental methods (lower half of the circle) that are more descriptive in nature and describe real-life effects and applicability. The latter can range from retrospective audit studies, prospective case series to one armed to multiple armed cohort studies. Matched pairs studies can be conducted as experimental studies, by forming first pairs and then randomizing them, or as quasi-experimental studies by forming pairs from naturally occurring cohorts according to matching criteria. Shading indicates the complementarity of experimental and quasi-experimental methods, of internal and external validity.

FIGURE 1: From a hierarchical to a circular model of evidence (Adapted from[26]).

15.1.5 THE EDUCATIONAL TASK OF PERSON-CENTRED MEDICINE

Person-centred medicine has the educational task to facilitate professional development in the directions described above, for each professional role, from as early as undergraduate training. Training should include courses and exercises in epistemology, holistic or multi-perspective thinking to enable the development of independent thought. The development of agile thinking abilities that are able to conceptualise changing processes can be achieved through the exercise of artistic activities practised according to specific methods.

Health-care professionals need to be equipped with knowledge and competencies that will enable them to work efficiently in health-care systems where organisational assets are changing across the world. This is particularly important if they hold managerial positions. All over the world, health-care systems are falling in line with each other. Practice and procedures are becoming standardised with a tendency towards centralisation of services into regional centres of excellence. Increasing importance is also being placed on TCAM systems. Current and future health-care professionals need to acquire knowledge about national health-care systems and about national health-care structure networks as well as an understanding of how the rest of the world's health-care systems work. This will enable them to deal with new pandemic diseases and chronic and invalidating illnesses and to develop measures for health promotion at a global level. New competencies are needed to provide care to migrant patient populations, many of whom come from cultures with specific and different medical approaches. Knowledge and skills are also necessary to meet the growing demand from citizens who wish to be able to choose treatment pathways, interventions and health-care practices that come from TCAM systems.

During their undergraduate and postgraduate education, health-care professionals need to be given the tools to understand the social changes that are taking place, including in the health-care system, and to address them with adequate sanitary responses and coherent political proposals [27]. People with decision-making power at all levels of the welfare system, of health-care organisations and of organisations in the public sector, free market or tertiary sector that provide services aimed at improving wellbeing are being called upon to give new solutions regarding health and health care. Current and future managers need to develop the skills that will enable them to plan, achieve and manage socio-sanitary initiatives in an innovative way, developing the public sphere with a system that considers the person as the core element and which aims towards health and wellbeing.

In order to have a person-centred approach, technological proficiency, solid grounding in EBM and knowledge of international protocols need to be complemented by knowledge of the epistemological systems and practical tools of TCAM. Doctors and other health-care workers need to be taught clinical judgment to become an accurate decision-making tool [28]. This complements the application of EBM and protocols, which are based on large numbers and therefore not always applicable to particular cases. Clinical judgment allows personalisation of guidelines and protocols to each case. It leads to more accurately placed resources and less waste. Learning and teaching about salutogenetic practices means that health-care workers may adopt healthier lifestyles for themselves. Greater work satisfaction and active involvement strengthen a health-care worker's resilience and sense of coherence, ultimately improving his or her health as well as that of his or her patients [15].

15.1.6 DEVELOPING SALUTOGENETIC HEALTH CARE

TCAM systems emphasise all aspects that influence the choice of lifestyle, the overall situation, patient outcome, therapy response, wellbeing and treatment compliance. These depend on multiple and interacting cofactors such as correct nutrition, regular exercise, adequate rest, biographical features, family, socioeconomics, health inequalities, the social gradient of health, the gender gradient, coming from a particular cultural or religious background and having a particular spiritual vision of life [17]. Although some TCAM caregivers have lost the link with the spiritual dimension of their discipline, traditionally this forms an essential part of the philosophical background that underpins TCAM systems. With variations, the human being is seen as the bearer of a sacred, incarnated spiritual element.

The pursuit of health in all its aspects is instrumental to allow the human being to unfold his or her incarnation and aims in this life.

Lifestyle changes form an essential, cost-effective part of generating health, preventing disease, treating illness and reducing mortality. They are also important in giving people responsibility for maintaining their own health. In a person-centred approach, lifestyle intervention needs to take into consideration all aspects of the human being and be personalised by tailoring it to the individual. Health promotion is a form of disease prevention. The first topic to be addressed in health promotion and health education is diet and the quality of foodstuffs. If diet were a better used resource in health care and people were taught its principles and practical applications, this may decrease the need to use medication in some cases. The care of biorhythms is another aspect to be addressed. Altered sleeping patterns, eating rhythms and patterns of physical activity are both a measure and a cause of pathology and health. The benefits of regular exercise are well known to everyone. It is important for people to become aware of their own biorhythms, which alter with age, gender, state of health and personal and constitutional characteristics. With the help of education, improved environmental conditions and appropriate care during illness, people can adjust or at least compensate for altered biorhythms and therefore actively improve their health. The emotional factors that contribute to health and illness can also be addressed. Negative emotions increase the incidence of physical illness. Conversely, positive emotions and humour improve health and wellbeing. Chronic stress can strengthen or weaken a person depending on how strong or weak his or her resilience and sense of coherence are [15,29]. Chronic stress and social deprivation have been shown to be similar risk factors for developing ischaemic heart disease compared to hypertension or hypercholesterolaemia [30]. Emotions can have adverse effects on the incidence of complication and prognosis during an acute cardiac event. Emotional resilience and SOC can be strengthened through artistic activity in the form of painting, music, dance, drama and creative writing. Through artistic activities, people learn new skills and their achievements have a positive effect on their self-esteem. This can be applied to overcome future challenges or unknown life situations with strengthened sense of coherence [15].

It has been shown that in some areas, we can obtain better therapeutic results with lifestyle changes compared to drug therapy. The influence of these factors on widespread disease such as diabetes, hypertension and coronary disease is immense and, in some areas, larger than the effects of drug treatments [30-33]. The INTERHEART study showed a more than 90% reduction in the risk of developing MI by adopting a healthier lifestyle, whereas high-cost interventional procedures do not show additional benefits in RCTs [34]. Another study in a cohort of apparently healthy men showed how adherence to healthy lifestyles was associated with lower risk of developing heart failure later in life [35].

To induce sustainable motivation for change, we cannot simply inform patients about risk factor reduction, which can be experienced as boring or abstract, or risk of death, which can frighten patients and therefore block off their further listening. The challenge is to develop individualised therapy concepts to activate the person's own resources considering his or her potential, values and environment. Strategies of lifestyle change must be tailored to the individual patient in order to be feasible and to cause him or her to quickly feel better and satisfied [17]. This is the key to long-term compliance. The other core aspect is human contact. Any lifestyle change requires questioning of values and sometimes deeply engrained habits. It is difficult to change them; there will be frustration, rebellion, refusal and relapse. The physician or caregiver needs to have the tools to deal with this, taking time to support patients at these times, encouraging and advising, and providing additional therapies if necessary. Giving information leaflets can be informative, but it cannot replace the importance of the doctor-patient relationship, which requires competence, patience and a profound conviction on the part of the physician or health-care professional.

15.1.7 DEVELOPING A THERAPEUTIC RELATIONSHIP BASED ON EMPATHY

The clinical encounter, born out of a more or less explicit request for help on part of the patient, is a chance to develop a therapeutic relationship. This is not an automatic transition. The time for paternalism may be over, but merely giving information, personally, through leaflets or computer-based systems is only part of the answer. It is through empathy that the thera-peutic relationship can be established. Generically, empathy is defined as the ability to understand and share the feelings of another [36]. Edith Stein goes even further to describe empathy as the way in which we perceive the experiences lived by another human being. Feelings become quali-fied as a tool for perception, like judgment which is a tool for cognitive understanding. 'Other human beings are not given to my perception as physical bodies, but as a sensitive, living body belonging to an "I". An "I" that senses, thinks, feels and wills. The living body of this "I" not only fits into my world of phenomena but it is itself the orientation point of such a world of phenomena. It faces this world and communicates with me. The other human being is another living being, structurally akin yet foreign to me. Yet I can perceive his or her experiences through empathy' [37]. This adds an element of understanding a deeper cognitive process to the state of sympathy, where we are purely feeling what another person feels without discernment [38].

Empathy does not mean feeling the happiness or sorrow of another hu-man being. It means widening our experience, enabling it to comprehend another person's joy or sorrow and maintaining the distinction between our self and the other. 'Empathy calls on the essential aspect of creating a relationship: going from the continuity of being one with another person, to the contiguity of being with the person' [39].

Empathy does not cloud clinical judgment; on the contrary, it improves the latter because the underlying feeling is one of understanding in the broader sense. Empathy does not necessarily make the clinical encounter longer. There is research to suggest the opposite [40] because develop-ing empathy allows the caregiver to grasp the core of the problem more quickly; this includes how the patient experiences illness as well as the subtle and contextual causes that have contributed to it. This in turn is the basis on which individualising advice and therapies can occur.

Empathy is a quality that is present in those with a 'flexible, mature and well-established personality' [41]. Stein goes further to say that 'empathy is possible if there is a fundamental correspondence between my being and the being of the other, if the "typus" is the same. However, as spiritually every person is a unique "typus", I will only be able to empathise with another person by the degree in which I have also become a "person", a totality, a whole with a purpose and meaning. Only then can I hope to understand another person. Otherwise we close ourselves off in our peculiar nature and other people become foreign to us or worse, we model them on our image distorting reality' [37].

Empathy requires training during higher education and continuous development during professional life in order to grow and become more skilfully used, but empathy cannot be identified with a particular habitus and even less as a communication technique. It is a way of being, of 'being available', which has its structure in the ontological and cognitive structures of the human being.

Educating ourselves to empathy as physicians means keeping our perception always alert, not letting ourselves being carried away by the illusion that knowledge of the patient's physical condition automatically means knowledge of his or her personal experience and of his or her personal reality. It means taking healing and cure back to their original source where they are services and not merely interventions or outcomes, in which they are answers before they are questions. It is the ability to be, which comes before and above the ability to do[39].

TCAM systems give practical, cognitive and meditative tools to physicians and caregivers to better develop these aspects. MCP requires that empathy be continuously renewed, deepened and refined for the good of patients and health-care professionals alike. Empathy adds a spiritual element to medicine because it intrinsically includes the most authentically human experience there is: that is the encounter between people. Through empathy, we perceive the other person in his or her intrinsic value, with his or her world of values, not because he or she does good in the world, but because his or her existence is intrinsically valuable to the world.

Studies that evaluate the success of lifestyle changes as therapeutic interventions to improve illness show that the main reason for failure is maintenance over time. For example, diet schemes, with a lot of human contact, are as good as bariatric surgery for treating obesity in some cases, but bariatric surgery shows better results in maintaining weight loss at long-term follow-up several years later. Lifestyle changes are difficult to undertake; they require active involvement to challenge habits and beliefs. A therapeutic relationship based on empathy, which has the flexibility to be continued over long periods of time, gives more opportunities for these interventions to be successful. A therapeutic relationship based on empathy can be cost-effective [40], improve adherence to treatment plans [42] and enhance patient health outcomes [43].

15.2 CONCLUSIONS

15.2.1 RECOMMENDATIONS FOR THE FUTURE DEVELOPMENT OF PERSON-CENTRED MEDICINE

PCM needs to be developed by broadening biomedicine with the epistemological basis, the diagnostic and therapeutic tools of TCAM systems, which stems from citizens, patients and health-care professionals alike. In this process, a balance needs to be struck between overcoming global health inequalities and individualising care.

TCAM systems offer a vision that considers the human being in his or her bio-psycho-spiritual aspects. They broaden the paradigm of personalised, preventive and predictive medicine. They are inclusive and participatory medical systems.

Personalisation in medicine needs to consider the individual as a unique being where the whole is more than the sum of its parts. Prediction needs to take into consideration dynamic understanding of the relationship between the physical, psychological and spiritual aspects of the human being, which allows the identification and treatment of pathological tendencies before they become overt organic disease.

Prevention needs to include health education and salutogenetic interventions aimed at all aspects of the human being that give patients the tools to take better responsibility for their own health. This has long-term effects and a low economic impact for the development of more sustainable health care. The medication and non-medication therapies of TCAM systems are also salutogenetic by strengthening physiological innate self-healing abilities. They complement the symptomatic and disease-based approach of biomedical interventions.

The basis to develop salutogenetic lifestyle changes that can last over time or change according to changing circumstances needs to be a therapeutic relationship based on empathy. TCAM systems can give the practical, epistemological and meditative tools to develop this. A therapeutic relationship based on empathy is a requirement for developing true participatory medicine.

PCM needs evaluation tools that go beyond EBM to include a circular model of evidence to evaluate the complexities of TCAM systems. The method of cognition-based medicine can give additional research tools for the scientific evaluation of individualised interventions. Patient-based outcomes need to become a core aspect of clinical evaluation. Health-care education needs to be broadened accordingly to give doctors and health-care workers of the future the tools to act in innovative and highly differentiated ways, always guided by deep respect for individual autonomy, personal culture, religion and beliefs.

REFERENCES

1. Leuenberger P, Longchamp C: Was erwartet die Bevolkerung von der Medizin? Ergebnisse einer Umfrage des GfS-Forschungsinstitutes, Politik und Staat, Bern, im Auftrag der SAMW. [What does the population expect from medicine? Results of a survey of the GfS-Research Institute, Politics and State, Bern commissioned by the Swiss Academy of Medical Sciences]. In Zukunft der Medizin Schweiz. Edited by Stauffacher W, Bircher J. Basel: Schweizerischer Arzteverlag; 2002::181.
2. Little P: Preferences of patients for patient centred approach to consultation in primary care: observational study. BMJ2001, 322:468.
3. Rakel D: The salutogenesis oriented session: creating space and time for healing in primary care. Explore 2008, 4:42-47.
4. Golubnitschaja O, Costigliola V, EPMA: General report & recommendations in predictive, preventive and personalised medicine 2012: White Paper of the European Association of Predictive. Preventive and Personalised Medicine. EPMA J 2012, 3:14.
5. Mezzich JE: Building person-centered medicine through dialogue and partnerships: perspective from the International Network for Person-centered Medicine. International J Pers Centered Medicine 2011, 1(1):10-13.
6. Maizes V, Rakel D, Niemiec C: Integrative medicine and patient-centered care. IOM Summit on Integrative Medicine and the Health of the Public. http://www.iom. edu/-/media/Files/Activity%20Files/Quality/IntegrativeMed/Integrative%20Medicine%20and%20Patient%20Centered%20Care.pdf

7. Virchow R: Alter und neuer vitalismus. Archiv f pathol Anat u Physiol U f klin Medizin, Bd 1856, 9:3-55.
8. Roberti di Sarsina P, Morandi A, Alivia M, Tognetti Bordogna M, Guadagni P: Medicine Tradizionali e non convenzionali in Italia. Considerazioni per una scelta sociale per la Medicina Centrata sulla Persona [Traditional and non conventional medicine in Italy. Considerations for a social choice of person centred medicine]. Advanced Therapies 2012, 1:3-29.
9. Virchow R: Die naturwissenschaftliche Methode und die Standpunkte der Therapie. Archiv f pathol Anat u Physiol U f klin Medizin, Bd 1849, 2:3-37.
10. Campbell AW: The art of medicine. Alternative Therapies 2012, 18(4):8-9.
11. Roberti di Sarsina P, Alivia M, Guadagni P: Widening the paradigm in medicine and health: person centred medicine as common ground of traditional and non conventional medicine. In Healthcare Overview: New Perspectives. Edited by Costigliola V. EPMA/Springer, 2012. [Golubnitschaja O (Series Editor): Advances in Predictive, Preventive and Personalised Medicine], Dordrecht; in press
12. Roberti di Sarsina P, Ottaviani L, Mella J: Tibetan medicine: a unique heritage of person-centred medicine. EPMA J 2011, 2:385-389.
13. Morandi A, Tosto C, Roberti di Sarsina P, Dalla Libera D: Salutogenesis and Ayurveda: indications for public health management. EPMA J 2011, 2:459-465.
14. WHO: Declaration of Alma-Ata International Conference on Primary Health Care, Alma-Ata, USSR. Geneva: WHO; 1978.
15. Alivia M, Guadagni P, Roberti di Sarsina P: Towards salutogenesis in the development of personalised and preventive healthcare. EPMA J 2011, 2:381-384.
16. Jonas WB: Optimal Healing Environments. Alexandria: Samueli Institute; 2002.
17. Kienle GS, Albonico HU, Fischer L, Frei-Erb M, Hamre HJ, Heusser P, Matthiesen PF, Renfer A, Kiene H: Complementary therapy systems and their integrative evaluation. Explore 2002, 7:175-187.
18. Kleinman A: The art of medicine. Catastrophe and caregiving: the failure of medicine as an art. Lancet 2008, 371:22-23.
19. Montgomery K: How Doctors Think: Clinical Judgement and the Practice of Medicine. New York: Oxford University Press; 2006.
20. Hood L, Flores M: A personal view on systems medicine and the emergence of proactive P4 medicine: predictive, preventive, personalized and participatory. New Biotechnol 2012, 29:613-624.
21. Sobradillo P, Pozo F, Agustì A: P4 medicine: the future around the corner. Archivos de bronchoneumologia 2011, 47(1):35-40.
22. Bardes CL: Defining "patient centered medicine". NEJM 2012, 366(9):782-783.
23. Reuben DB, Tinetti ME: Goal-oriented patient care—an alternative health outcomes paradigm. NEJM 2012, 366(9):777-779.
24. Bebb C, Kendrick D, Coupland C, Madeley R, Stewart J, Brown K, Burden R, Sturrock N: A cluster randomised control trial of the effect of a treatment algorithm for hypertension in patients with type 2 diabetes. Br J Gen Prac 2007, 57:136-143.
25. Kiene H: Was ist Cognition-based Medicine? [What is cognition-based medicine]. Z artztl Fortbild Qual Gesund Wes 2005, 99:301-306.

26. Walach H, Falkenberg T, Fonnebo V, Lewith G, Jonas W: Circular instead of hierarchical methodological principles for the evaluation of complex interventions. BMC Med Res Methodol 2006, 6(29):6-9.
27. Roberti di Sarsina P, Tognetti Bordogna M: The need for higher education in the sociology of traditional and non-conventional medicine in Italy: towards a person-centred medicine. EPMA J 2011, 2:357-363.
28. Kienle GS, Kiene H: Clinical judgement and the medical profession. J Evaluation Clinical Practice 2011, 17(4):621-627.
29. Roberti di Sarsina P: The social demand for a medicine focused on the person: the contribution of CAM to healthcare and healthgenesis. Evidence-Based Complementary and Alternative Medicine 2007, 4(S1):45-51.
30. Giallauria F, Battimiello V, Veneziano M, De Luca P, Cipollaro I, Buonincontro M, Vigorito C, Del Forno D: Psychosocial risk factors in cardiac practice. Monaldi Archives Chest Dis 2007, 68:74-80.
31. IOM (Institute of Medicine): Integrative Medicine and the Health of the Public: A Summary of the February 2009 Summit. Washington, DC: National Academies; 2009.
32. Diabetes Research Programme Research Group: Reduction in the incidence of type 2 diabetes with lifestyle intervention or metformin. NEJM 2002, 346:393-403.
33. Chobanian AV, Bakris GL, Black HR, Cushman WC, Green LA, Izzo JL Jr, Jones DW, Materson BJ, Oparil S, Wright JT Jr, Roccella EJ: Seventh report of the Joint National Committee on Prevention, Detection, Evaluation and Treatment of High Blood Pressure. Hypertension 2003, 42:1206-1252.
34. Yusuf S, Hawken S, Ounpuu S, Dans T, Avezum A, Lanas F, McQueen M, Budaj A, Pais P, Varigos J, Lisheng L, INTERHEART Study Investigators: Effect of potentially modifiable risk factors associated with myocardial infarction in 52 countries (the INTERHEART study) case–control study. Lancet 2004, 364:937-952.
35. Djoussè L, Driver JA, Gaziano JM: Relation between modifiable lifestyle factors and lifetime risk of heart failure. JAMA 2009, 302(4):394-400.
36. Oxford Dictionary Online. http://oxforddictionaries.com/definition/english/empathy?q=empathy
37. Stein E: On the Problem of Empathy. 3rd edition. Washington: ICS; 1989.
38. Adams R: Clinical empathy: a discussion on its benefits for practitioners, students of medicine and patients. Journal of Herbal Medicine 2012, 2:52-57.
39. Venuti G: Il rapporto paziente-medico: la capacità di essere con il paziente [The doctor patient relationship: the ability to be with the patient]. In Il medico e l'arte della cura [The Doctor and the Art of Healing]. Edited by Gensabella Furnari M. Soveria Mannelli: Rubbettino; 2005::94.
40. Bellet P, Maloney M: The importance of empathy as an interviewing skill in medicine. JAMA 1991, 266(13):1831-1832.
41. Kolb CL: Modern Clinical Psychiatry. 10th edition. Philadelphia: Saunders; 1991.

42. Buckman R, Tulsky J, Rodin G: Empathic responses in clinical practice: intuition or tuition. CMAJ 2011, 183(5):569-571.
43. Neumann M, Bensing J, Mercer S, Ernstman N, Ommen O, Pfaff H: Analysing the nature and specific effectiveness of clinical empathy: a theoretical overview and contribution towards a theory–based research agenda. Patient Educ Couns 2009, 74(3):339-346.

AUTHOR NOTES

CHAPTER 1

Competing Interests
The author declares that they have no competing interests.

Acknowledgments

This article was presented as a plenary lecture on the 11th Congress of the International Society of Ethnopharmacology (21 September 2010, Albacete, Spain). I thank participants for their useful comments. M. Henrich, D. Moerman, M. Pardo-de-Santayana, A. Pieroni, and J. Vallès read a previous version of this article and provided useful comments and bibliographical leads. Thanks also go to F. Zorondo-Rodriguez for editorial assistance and to GT-Agroecosistems (ICRISAT-Patancheru) for office facilities.

CHAPTER 2

Competing Interests
The authors declare that they have no competing interests.

Author Contributions
FSP: Was responsible for conception and design, acquisition of data, analysis and interpretation of data and drafted the manuscript. MAF: made substantial contribution to conception and design, interpretation of data and revised it critically for important intellectual content. JEC: made substantial contribution to conception and design of the antiproliferative assay, interpretation of data and revised it critically for important intellectual content. ALTGR: made substantial contribution to conception and design of the antiproliferative, DPPH and total phenolic content assay, interpretation of data and revised it critically for important intellectual content. All authors read and approved the final manuscript.

Acknowledgments

Ms Fabricia de Souza Predes is supported by a scholarship from Fundação de Amparo à Pesquisa do Estado de São Paulo (FAPESP: proc. 2006/06142-8) and by CAPES, an entity of the Brazilian Government for the training of human resources. MAF wishes to thanks CNPq for research fellowship. The Authors thank Prof. Dr. Marcos N. Eberlin and Dr. Regina Sparrapan from Thomson Laboratory from IQ-Unicamp for acquiring HRESI-MS data services and Elaine Cabral.

CHAPTER 3

Competing Interests

The authors declare that they have no competing interests.

Author Contributions

NAS, RAE and RGS carried out the isolation and identification of plant extracts. RST, FRH, SFF and JAA performed in-vitro studies on SCp2 (RST and SFF) and Mode-K cells (FRH and JAA) and outlined mechanisms of action. RST, FRH and NAS were the primary investigators who designed the experiments. SFF carried out the statistical analysis and prepared the manuscript. All authors read and approved the final manuscript.

Acknowledgments

This work was supported by grants from HITECH, FZE, Dubai, UAE, and the research was conducted at the "Nature Conservation Center for Sustainable Futures (IBSAR)" at the American University of Beirut, Beirut, Lebanon.

CHAPTER 4

Competing Interests

GH filed a patent application (WO2005/065063: "Use of the mushroom Agaricus blazei Murill for the production of medicaments suitable for treating infections and allergies") with priority Jan 2004, based on preliminary anti-infection and anti-allergy experiments in 2003. LKE has no competing interests.

Author Contributions

LKE supervised the animal experiments and the Ig, cytokine and other measurements that were performed together with technicians. GH had the idea for the project and did most of the data analysing and writing, and both authors collaborated on the study design.

Acknowledgments

We thank Else-Carin Groeng, Åse Eikeset, Bodil Hasseltvedt and Berit Steinsby and personnel at The animal facilities, Norwegian Institute of Public Health, Oslo, for excellent technical assistance. The Norwegian Ashma and Allergy Foundation and The Foundation for Health and Rehabilitation, Norway, supported this work financially.

CHAPTER 5

Competing Interests

The authors declare that they have no competing interests.

Author Contributions

TTXD, JJC, ZTW and KWKT designed the experiments. RCYC, ZYJ, HQX, AWHC, DTWL and QF conducted the experiments. All authors read and approved the final version of the manuscript.

Acknowledgments

This research was supported by grants from the University Grants Committee (AoE/B-15/01), Research Grants Council of Hong Kong (HKUST 6419/06M, 662608, N_HKUST629/07) and Croucher Foundation (CAS-CF07/08.SC03) to KWKT.

CHAPTER 6

Competing Interests

The authors declare that they have no competing interests.

Author Contributions

RN: Performed the study, collected plant material, evaluated the MS/MS data and prepared the manuscript; MWC: Carried out the study on cell lines, performed the statistical analysis and helped to draft the manuscript; WB: Isolated and purified proteins from plant extracts on a heparin column; DW: Participated in protein isolation and purification and in cell line analyses, helped in MS/MS data analysis; SB: Participated in design and coordination of the study, helped to collect the plant material; AGJ: Supervised the work, participated in its design and coordination and corrected the manuscript for publication. All the authors have approved the final manuscript.

Acknowledgments
This work was financed by the AMU-UMS-ULS inter-universities grant no. 512-00-073 (2009, Poznań, Poland) and Polish Minister of Science and Higher Education grant no. 0872/B/P01/2008/34.

CHAPTER 7

Competing Interests
The authors declare that they have no competing interests.

Author Contributions
WJT and CTC designed and conducted the experiments. GJW and THL isolated and purified AC fromA. lappa. SFC and SCL constructed pGL4.30 (luc2P/NFAT-RE/Hygro) plasmids. YCK supervised the study and revised the manuscript. All authors read and approved the final version of the manuscript.

Acknowledgments
This study was partially supported by grants from Council of Agriculture (97-1.2.1-al-22), National Science Council (NSC96-2320-B-030-006-MY3; NSC 99-2320-B-030-004-MY3), Committee on Chinese Medicine and Pharmacy (CCMP96-RD-207) and Fu-Jen University (9991A15/10993104995-4), Taiwan.

CHAPTER 8

Competing Interests
The authors declare that they have no competing interests.

Author Contributions
HSP drafted and wrote the manuscript. MQW revised the manuscript critically for important and intellectual content. GL provided translation of articles written in Chinese and revised the manuscript for intellectual content. All authors read and approved the final manuscript.

Acknowledgments
The authors thank Dr Kathryn Steadman, School of Pharmacy, University of Queensland for proof-reading the manuscript and valuable feedback; Helen Xia for providing plant & root photographs.

CHAPTER 9

Competing Interests
The authors declare that they have no competing interests.

Author Contributions
GS and TD contributed to the discussion and preparation of this manuscript. Both the authors read and approved the final manuscript.

Acknowledgments
This work was supported by research grants from DST and ICMR, Govt. of India.

CHAPTER 10

Competing Interests
The authors declare that they have no competing interests.

Author Contributions
BH and RS both have performed the study such as extract preparation, antioxidant evaluation and animal experiments. They also have been involved in analysis of data and preparation of manuscript. SB has helped in the acquisition and statistical analysis of data. NM has been involved in study design, revising the manuscript and final approval of manuscript for submission. All authors have read and approved the final manuscript.

Acknowledgments

The authors would like to thank Mr. Ranjit Das for technical assistance in sample preparation, handling of lab wares and animals in experimental procedures.

CHAPTER 11

Competing Interests

The author(s) declare that they have no competing interests.

Author Contributions

MC, EEP, and DYWL participated in the design of experiments.MC, EEP, XL, and DYWL participated in the interpretation of the results.MC and EEP prepared the manuscript.EEP, XL, WL, ER, RC, EKY, WBC, JCV, and YL performed the experiments.

Acknowledgments

We thank Dr. Carlos de Noronha for technical help with cell-to-cell fusion experiments, useful comments and discussion, and editorial help. This work was supported by NIH grant RO1-NS-40666, and The Campbell Foundation grant to MC.

CHAPTER 12

Funding

The study was funded through a John Spedan Lewis Fellowship award to CHSL. The funders had no role in study design, data collection and analysis, decision to publish, or preparation of the manuscript.

Competing Interests

The authors have declared that no competing interests exist.

Acknowledgments

The authors would like to thank Laszlo Csiba (RBG Kew) and Sue Rumsey (University of Reading) for their technical assistance, Gwilym Lewis (RBG Kew) for his assistance at the RBG Kew Herbarium, and Mark Chase (RBG Kew) for his assistance and comments during this study. Matt

Lavin (Montana State University) and an anonymous reviewer provided comments that enhanced the quality of this manuscript.

Author Contributions

Conceived and designed the experiments: CHSL JAH VS BBK EMW. Performed the experiments: CHSL LF. Analyzed the data: CHSL. Contributed reagents/materials/analysis tools: BBK FF. Wrote the paper: CHSL JAH. Reviewed ethnobotanical uses from the literature: EMW.

CHAPTER 13

Competing Interests

The authors declare that they have no competing interests.

Author Contributions

SGN conceived and designed the study, carried out analysis and writing of the manuscript. SR carried out the field and lab work, contributed to the study design and writing of the manuscript. both authors read and approved the final manuscript.

Acknowledgments

This project is funded by a SSHRC Standard Research Grant to Dr Newmaster, the Canadian Foundation for Innovation, and the financial support of the Shastri Indo-Canadian Institute. We would like to thank Dr. V. Balasubrmaniam and Dr. M. Murugesan at the Kongunad Arts and Science College, Coimbatore, India offered valuable time to time help and advice regardingBiophytum and Tripogon ethnotaxa and members of the Biodiversity Institute of Ontario Herbarium: Jose Maloles for editing an earlier version and Dr. Aron Fazekas and Royce Steeves for their assistance at our Centre for Biodiversity Genomics, University of Guelph.

CHAPTER 14

Funding

This work was funded in part by the National Science Council, Taiwan (Republic of China) grant # 97-2112-M-008-003-MY3. The funders had no role in study design, data collection and analysis, decision to publish, or preparation of the manuscript. No additional external funding received for this study.

Competing Interests

The authors have declared that no competing interests exist.

Acknowledgments

This study is based in part on data from the National Health Insurance Research Database provided by the Bureau of National Health Insurance, Department of Health and managed by National Health Research Institutes. The interpretation and conclusions contained herein do not represent those of Bureau of National Health Insurance, Department of Health or National Health Research Institutes.

Author Contributions

Conceived and designed the experiments: SCW. Performed the experiments: HYH. Analyzed the data: PHC SCW. Wrote the paper: SCW.

CHAPTER 15

Competing Interests

The authors declare that they have no competing interests.

Author Contributions

The authors worked together on the article, reflecting on the paradigm, planning the article and writing it. All authors read and approved the final manuscript.

Author Information

PRdS is the Expert for Non-conventional Medicine in the High Council of Health, Ministry of Health, Italy; the President of the Charity Association for Person Centred Medicine, Bologna, Italy; and the Director responsible for Complementary and Alternative Medicine and Contacts to Patient Organisations, National EPMA Board in Italy. MA is the Vice President of the Charity Association for Person Centred Medicine, Bologna, Italy, and the former President of the Italian Society of Anthroposophic Medicine (SIMA). PG is affiliated to the Charity Association for Person Centred Medicine, Bologna, Italy, and to the SIMA.

INDEX

V

vascular endothelial growth factor
  (VEGF), 138–140, 146–147, 170,
  300
virus synthesis, 227
Viscum album, 108, 110, 148
Vitamin C, 83, 85–88, 90–91, 93, 182

W

World Health Organization (WHO),
  xi, xxi, 2, 4–5, 17, 19–20, 64, 161,
  299, 290, 299, 303, 320, 325–326,
  331, 335, 343, 348

X

xanthine oxidase, xxv, 83–86, 90

For Product Safety Concerns and Information please contact our EU
representative GPSR@taylorandfrancis.com
Taylor & Francis Verlag GmbH, Kaufingerstraße 24, 80331 München, Germany